MEN'S
HEALTH
TODAY
2002

Life-Changing Tools for Taking Charge
of Your Health, Mind, and Body

Edited by Leah Flickinger, Men'sHealth. Books

RODALE

© 2002 by Rodale Inc.

Cover photograph © by Darryl Estrine

Interior photographs on pages 2–4 © by Mitchel Gray; pages 6, 11, and 12 © by Ron Amato

Illustrations on pages 5, 7, 8, and 9 © by Shawn Banner; pages 124–25 © by John Hull

Men's Health is a registered trademark of Rodale Inc.

Printed in the United States of America
Rodale Inc. makes every effort to use acid-free ∞, recycled paper ♻.

ISBN 1–57954–513–0 hardcover

Distributed to the book trade by St. Martin's Press

2   4   6   8   10   9   7   5   3   1   hardcover

Visit us on the Web at www.menshealthbooks.com, or call us toll-free at (800) 848-4735.

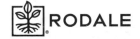

WE **INSPIRE** AND **ENABLE** PEOPLE TO IMPROVE
THEIR LIVES AND THE WORLD AROUND THEM

Men's Health Today 2002 Staff

EDITOR-IN-CHIEF,
MEN'S HEALTH MAGAZINE: David Zinczenko

EDITOR: Leah Flickinger

ASSOCIATE EDITOR: Kathryn C. LeSage

CONTRIBUTING WRITERS: Matthew Barbour; Norman Berlinger; Brian Boyé; Mike Butler; Adam Campbell; Kristen Chanley; Tom Clark; Jeff Csatari; Shannon Davis; Deb Dellapena; Don Donoho; Amy Donohue; Shelley Drozd; Tracy Erb; Gavin Evans; Jenny Everett; Leigh Farr; Kimberly Flynn; Linda Formichelli; Pam George; Ron Geraci; Brian Good; Melissa Gotthardt; Bill Gottlieb; Steve Gourley; Robert Greene; Warren Greene; Kimberly Haas; Jennifer Haigh; Kristen Harmel; Janine Hazlewood; Terrance Henderson; Brian Hickey; Kerry Holland; Robert Huber; Jean Ignatuk; Theresa Iknoian; Thomas Incledon, R.D., C.S.C.S.; Alex James; Mark Jolly; Lisa Jones; Larry Keller; Ian King; Chris Kita; Joe Kita; Rebecca Kleinwaks; Mike Krzyzewski; Kristyn Kusek; Jennifer LeClaire; Andy Lippstone; Erin Loos; James Mack; Matt Marion; Kim Maxwell; Steve Mazzucchi; Jim McCommons; Katrin McDonald; Mike Mejia; Eric Metcalf; Christian Millman; Peggy Noonan; Joe Nye; Hugh O'Neill; Marty Padgett; Francine Parnes; Donald T. Phillips; Carol Potera; Joe Queenan; Donna Raskin; Jessica Rossi; Lou Schuler; Nicole Serr; Ken Settar; Ted Spiker; Vince Steinman; Bill Stieg; Bill Stump; Duane Swierczynski; Andrew Taber; John Thompson; Margo Trott; Amanda Ursell; Mariska Van Aalst; Zachary Veilleux; Elizabeth Ward, R.D.; Debra Wein; Gene Weingarten; Fred Zahradnik; Tom Zoellner

ART DIRECTOR AND DESIGNER: Charles Beasley

RESEARCH EDITOR: Deborah Pedron

SENIOR RESEARCHER: Deanna Portz

LAYOUT DESIGNER: Jennifer H. Giandomenico

PRODUCT SPECIALIST: Jodi Schaffer

Rodale *Men's Health* Books

VICE PRESIDENT, WORLDWIDE PUBLISHER: Edward J. Fones

CUSTOMER MARKETING MANAGER: Matt Neumaier

CONTENT ASSEMBLY MANAGER: Robert V. Anderson Jr.

OFFICE MANAGER: Alice Debus

ASSISTANT OFFICE MANAGER: Marianne Moor

ADMINISTRATIVE ASSISTANT: Pamela Brinar

Contents

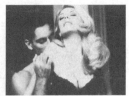

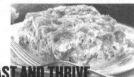

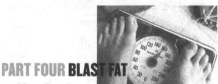

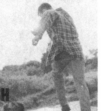

Introduction

Live for tomorrow

People will tell you that each passing day brings you that much closer to old age and a less fulfilling lifestyle. Maybe you've seen the not-so-subtle signs: that stubborn gut that moved in and now calls you home. The wad of graying hair that collects in the shower drain each morning. The slightly-less-than-rock-hard erection. Sore joints and muscles. Those vague pains that make you wonder, "Is it just heartburn . . . or something worse?"

And each day that passes, you say, "Tomorrow. I'll do something about it tomorrow."

Or maybe you haven't actually seen these signs yet, but you expect them at any moment. In which case you dread tomorrow and what it may bring.

Whichever camp you fall into, here's a newsflash: It's tomorrow. It's been tomorrow for years. So don't wait any longer—take control of your life today.

Think of this book as a vehicle that will steer your body clear of those nasty aging potholes and slam the brakes on your lifestyle's decline. *Men's Health Today 2002* will help you navigate a smooth ride to the body, the life, the mindset you want. It'll park you safely in the "no-doctor" zone.

The best part? It's fully loaded with standard features even cooler than a V-8 engine and dual moon roof: We've selected the best and most promising advice from medical experts, researchers, NBA veterans, NFL coaches, fitness professionals, and others. We've culled vital information from cutting-edge research, groundbreaking books, and leading professional journals. And we've made it entertaining and readable for guys like you who want to read English, not medical-ese.

Some highlights:

- **Do the best exercises of all time.** We sorted through all the fitness fads that have tempted men over the past few decades and chose the best, most powerful exercises for you. Then we whipped 'em into a workout. Let it whip you into shape.
- **Eat the best foods of all time.** Not to be outdone, nutrition wanted its share of the credit for changing your life. We'll show you how to make your groceries work for you—from healing a hangover to building muscle to warding off prostate cancer.
- **Read baseball-themed sex advice.** What more do you want—x-ray vision? Okay, then . . .
- **Get x-ray vision.** Or at least take a peek into her head to see what she's thinking in bed. You'll have the hottest sex ever. Check it out.

• **Eat well the easy way.** For those of you too busy to spend an hour at the supermarket, we offer an aisle-by-aisle guide to stocking up at the convenience store. We even toss in a recipe for a can't-miss meal she'll love.

• **Lose your hair.** Where you want to, that is. We rate the best and the worst body-hair removal techniques for men—in terms of cost and pain.

• **Get the most from the test you hate.** Your yearly prostate exam. Read our tactics to help you get the most accurate and relevant results in the quickest amount of time. That means less suffering for you.

• **Sail through flu season unscathed.** Tired of being exiled to the guest room, where it's just you, the lumpy mattress, and the 13-inch TV without cable? What could be worse when you already feel like crap? With these tips for beating the bug, we'll give you unlimited access to 157 big-screen channels all winter.

• **Never have a heart attack.** Read what guys like you learned from their brushes with this top man killer. Then do what they did to give it the brush-off.

• **Win every fight.** Battles are a part of life. Losing them doesn't have to be. Try our advice for beating the other guy. You can't lose.

Let *Men's Health Today 2002* transport you along life's highway. We'll give you better tomorrows—maybe even more of them.

—Leah Flickinger

Editor

PART ONE
MUSCLE UP

MUST READS

Stretch Test

Find out where your body needs improvement

By Adam Campbell

Our idea of stretching? Bending over to tie our shoes every morning. But a lack of flexibility causes injuries and prohibits lifting a lot of weight. That's why we recommend this 10-second flexibility test from Jim Liston, C.S.C.S., a state director for the National Strength and Conditioning Association.

To start, get into the position shown below.

THE TEST

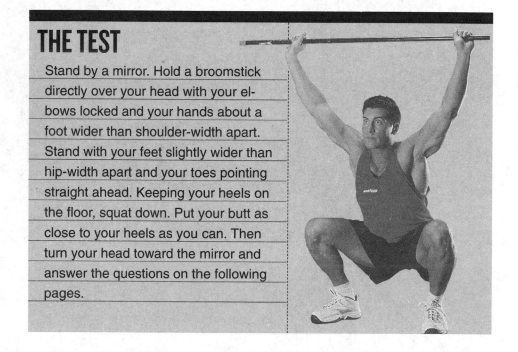

Stand by a mirror. Hold a broomstick directly over your head with your elbows locked and your hands about a foot wider than shoulder-width apart. Stand with your feet slightly wider than hip-width apart and your toes pointing straight ahead. Keeping your heels on the floor, squat down. Put your butt as close to your heels as you can. Then turn your head toward the mirror and answer the questions on the following pages.

POUNDS OF MUSCLE COLLEGE-AGE MEN BELIEVE THEY MUST ADD TO THEIR BULK TO IMPRESS WOMEN: 27

PERCENT OF MUSCLE MASS AND STRENGTH THE AVERAGE 30-YEAR-OLD WILL LOSE BY AGE 70: 25

1. Can you keep your heels touching the floor until you complete the squat?

If not, you have tight Achilles tendons. To improve your flexibility, put one knee on the floor and one knee in front of you. Place both hands on the floor and lean forward to stretch the tendon of your front leg. Switch legs after 20 to 30 seconds. Do this twice daily.

2. Is your upper body straight, and can you lower your butt to your heels?

No? You need to stretch your hip flexors (on the sides of your upper legs). Kneel on one knee and keep the other leg in front of you, bent at 90 degrees. Lean your torso forward until you feel a stretch in the hip flexor of your kneeling leg. Hold for 20 seconds, then switch legs.

(continued)

3. Can you lock your elbows and keep your head up?

If not, your chest and shoulders are too tight. After warming up, loosen them by placing one arm along a door frame with your elbow bent 90 degrees. Lean forward until you feel a stretch in the front of your shoulder. Hold for 20 seconds and repeat; do the same with your other arm.

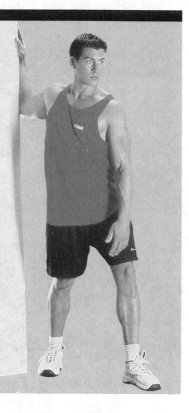

Get Your Body Back

Want a classic physique? Then do these classic exercises. Here's our ranking of the best workout moves of all time

By Lou Schuler

Exercise trends are called trends for a reason: They last about as long as a head of lettuce and offer about as much benefit as, well, a head of lettuce. But there are some exercises that have been around since the birth of Larry King. And that's because they work. But which are the best of the best?

We polled the people whose opinions matter—exercise researchers, strength coaches, physical therapists, top trainers, an entire C.S.C.S. convention, and a few thick-necked guys who watch the door at our favorite bar—and made them vote on the most effective exercises you can do in a dozen different categories, plus the single best one of all time.

We didn't bother coming up with a catchy name for these awards. As long as you add them to your workouts, we'll be happy. And once you see the results, so will you.

Best No-Weight Exercise: THE PUSHUP

What's great about pushups is that you can do them even though you may be weaker than the Russian ruble. You can start with a few and, over time, increase repetitions at a good, even pace that builds muscle in the places that count (chest, shoulders, triceps). Different variations of the exercise can work the abdominals as well, says Eric Ludlow, C.S.C.S., senior trainer at World Gym in New York City.

The pushup that impresses: Only the strongest and bravest should attempt a one-arm pushup. Don't even try it unless you can bench-press your own body weight 8 to 10 times.

To do a one-arm pushup with your right arm, widen your feet and place your right hand on the floor beneath the middle of your chest. Tuck your left arm behind your back. As you lower yourself, you'll realize that this isn't a straight-up-and-down movement like a regular pushup. You'll twist on the ball of your left foot and untwist as you push yourself back up (if you can). You'll feel muscles working all up and down the right side of your body. Do an equal number with each arm.

Best Exercise No One Does Anymore: THE CLEAN AND JERK

The clean and jerk used to be a staple move in hard-core gyms where guys named Tiny threw around weights the size of Toyotas.

"It's making a comeback in collegiate training rooms," says Dave Pearson, Ph.D., an exercise physiologist at Ball State University in Muncie, Indiana.

"It requires a combination of speed, strength, skill, and balance that few exercises match," raves Thomas Incledon, Ph.D., C.S.C.S., president and director of sports nutrition at Human Performance Specialists in Plantation, Florida.

Go ahead and jerk: Juan Carlos Santana, C.S.C.S., recommends this version using dumbbells instead of a barbell. Start with light weights, and focus on building speed more than building strength. Add weight only when your form is fluid and the move feels natural.

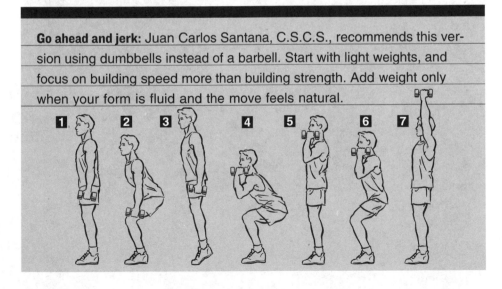

Best Exercise for the Beach: THE ARM-BLASTER CURL

The arm blaster—a thin strip of metal that hangs from your shoulders and prevents your elbows from moving forward and back during a curl—forces your biceps to work much harder than they would if allowed to swing a little. Consequently, this curl is the best single exercise for working all parts of the biceps with maximum intensity, according to *Target Bodybuilding* author Per Tesch, Ph.D.

And the biceps are the best muscles to display on the beach, according to our experts, especially if a rumble breaks out over blanket space. "The stronger your biceps, the faster you can punch," says *Complete Cardiokickboxing* author Tom Seabourne, Ph.D., a sports psychologist and martial artist.

Best Strength Exercise: THE SQUAT

If you aren't doing squats in your workout, you don't have a workout. Squats shape the body and develop performance power, asserts Olympic trainer Don Chu, Ph.D., P.T., C.S.C.S., director of the physical-therapist-assistant program at Ohloney College in Newark, California.

"It's the easiest power move to learn, and you'll see the fastest results" in both strength and muscle size, adds Jason Pulido, personal-training manager at the Crunch gym in lower Manhattan.

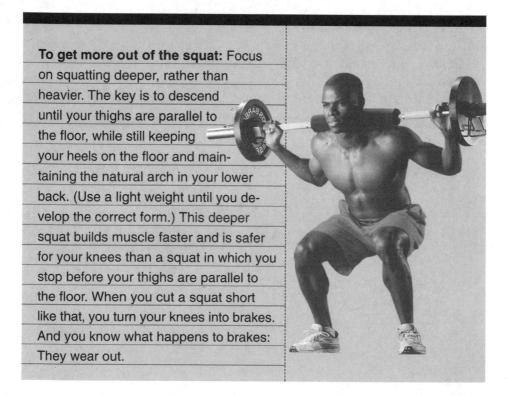

To get more out of the squat: Focus on squatting deeper, rather than heavier. The key is to descend until your thighs are parallel to the floor, while still keeping your heels on the floor and maintaining the natural arch in your lower back. (Use a light weight until you develop the correct form.) This deeper squat builds muscle faster and is safer for your knees than a squat in which you stop before your thighs are parallel to the floor. When you cut a squat short like that, you turn your knees into brakes. And you know what happens to brakes: They wear out.

Best Exercise You Won't Want Your Co-Workers to Know You Do: PILATES

At least it's not Suzanne Somers's Buttmaster. But what the hell is Pilates? It's a form of exercise designed by the dancer Joseph Pilates back in the 1920s. (You remember him, right?) The idea is to make your body more stable and injury-resistant by strengthening muscles when they're in fully lengthened positions, since those tend to be the points at which injuries occur in athletes.

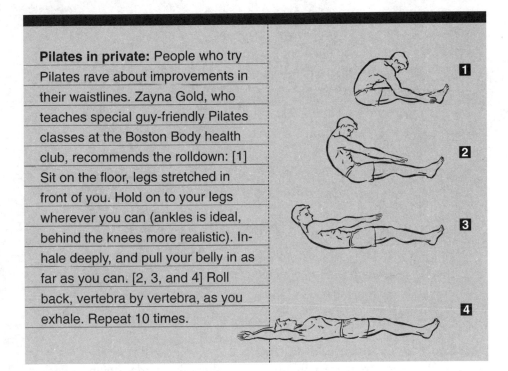

Pilates in private: People who try Pilates rave about improvements in their waistlines. Zayna Gold, who teaches special guy-friendly Pilates classes at the Boston Body health club, recommends the rolldown: [1] Sit on the floor, legs stretched in front of you. Hold on to your legs wherever you can (ankles is ideal, behind the knees more realistic). Inhale deeply, and pull your belly in as far as you can. [2, 3, and 4] Roll back, vertebra by vertebra, as you exhale. Repeat 10 times.

Best Exercise for Health and Longevity: CIRCUIT WEIGHT TRAINING

The beauty of circuit weight training—moving from one exercise to the next with little rest in between—is that you can modify it to achieve lots of different goals. Going faster and using lighter weights can improve heart health and muscle endurance, while doing a slower circuit with heavier weights can build strength, muscle size, and a faster metabolism. Research has shown that for men recuperating from heart surgery, circuit training is the safest and most effective rehabilitation exercise.

You can turn any workout you do into a circuit. It's simple: Do all your exercises one after the other, with 15- to 30-second rests in between. Repeat the circuit three times.

Best Exercise Class for Men: BOOT CAMP

If you're going to train men to kill, you're not going to teach them Tae-Bo. "Boot camp develops willpower and determination, which can really help a man achieve in life," says *Get Buffed* author Ian King, a strength coach who works with Olympic and professional athletes.

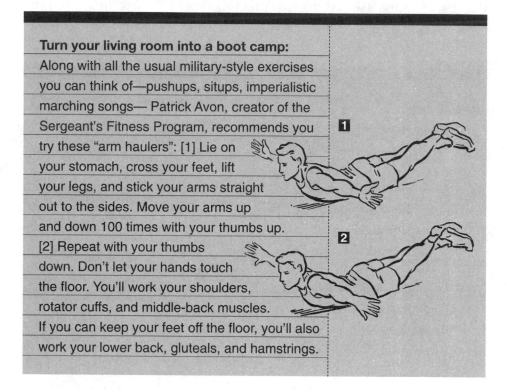

Turn your living room into a boot camp: Along with all the usual military-style exercises you can think of—pushups, situps, imperialistic marching songs— Patrick Avon, creator of the Sergeant's Fitness Program, recommends you try these "arm haulers": [1] Lie on your stomach, cross your feet, lift your legs, and stick your arms straight out to the sides. Move your arms up and down 100 times with your thumbs up. [2] Repeat with your thumbs down. Don't let your hands touch the floor. You'll work your shoulders, rotator cuffs, and middle-back muscles. If you can keep your feet off the floor, you'll also work your lower back, gluteals, and hamstrings.

Best Sport for Exercise: BASKETBALL

Basketball players are in great shape because they never stop moving. "Basketball allows you to run, sprint, jump, slide, stop, and then start all over again," says E. J. "Doc" Kreis, strength coach at the University of Colorado in Denver.

Another benefit: Basketball requires both "power and power endurance—the ability to repeatedly jump up and down for rebounds and putbacks," adds New York City trainer Michael Mejia, C.S.C.S.

Power up your rebounding: The rebound doesn't always go to the player who can jump the highest—it goes to the man who can keep jumping the same height three or four times in a row. Try these rim jumps: Stand beneath a basket, leap up, and slap both hands on the backboard, if you can. If not, just grab some net. (If you can't do that . . . well, we hear racquetball is fun.) Land, then immediately hop back up. Keep going for 30 seconds. Rest 3 to 5 minutes, then repeat. Do a total of two to four sets, and do these only twice a week.

Best Exercise That's Also Fun: MOUNTAIN BIKING

Mountain biking uses tons of energy and muscles, takes a ton of balls—and you don't even notice what it does for your body: A 180-pound guy mountain biking for an hour burns almost 700 calories.

Bring the mountain to you: Mountain biking has a fitness payoff even when you have no mountain handy. Hit the flat road. Riding a mountain bike takes about a third more effort than riding a road bike, largely because of the increased rolling resistance from the fatter tires and the heavier bike. So if your time is limited and you have a choice of bikes, it's always better to choose the mountain bike, even if you'll be riding it on the road. Riding 12 miles on fat tires is the equivalent of doing 15 on the skinny rubber.

Best Exercise That Produces a Useful End Product: CHOPPING WOOD

"Chopping wood is the only real-life exercise that we try to replicate in the gym," says Alwyn Cosgrove, C.S.C.S., owner of Cosgrove Fitness and Sports Training Systems in Santa Clarita, California. And Avon notes that no other activity burns as many calories as wood chopping: up to 23 per minute for a 180-pound man going all-out. Plus, he adds, "chicks dig a man with a flannel shirt and an ax."

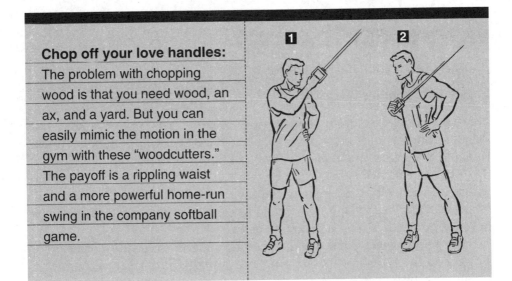

Chop off your love handles: The problem with chopping wood is that you need wood, an ax, and a yard. But you can easily mimic the motion in the gym with these "woodcutters." The payoff is a rippling waist and a more powerful home-run swing in the company softball game.

Best Aerobic Exercise: RUNNING

It's the most basic exercise you can do, but it's also the most intense, says Santana. Become good at it, and you'll be the only person smiling through the oil crisis.

Be a better runner: Focus on improving the speed of your strides rather than their length, says Tom Miller, Ph.D., a biomechanics specialist in Salt Lake City. Your front foot should land under your body—rather than out in front of it—and you should push off the toes of your rear leg for propulsion. Another key is to keep your forearms high throughout the run. You should be able to brush your nipples with your thumbs. (And you may possibly enjoy it.)

Best Exercise of All Time: A Tie between RUNNING and the SQUAT

Our esteemed group chose running because you can do it anywhere, and it doesn't cost anything except what you pay for shoes. It also helps your heart while burning away flab. Our experts suggest you get out and walk, jog, or run three to five times a week. Or, better yet, do some of all three.

The squat, as we said before, builds the muscles of your lower body better than anything else can. And it builds them fast. So if you want a body that won't blow away in a gentle summer breeze, run to the weight room, settle under that bar, and do your squats. Three sets of 10, twice a week, is good for starters. Then mix it up. Use heavy weights and low repetitions for a few weeks to build strength. Use lighter weights and higher reps after that to build muscle endurance. And never forget: The man who squats has carte blanche to bellow and grunt. You'll be as strong as a caveman, with the freedom to sound like one, too.

Be Stronger Than Ever

Try this program for the next 12 weeks

By Lou Schuler

First we asked the experts to pick the best exercises, then we asked Dave Pearson, Ph.D., an exercise physiologist at Ball State University in Muncie, Indiana, to organize them into the best strength workout.

Pick a number. Decide how much you want to be able to lift by the time you're finished with this program. Improving your maximum bench press by 20 percent, for example, is both challenging and doable, especially if you've never done a pure strength program before.

See the goal line. Even if you don't reach your goal, stop after 12 weeks and go back to the type of workouts you were doing before. Heavy lifting is too tough on your body to do year-round.

Rest a lot. Give yourself 2 to 3 minutes between sets.

Don't sweat the small stuff. Exercises for your abdominals, arms, and calves won't help much when you're trying to get stronger. You'll still do them on this program, but if you're feeling wiped out from the heavy lifts, you can skip the small-muscle moves and not notice much difference in your strength.

The Strength Schedule

Exercise	Sets	Reps
Monday		
Clean and press	3	4–6
Lat pulldown	3	6–8
Cable row	3	6–8
Squat	3	6–8
Leg curl	3	6–8
Calf raise	1–3	10–12
Tuesday		
Flat barbell bench press	3	4–6
Incline dumbbell bench press	3	4–6
Lateral raise	1–3	6–8
Biceps exercise (your choice)	1–3	6–8
Triceps exercise (your choice)	1–3	6–8
Abdominal exercise (your choice)	1–3	10–12

Exercise	Sets	Reps
Thursday		
Clean and press	3	4–6
Lat pulldown	3	6–8
Cable row	3	6–8
Squat	3	4–6*
Leg curl	3	6–8
Calf raise	3	10–12
Abdominal exercise (your choice)	1–3	10–12
Friday		
Deadlift	3	4–6
Flat barbell bench press	3	6–8**
Lateral raise	1–3	6–8
Biceps exercise (your choice)	1–3	6–8
Triceps exercise (your choice)	1–3	6–8

*Use more weight than you did Monday.
**Use less weight than you did Tuesday.

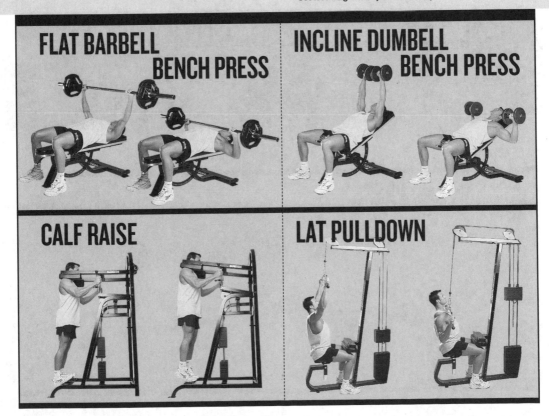

FLAT BARBELL BENCH PRESS

INCLINE DUMBELL BENCH PRESS

CALF RAISE

LAT PULLDOWN

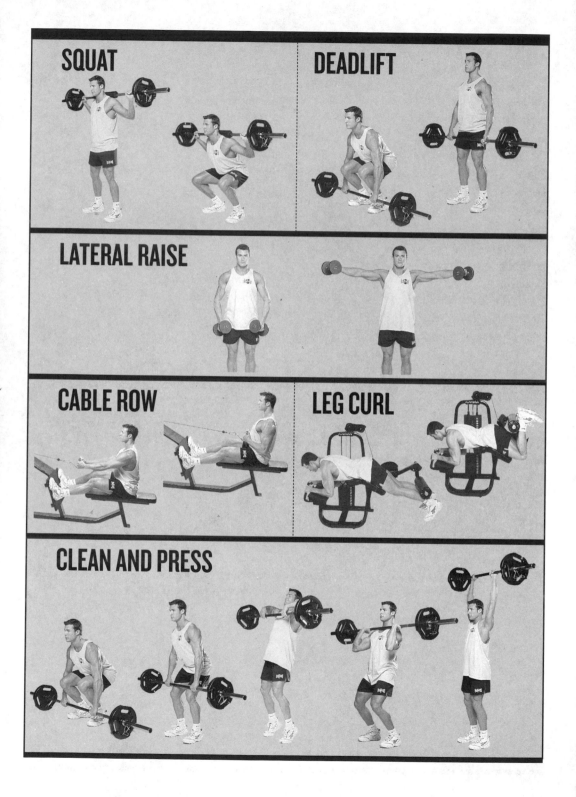

SQUAT

DEADLIFT

LATERAL RAISE

CABLE ROW

LEG CURL

CLEAN AND PRESS

Maximize Your Workout

Seven instant ways to tell if you're building muscle or just wasting time

By Michael Mejia, C.S.C.S., and Lou Schuler

Few areas in life offer you immediate feedback. The only job we can think of in which you know exactly how well you're doing is piloting an airplane. You're either up in the air or spread out over miles of marshland. It's been especially hard to get that kind of feedback in the gym—until now.

We interviewed the experts and found seven immediate signals that tell you how well you're doing when you exercise. Now you'll be able to find out sooner—rather than later—whether your workout is actually working.

If these signs are there, you're getting the most from your muscle. So now a really great workout can be just like flying a plane. And here's your instrument panel.

You feel the exercises where you're supposed to. You may feel a little discomfort in your joints on the first set of an exercise. But the discomfort should disappear on subsequent sets, says Scott Reale, M.D., a sports-medicine specialist in Manhattan.

After that, you should notice it right in the belly of the muscle. Here are the exercises you're likely to feel in the wrong places.

Exercise	Feel It in Your . . .	But Not in Your . . .
Abdominal crunch	Midsection	Lower back, neck
Bench press	Chest, triceps	Shoulder joints
Biceps curl	Upper arms	Elbows, wrists
Lateral raise	Shoulders, upper back	Elbows, neck
Lat pulldown	Upper back	Shoulder joints, arms
Leg curl	Hamstrings	Lower back, gluteals
Leg extension	Quadriceps	Knees
Row	Upper back	Lower back, arms
Squat, deadlift	Thighs, gluteals	Knees, lower back
Triceps extension	Upper arms	Elbows

You're pumped. After a couple of sets, the muscles you're targeting should feel full and hard. This is the pump, the best feeling you can have in a weight room without getting arrested. "You see the results of your work. You look better already," says Tom Baechle, Ed.D., chairman of the exercise-science department at Creighton University in Omaha, Nebraska.

The pump also serves an important physiological purpose. The movements that trap blood in your muscles also generate lactic acid. Lactic acid helps produce growth hormone. Growth hormone is thought to help your muscles grow bigger and your fat cells shrink, since it mobilizes fat for energy.

You don't feel hungry. The last thing you want is for hunger to kick in before your workout is over. "That's a sign your blood-glucose levels are dropping—muscle glycogen is being used at a really rapid rate, and you're about to use muscle protein for energy," says Jacqueline Berning, Ph.D., R.D., a sports nutritionist who works with the Denver Broncos and Colorado Rockies. When you use muscle protein for energy, you make your muscles smaller instead of bigger. We can't support you in that endeavor.

You're nearly as strong from one set to the next. This tells you three good things: You're using the right weight, you're resting enough between sets, and your body is properly fueled. But if your strength drops rapidly between sets, a bunch of stuff is going wrong: You didn't warm up enough, you're using too much weight, or you rushed through your sets—for most purposes, a minute or two between sets is enough time to recover.

Your body feels worked but not trashed. Your muscles will let you know when you've hit it just right. "Muscle spasms may occur in a fatigued muscle, most obviously in the small muscle groups," says Dr. Reale. For example, if your arm shakes a little when you comb your hair after an upper-body workout, that's a sign you really challenged the muscles without overdoing it. (If you can't lift the arm, go to a hospital.)

You feel as if you were on Prozac. For the first couple of hours after a great workout, nothing should bother you. "You should experience an elevation in mood and a decrease in anxiety," says Dr. Reale, who attributes this surge in well-being to hormones called endorphins. "You should also feel more mental energy after a workout." Go ahead, tackle that dissertation you've been putting off.

You can't wait to return. "If you see that you've improved in this workout, that creates a mindset that next week will be even better," says Baechle. Record what you lifted and the number of times you lifted it. You may even feel motivated enough to write down what you expect to hoist in your next workout. You'll be more excited about training, says Baechle, which lays the groundwork for another perfect workout.

YOUR WORKOUT ISN'T WORKING IF...

You can't wait to leave the gym. The opposite of an endorphin release is boredom.

You feel exercises in places you shouldn't feel them. Joint pain signals an impending injury, and only the dumbest keep going.

You're weaker than you were last workout. You should make progress in every workout. If you start to go backward, your body is telling you it's time to try something new.

You feel lousy afterward. If you go into the locker room with nausea, muscle cramps, cold sweats, or a rapid heartbeat, you know you've pushed yourself too far—or you're sick and you shouldn't have been in the gym in the first place.

Game Essentials

25 basic sports skills it's never too late to learn

By Bill Stump

Watch a ball game on TV and you'll inevitably hear one of the announcers say, "You know, Kenny, this team is really well-schooled in the fundamentals."

Here's a surprise: This isn't total blather. There really are such things as fundamentals in sports, and you really can be well-schooled in them. Well, at least you could be if *schooled* were actually a word we used.

But how do you get an athletic education if you're over the age of 7 and not playing in your local Pee Wee League? You keep reading this article. We talked to seasoned basketball, football, and baseball experts and asked them for the insider tips and tactics most pros know and most amateurs don't. Here are 25 reasons you didn't make the team in high school.

BASKETBALL

How to guard a man: Never play him straight up. Find out your guy's weaknesses, then exploit the hell out of them. Is he a horrible outside shooter? Back off and make him fire threes all night. Can he use only his right hand? Overplay him and make him go to his left. "Never play two guys the same way," says Barry Clemens, an 11-year NBA veteran and now the best 51-year-old player on the planet.

How to block a shot: Use the hand opposite the one the shooter is using— if he's a righty, swat away his shot with your left hand, says Clemens. By not having to reach across your body, you gain an extra 6 inches, and you're less likely to get tangled up with the shooter and whistled for a foul.

Another tactic: Swat at the ball as your opponent raises it from hip level to shoot. "I can't jump anymore, so I take a swipe at the ball when it's lower," Clemens says. "Even if I just graze it, I can affect his timing."

How to sink a free throw: The key is consistency: You need to grip and release the ball the same way every time you shoot. To hold the ball in the same place every time, put the middle finger of your shooting hand on the ball's black air valve, which is conveniently positioned in the middle of the ball. The fact that the air valve is slightly raised above the surface of the ball will give your shot a

THE NUMBER OF SITUPS
THE AVERAGE MAN IN HIS 20s CAN DO IN I MINUTE: 40

THE NUMBER OF SITUPS
THE AVERAGE MAN IN HIS 50s CAN DO IN I MINUTE: 26

little more spin, which helps those rim shots fall in, not out. Use your other hand as a guide, but don't let it push the ball in one direction or another.

How to shoot in traffic: Fake one shot, then shoot another by changing your angle, the hand you're using, or your position on the court relative to the rim. Otherwise, you're giving the defender a chance to gather himself and stuff the ball down your throat.

And don't be afraid to use the backboard. "When I'm being harassed by the defense, I tend to shoot harder," Clemens says. "A hard shot has a better chance of going in if you use the glass."

How to create a shot: To create more room to shoot, dip your shoulder into your opponent or gently push him with your forearm. "You have to be subtle," Clemens says. "But when a defender's on his heels, he can't jump. That gives you the room you need."

How to make a steal: Swipe up, not down. Refs and whiny opponents are just waiting for you to hack down on the ball. Flicking up is more surprising— and if you do poke the ball away, it will be higher and easier to grab.

How to avoid a steal: Always hold the ball tightly, with both hands at chest height. If you keep it at your waist, you have to lift it higher to pass or shoot, which telegraphs your move and makes a steal more likely. When you're on the move, the lower you dribble the ball, the harder it is to steal.

How to raise your scoring average 10 points: Master the lost art of the midrange jump shot, Clemens says. It can double your offensive effectiveness, since the 3-point line and the area under the basket are usually clogged.

The following drill can help you perfect your midrange jumper: Using a wall, a bounce-back net, or a buddy to feed you, sprint across the lane at the free-throw line, plant your inside foot with the toe pointed at the basket, and pivot on that foot as you catch the ball. When your shoulders are square to the rim and you're at the apex of your jump, squeeze off the shot.

FOOTBALL

How to get open for a pass: First, close the cushion of space between you and the defender before you change direction. "Get near enough to shake his hand, and don't slow down," says Jim Zorn, former all-pro quarterback with

PERCENTAGE OF AMERICAN MEN
OVER AGE 74 WHO ARE COMPLETELY INACTIVE: **66.6**

PERCENTAGE OF ALL ADULT
AMERICANS WHO ARE COMPLETELY INACTIVE: **25**

PERCENTAGE OF CHILDREN
WHO PARTICIPATE IN VIGOROUS PHYSICAL ACTIVITY: **70**

the Seattle Seahawks and now an assistant coach with the Detroit Lions. "The closer he is when you break, the easier it is to blow past him." Second, as you make your first break, take shorter strides and flex your knees to lower your center of gravity. Both actions will help you make sharper cuts.

How to take off somebody's head: Face the runner as squarely as you can. Stay low by bending your knees (not your waist), and keep your head up to avoid injuring your neck or being faked out. When you get closer, keep your feet directly under your shoulders and take short, choppy steps. Make contact with your chest and outside shoulder, and wrap your arms behind the runner's legs. Try to lift and push the runner backward.

How to catch anything: This receiving drill will turn you and your quarterback into Jerry Rice and Steve Young: Have the QB stand 15 yards away with the ball. Turn your back to him. As he throws the pass, have him yell, "Ball." When you hear the word, turn around, pick up the pass, and snag it. "That's what it's like in a game," Zorn says. Gradually reduce the warning time the QB gives you.

How to rush the passer: Never jump to block a pass; just put your arms up. Why? Because jumping is how guys like Zorn buy time in the pocket. Forcing a defender into the air gives the QB a couple of extra seconds to find a receiver or to take off and run.

How to throw a spiral: To make your missiles hit the mark, follow these tips from Zorn.

1. Stand with a wide, balanced stance, sideways to your target.
2. Step forward with your front foot and point your toe toward your target.
3. Make sure your elbow is higher than your shoulder as you prepare to throw.
4. Follow through by flicking your thumb down and away.

How to break up a pass: The problem with diving in front of the receiver to break up a pass? If you miscalculate, it's a touchdown. To hedge your bet, reach across the receiver's body with your outside arm to knock down the ball, but put your inside arm behind his back. That way, if you miss the ball, you still have the player.

BASEBALL

How to field a grounder: Put your mitt on the ground and adjust upward if the ball takes a hop. "It's impossible to move down on a ball," says Andy Nieto, a baseball coach at the University of Southern California in Los Angeles. Also, be sure to keep your feet wider than your shoulders, flex your knees, and "put a lid on it" with your off hand.

How to throw to first on the run: On softly hit grounders, infielders often have to charge the ball and throw sidearm to first base. The problem: Sidearm throws tend to tail to the right. The solution: Aim to the left of the first baseman, adjusting more for longer throws and not at all for ones within 20 feet.

How to catch a pop fly in the sun: Use your glove to shade your eyes. It's bigger than your free hand and puts the leather in perfect position to snag the ball. "And wear your hat right," says Nieto. "Pull it down over your eyes tightly so that it won't fall off when you run after a fly."

How to field a ball in the outfield: Play the ball to the glove side of your body. "If you try to field it in front of you like an infielder, you'll get tangled up because your feet are moving. That means it will take you longer to throw," says Nieto.

How to take batting practice when you don't have the time or space to take batting practice: Grab a bat, a buddy, and three softballs. Stand so you'll hit the balls into the backstop but have enough room to swing. Your buddy should stand off to the side and slightly ahead of you. Have him toss a ball softly in front of you. Try to drive the ball solidly into the screen. Take 10 swings, then switch and let your buddy take a turn.

How to hold the bat: Put it in your fingers; don't jam it into your palms. "Your fingers are stronger and more flexible, giving you more snap. Gripping it in your palm slows your bat speed," Nieto says. Speed is the key to really tagging the ball.

How to swing at a pitch: Put your feet at shoulder-width, parallel to one another and perpendicular to the mound. "Everything should be in nice straight lines," Nieto says. To swing, stride toward the pitcher with your lead foot and pivot on the ball of your back one. When you make contact, snap your wrists, rolling your dominant hand over. "Guys with funky stances reduce their reaction times," Nieto says. "That's not smart when an 86-mph pitch gives you only 0.4 second to react."

How to hit to the opposite field: Wait a little longer on the pitch so that it's deeper in the strike zone. That will allow you to get "inside" the pitch by keeping your right elbow in. To avoid popping up, concentrate on hitting down on the ball. Keep your front shoulder pointing to the opposite field and follow through.

How to run the bases: When you round a base, tag it with whichever foot you need to in order to ensure you don't break stride. "Coaches used to tell you to use your inside foot, but then you'd see guys stutter-stepping and losing speed," Nieto says. When you hit the bag, use it as a sprinter would use a starting block: Push off to give yourself more speed heading to the next base.

How to slide into a base: Always go feet first, not head first. You're less likely to be injured, and you can stand up more quickly and run to the next base if there's an overthrow. And never slide into first base, except to avoid a tag. "If it's faster, then why didn't Carl Lewis slide across the finish line of his races?" Nieto asks.

KNOW THIS

Lift for Longevity

We've known for a while that aerobic exercise protects you from the cellular damage caused by free radicals, highly reactive molecules that cause oxidation, a cell-damaging process linked to heart disease, among other age-related health problems. A University of Florida study is the first evidence that resistance training offers free-radical protection, too. Though the mechanism of protection was unclear, the results were decisive, according to Kevin Vincent, Ph.D., the study author. Older people who did resistance exercises three times a week for 6 months showed less oxidative cell damage than nonlifters. One explanation: Lifting boosts both the levels of free radicals in your body and the levels of enzymes that combat them, which increases your antioxidant defenses.

Avoid Sideline Infection

Athlete's foot isn't all you can catch in the locker room. According to Japanese researchers, one player on an American football team accidentally infected 10 of his teammates with hepatitis B. The virus was likely transmitted during training, through exposure to open wounds. If you play contact sports that can cause bloody injuries, ask your doctor about a hepatitis-B vaccination. You can also make sure that bandages stay in place on the court or field by covering them with prewrap and tape, just as you would a strained muscle.

Vitamin Ease

Antioxidants like vitamin E reduce muscle soreness caused by lifting weights, according to research from Ball State University. In the study, 11 college-age men took either a placebo or 1,200 international units of vitamin E and went on a weight-lifting regimen for 3 weeks. "The vitamin-E users showed statistically lower levels of free radicals after working out, which translated to less soreness after lifting," says Bruce Craig, Ph.D., the physiologist who conducted the research.

Shoe Mileage

Wearing out the rubber in your shoes can be almost as dangerous as wearing out the one in your wallet. Perry Julien, D.P.M., of the American Academy of Podiatric Sports Medicine, estimates that 15 percent of overuse injuries to the foot are caused by worn-out or wrong footwear. Here's how long to keep your treads.

Running: 300 to 500 miles

Walking: 300 to 600 miles

Hiking: 500 miles

Basketball: 6 months, playing twice a week for 1 hour

Tennis/racquetball: 6 to 9 months, playing 1 hour a week

All-purpose cleats: 1 year, playing once or twice a week

Fit Beats Thin

Don't envy your skinny co-worker's fast metabolism. He's headed toward the grave faster than you are. An 8-year National Institute on Aging study of 22,000 men found that men who were thin but not aerobically fit had a higher death rate from heart disease than overweight guys who exercised regularly. "Leanness is no guarantee of good health. Being fit is more important in predicting mortality," says study author Steven N. Blair, P.Ed. So quit worrying about how your pants fit, and start running—or some other pudgy guy might retire with your wife.

Nature's Carb Gel

Honey is a cheaper alternative to preexercise sports drinks and carbohydrate gels. Researchers at the University of Memphis gave people about 3 tablespoons of honey just before their workouts. Turns out that the honey was just as good a source of energy as commercially available gels and sports drinks. "You'd have to drink about a liter of a sports drink to get the same effect you get with the honey," according to Richard Kreider, Ph.D., the lead researcher.

DOWN THE PIKE

Try This Gel and Call Me in the Morning

Say goodbye to bottled aspirin: Rutgers University researchers recently found that a new aspirin gel reduces pain almost immediately after being rubbed on joints or muscles. The gel activates when it comes into contact with water in the skin. "The difference is that this form of aspirin may not cause problems such as stomach irritation, since it isn't taken internally," says study author Kathryn Uhrich, Ph.D. The gel—called PolyAspirin—is expected to be on the market in 2004.

NUMBER OF AMERICANS BETWEEN THE AGES OF 18 AND 64 WHO DO STRENGTH-BUILDING EXERCISES: 1 IN 6

NUMBER OF MEN TREATED IN THE ER FOR WEIGHT-LIFTING INJURIES OVER THE PAST 20 YEARS: 1 MILLION

POUNDS THE AVERAGE 175-POUND MAN IN HIS 20s CAN BENCH-PRESS ONE TIME: 180

POUNDS THE AVERAGE 175-POUND MAN IN HIS 50s CAN BENCH-PRESS ONE TIME: 128

DOES IT WORK?

Ankle Weights

A quick way to lose 20 pounds?

 Besides clashing with your bunny slippers, 20-pound ankle weights could cause ankle sprains and shinsplints because the weight is supported by your feet, not your muscle. Use them under supervision for rehab purposes only.

Dunlop's Abzorber Tennis Ball ($4 for Three)

The claim: The ball (which is made of a variety of lightweight materials) generates less impact on your forearm and elbow than a regular ball.

 The ball can help a little. But "reducing vibration on your arm isn't nearly as effective in preventing tennis elbow as building up strength in your arm so that it absorbs the impact of the torque forces on its own," says Robert Nirschl, M.D., medical director of the Nirschl Orthopedic Sports Medicine Clinic.

Kelty's Back Balancer Abdominal Support System ($30)

The claim: Strap the Balancer in place over your belly and you'll convert your backpack into a back brace that prevents back strain and allows you to carry more weight for a longer period of time without getting tired.

 The Balancer does make your pack function like a back brace, but that won't actually help reduce back pain while you're hiking.

We had William Marras, Ph.D., a bioengineer at Ohio State University in Columbus, try out the Back Balancer in his lab. His finding: "The Back Balancer had virtually no effect on the amount of force a pack places on your spine." In fact, in two different tests Marras performed using a 35-pound backpack, the Balancer was not able to reduce force on the spine at all.

COOL STUFF

Summertime Skis

Here's something for the snow junkie who's been transferred to Florida: The new Crosskate 616 BackCountry Skates ($1,200) work like cross-country skis but have mountain bike–style tires to rumble over rough, snowless terrain. To turn, just lean in the direction you want to go. They won't roll backward, so it's easy to climb hills. Check www.crosskate.com or call (877) 276-7758.

Get It off Your Chest

Wearing a heart-rate monitor that wraps around your chest makes you feel as if you're working out in a bra (sure, we know how that feels!). Thankfully, newer watchlike monitors have sensors that pick up the pulse from your fingers. Our testers liked both the Pulse Pro ($99) and the Mio ($119) monitors, but warned that they didn't always register heart rates on uneven terrain—which means there's no point in wearing one while you're mountain biking or giving her a massage.

Dumbbells for Dummies

Adjustable dumbbells have been around for years, but most sets are harder to adjust than the water temperature in the gym showers. Thankfully, Probell dumbbells are easy. Turn the dial on the side of the holder to pick a weight from 5 to 30 pounds; this locks the unused weights in place while you curl away. These are good for a circuit that calls for different weights. You can

**PERCENTAGE OF AMERICANS IN 1999
WHO MADE A DAILY EFFORT TO HELP KEEP THEMSELVES FIT: 60**

**PERCENTAGE OF AMERICANS IN 1961
WHO MADE A DAILY EFFORT TO HELP KEEP THEMSELVES FIT: 24**

quickly adjust the dial to do a round of shoulder presses (heavy weight), lateral raises (medium weight), and rear raises (light). The convenience of a six-in-one weight set will cost you $330. Check www.probell.com to order.

Comfort in a Nutshell

The new Bike Pro-Fit Adjustable Supporter has a large Velcro pad that lets you adjust the support and ensures that the kick-resistant cup doesn't ride too high or low. Wear it to the next Million-Mom March—but under your pants this time. Pick one up for $16 at www.bikeathletic.com.

WHAT WORKS

At the end of the day, every guy's dream is a six-pack. And we're not just talking about the kind you down with pizza. It'd be nice if getting a hard body weren't so, well, hard. (It's a lot easier to down that six-pack than it is to achieve one.) Here, we make it easier to get ripped with a slew of tips to sculpt you from head to toe, not to mention pointers to prevent injuries and recover from them fast.

Once you get and stay fit, you'll be at the top of your game, looking and feeling years younger—and maybe even turning the heads of younger women. So don't give up that dream of dating a cheerleader just yet (though you might have to give up the liquid six). Oh yeah, we almost forgot: You'll likely live longer, too. That's what we call true survival of the fittest.

I. Drink this for more muscle. It's true that you go to the gym to build muscle, but that's not where the stuff is really made. It's made later, when you're collapsed on the sofa, watching reruns of *Chico and the Man* and wondering where your life went wrong. As you rest, your body is busy repairing and rebuilding the muscle tissue you flexed all afternoon. You can maximize the process by taking in the right mix of protein and carbohydrates within 3 hours of your workout. Your body builds muscle faster during this time, and that optimum nutrient combination stimulates the hormones needed to make it happen.

There's no simpler or more convenient muscle-building mix than a shake made with a pasteurized egg substitute, flavored soy milk, and fruit, says sports nutritionist Liz Applegate, Ph.D., R.D., of the University of California at Davis. Throw this stuff into a blender and you produce a 370-calorie shake with 25 grams of high-quality egg and soy protein, only 5 grams of fat, and plenty of healthy stuff like fiber, vitamin C, and other antioxidants. Plus, it tastes good, and it's festively pink.

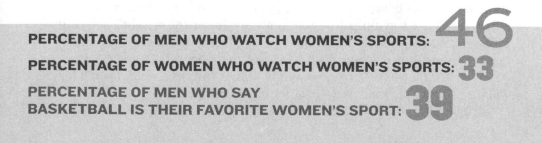

PERCENTAGE OF MEN WHO WATCH WOMEN'S SPORTS: **46**

PERCENTAGE OF WOMEN WHO WATCH WOMEN'S SPORTS: **33**

PERCENTAGE OF MEN WHO SAY
BASKETBALL IS THEIR FAVORITE WOMEN'S SPORT: **39**

Ingredients

1	cup ice cubes
¾	cup egg substitute, such as EggBeaters (It's found in the frozen-food section; use it partially thawed. Don't worry about cooking; since it's pasteurized, it's okay to use right out of the carton.)
¾	cup vanilla soy milk (found in the dairy or health-food section)
1	cup frozen strawberries
½	banana
½	cup cranberry juice

Put the ice, egg substitute, soy milk, strawberries, banana, and cranberry juice in a blender with a tight lid. Blend on high for 30 seconds. Drink it out of the blender cup so you don't have to wash another glass.

2. Climb stairs for a six-pack. We can turn just about anything into a way to work our abs (if we don't, we're fired). Next up: the stairclimber. This move from physical therapist Neil Chasan will fry your gut faster than a jar of habaneros. With the climber set on a fast setting and body weight set at 50 pounds, get into a pushup position behind the machine. Place your hands on the pedals, with your shoulders over them. Keep your legs straight and your feet shoulder-width apart. Step with your hands to keep up with the quick-moving pedals. Your abdominal muscles will be under constant strain while trying to keep your body balanced during the movement. Go for 30 to 45 seconds (or as long as you can), then rest for a minute. Try to do three to five sets.

3. For bigger biceps, do smaller reps. A few more inches in the right place can make a big difference. Women are always telling us that. But we're not just talking about your sex life—it applies to your workout, too. Add an extra one-fourth repetition to a biceps preacher curl, for example. The lower part of the curl is where most men are weakest, and that can limit the effectiveness of the exercise, says Alwyn Cosgrove, C.S.C.S., owner of Cosgrove Fitness and Sports Training Systems in Santa Clarita, California. The extra movement (described below) will put your muscles under tension for a longer time, which is crucial for muscle growth.

Here's how to do it: Sit at a preacher bench, rest your upper arms on the pad, and lower the barbell in an underhand grip until your elbows are almost straight. Without bouncing at the bottom of the move, slowly curl the weight a quarter of the way up. Pause momentarily, lower the weight back to the bottom position, then curl it all the way up. The entire sequence counts as one repetition; do anywhere from 6 to 10 of them per set.

(Tip: You may have to use less weight at first, but the strength you'll build will have you lifting more in your other biceps exercises.)

4. Build your ski legs. There's more to skiing than avoiding trees and women named Picabo. You need balance, endurance, and strength. These three exercises from *Get Buffed* author Ian King, C.S.C.S., a strength coach who works with Olympic and professional athletes, will prepare you for skiing—or for anything that requires you to move from leg to leg quickly, like basketball or bank robbery. Warm up for 5 minutes, then do these exercises, with only 1 minute of rest after each.

Single-leg balance squat (for balancing on one leg when your legs are fatigued). Stand sideways on a 6-inch block or step and move one foot off the edge. Bend the knee of the supporting leg so that the nonsupporting foot brushes the floor. Hold that position for 3 to 5 seconds; stand back up. When you can do 20 of these, increase the height of the block.

Single-leg ski squat (for balance and controlling your ski direction). Stand on one leg; place the other leg in front of you with your heel about 6 inches above the floor. Squat down until the thigh of your back leg is almost parallel to the floor. Do 10 repetitions. Rest for 15 seconds, then switch legs. Use two sturdy chairs only for balance. (Hey, like ski poles!)

Double-leg ski squat (for strength and endurance). Lean against a wall, with your feet about 2 feet away from it and shoulder-width apart. Bend your knees slightly and hold that position for 5 to 10 seconds. Bend deeper and hold. Repeat until you've hit five different positions; go as low as you can. Work up to 30 seconds in each position.

5. Angle for a bigger chest. Geometry students and pool hustlers aren't the only ones who benefit from understanding sharp angles. You can, too, by working your chest at different angles—with virtually no rest between sets, says New York City trainer Michael Mejia, C.S.C.S. The benefit of doing these "angled drop sets" is that by working from the hardest to the easiest press positions, you'll stimulate more muscle fibers in your chest in about half the time. To start, do a set of incline presses with a weight that will fatigue you after 8 to 10 repetitions. Rest for 10 seconds, drop the angle of the bench, and do a flat press with the same weight. Do as many repetitions as possible— usually three to five more than on the incline. Rest for 10 seconds, then do as many decline presses as you can. Rest for 2 minutes and repeat.

6. Maximize your sprinting power. Half a step can make a huge difference. Safe or out. Touchdown or incomplete. Clean escape or dog-nipped ankles. To squeeze the most out of every stride, listen to Monte Stratton, head sprinting coach at Texas Christian University in Fort Worth. Before you start, imagine your face is made out of jelly (we like grape). This helps keep your body relaxed, which will help you outrun anything on two legs.

Play the angle. As you push off with your dominant leg, lean 50 to 60 degrees forward. This low position will keep you as aerodynamic as possible at the start. Work into an upright position in the first 10 yards of your run.

Move your arms. Start to bring your shoulders back. Keep your arms at about a 90-degree angle; pump them so your hands move from your hips to your chin. Imagine your hands ripping through your pockets. They shouldn't cross your body.

Stay straight and strong. Keep your chest and shoulders still. Run with your upper body leaning slightly forward. This is the most efficient sprinting position. Don't look back until you make it to the getaway car.

7. To tighten your gut, improve your posture. Sitting straight will not only keep your nose out of your soup but also make your abdominal muscles look better. How? When you have good posture, your back supports more of your body weight, which in turn keeps your gut from spilling over your belt, says Cosgrove. The hard part is developing the muscles that'll help you maintain good posture all day: your lower back, hip flexors, and hamstrings. This exercise will help. Lie on your back with a rolled-up towel under your left knee. Raise your right leg straight up and hold it. Push down with your left leg while pushing up with your hips. Hold for 15 to 20 seconds, then switch legs. Repeat three times.

8. Strengthen your rotator cuffs with this move. Between golf and tennis, your arms swing more than Tarzan when Jane leaves town. That's why it's important to do the following move, courtesy of Cosgrove. It'll help strengthen your rotator cuffs—the muscles and tendons in the front, top, and back of your shoulders—so you can wield your club, racket, or machete with more power.

- Lie facedown on an incline bench. Hold dumbbells that weigh less than 10 percent of what you can bench-press. (Don't know that vital stat? Start with 12 to 15 pounds.)
- Drop your hands toward the ground with your knuckles facing the floor. Row your arms back until they bend at a 90-degree angle, keeping your hands in the same position.
- Rotate your forearms up—pivot at the elbow—until the dumbbells are even with your chin. Reverse the maneuver to return to the starting position. Do two sets of 6 to 10 repetitions.

9. Minimize workout heartburn. Have you ever finished working out, only to find your heart burning more than an Irish girl in the tropics? You might be suffering from exercise-induced acid reflux. A survey of 319 athletes by the Oklahoma Foundation for Digestive Research found that weight lifters reported suffering from heartburn three times more often than other athletes. When lifters hold their breath during repetitions, abdominal pressure increases and shoots extra stomach acid up the esophagus, says gastroenterologist Philip Schoenfeld, M.D. To reduce symptoms, don't eat for 1 to 2 hours before a workout and always exhale when you're pushing or pulling the weight.

10. Build abs that show. It takes more than crunches to make your abs look like speed bumps. You need to do exercises that incorporate added resistance or that extend your abdominals' range of motion, says Mejia. We can show you two exercises that do both at the same time.

Angled reverse crunch. Lie on a slant board with your head near the top. Place a medicine ball between your knees. Lift your legs and bring your knees toward your chest. Return to the starting position. Do three sets of 10 to 12 repetitions. At home, you can do the same exercise on the floor; try holding a phone book between your knees.

Weighted exercise-ball crunch. Lie with your back on an exercise ball and your feet planted in front of you. Rest a dumbbell (start with 10 pounds) on your upper chest, right under your chin. Crunch your abdominals as you lift your shoulder blades as high off the ball as you can. Hold for a second, then return to the starting position. Do three sets of 10 to 12 crunches. If you can't do that many with a dumbbell, start without weights, holding your hands behind your ears. No ball? Put a rolled-up towel under the small of your back.

11. Speed recovery from pulls, strains, and tears. Stretch with an ice pack on a sore muscle. When your muscle is cold, it's relaxed and stays elongated during stretching. This makes it easier for blood to get to the injury to heal it, says Olympic trainer Don Chu, Ph.D., P.T., C.S.C.S., director of the physical-therapist-assistant program at Ohloney College in Newark, California. When treating a pulled muscle, tape an ice pack to the tender part and stretch the muscle for 12 to 20 minutes a day. That can knock days or weeks off your recovery time.

12. Twist to prevent golf injuries. Golfers can develop small stress fractures in their lower ribs because their abdominal muscles constantly pull on their ribs as they swing, says Gail Wadley, A.T.C., an athletic trainer at the Ohio State University Medical Center in Columbus. If you have a persistent pain in your ribs that lasts longer than a month, ask your doctor about getting an x-ray to make sure no ribs are broken. You can avoid these cracks by strengthening your back and abdominal muscles during the off-season. Place a broom or bar across your shoulders. Drape your wrists over each side and do slow side twists. Work up to three sets of 30 turns, three times a week.

13. Save your golf balls to save your feet. If you're on the run more than Robert Downey Jr.'s parole officer, try rolling golf balls under your feet from heel to toe for 2 minutes each morning. It'll help prevent painful inflammation of the ligament in the sole of your foot.

ANY QUESTIONS?

Spare My Feelings

I've recently started to lift weights again, and my thumbs, index fingers, and middle fingers go numb. I can't narrow it down to any specific group of exercises, and it happens every time I lift. What is this?

—L. D., Louisville

It sounds like a form of repetitive strain injury, says Olympic trainer Don Chu, Ph.D., P.T., C.S.C.S., director of the physical-therapist-assistant program at Ohloney College in Newark, California. "This is typically a problem for people who use a computer all day or do other repetitive movements with their hands," he says. (Chu didn't choose to elaborate on that last one, for some reason.) When you grip the bar, you put pressure on the soft tissues of your wrists. This may compress the nerves around the carpal tunnel, an opening among the bones of your wrist. To ease the pressure, make the following adjustments.

Wear a pair of lifting gloves. This will allow you to relax your grip a little.

Warm up properly. Do 10 or so wrist circles, then stretch each wrist by pressing your fingers back lightly with the opposite hand. Hold for a few seconds, then repeat with the other hand.

Use a thumbless grip. Avoid wrapping your thumb around the bar when you lift.

If You Grunt in the Gym and No One Hears You . . . ?

Why do some men grunt when they lift weights? Does this really help, or is it just a way for these guys to show off to the whole gym?

—M. C., San Antonio

We know that grunting is appropriate at certain times—like when she asks you something during SportsCenter. But it can also help you in the gym, especially when you're lifting heavy weights. Try exhaling forcefully while lifting during a tough set of bench presses. This stabilizes your spine, which improves your form and enables you to lift heavier weights, says Mike Barnes, C.S.C.S., of the National Strength and Conditioning Association. That stabilization can help give you the last push you need to finish a difficult set.

Cut Your Weighting Time

I hate weight training. How much of it do I absolutely need? Did I mention that I hate it?

—T. B., Akron, Ohio

Three times a week is optimal; but you can get 70 percent of the benefit by training only once a week. It's a great return on a small investment. You can get away with a single exercise for each muscle group—about 15 in all. Do one set of 8 to 12 repetitions with a weight heavy enough that the last couple of repetitions are difficult. The whole session should take no more than 30 minutes. If you're a beginner, you'll gain significant strength. If you're more experienced, you'll at least maintain the strength and muscle mass you already have.

Saddle Damage

You always talk about how bike saddles can damage the penis and testicles. Exactly how much is too much?

—J. J., Kirkland, Wash.

If you ride less than 50 miles a week, it's unlikely you'll ever have a problem," says Marc Goldstein, M.D., an avid cyclist and director of the center for male reproductive medicine at New York Hospital–Cornell Medical Center. "But if you're riding 75 miles or more per week, you have reason to be concerned." The usual narrow bike saddle puts pressure on the nerves and arteries leading to your penis. The more time you spend this way, the greater the potential damage to your twig and berries, including impotence and lowered sperm counts. To prevent the unthinkable:

Get off on a regular basis. Every half-hour, dismount, walk around, and shake your legs out for a few minutes.

Let your boys breathe. Avoid spandex bike shorts, which keep your testicles at an elevated temperature and can lower sperm count.

Pick another seat. Several companies make bike seats designed to exert less pressure on the genitals. (One, the Oasis M.D. seat by Trek, was designed by Dr. Goldstein.) If you ride your bike a lot, this could be the best investment you'll ever make.

Take It Queasy

I sometimes feel nauseated after I work out. I don't think it's dehydration, because I drink gallons of water before and during my workout. What's going on?

—M. C., Pearl River, N.Y.

Sit down, put your head between your knees, and ask yourself these questions, courtesy of Lawrence Armstrong, Ph.D., of the University of Connecticut in Farmington.

1. "Am I exercising too soon after a meal?" If so, your muscles, skin, and gastrointestinal tract may be competing for blood, which can sabotage your workout and your digestion. Wait at least 2 hours after a light meal, 4 hours after a heavier one.

2. "Am I exercising like a demon?" This can cause lactic acid to build up in your blood, which can lead to nausea and vomiting. To avoid this, keep your workouts at 65 to 70 percent of your maximum heart rate. (A quick test: If you're so out of breath that you can't carry on a conversation, you're probably exercising above 70 percent.)

3. "Am I drinking too much at one time?" "The average person can empty $\frac{3}{4}$ to $1\frac{1}{2}$ quarts of fluid from the stomach per hour," says Armstrong. "If you're drinking more than that, the stomach is expanding and could make you feel sick." To be safe, drink no more than a quart an hour.

NUMBER OF CALORIES A GOLFER BURNS SHOOTING A 72 ON AN 18-HOLE COURSE: 1,473

NUMBER OF CALORIES A GOLFER BURNS SHOOTING A 110: 2,227

Aerobically Challenged

How much aerobic exercise do I absolutely need? I hate it. And do I have to do it all at once, or can I break it up?

—R. E., Flemington, N.J.

The least you can get away with is 20 minutes of aerobic exercise three times a week," says exercise physiologist Richard Cotton. "That's to maintain aerobic fitness—you won't transform your body with that little exercise."

If you're trying to lose body fat—or stay lean in spite of frequent beer-and-chicken-wing orgies—a more rigorous schedule is in order. For the fat-conscious, Cotton recommends four or five 45-minute sessions every week.

It's fine to break it up into a couple of shorter sessions during the day, says Cotton—just make sure you're doing a full 20 (or 45) minutes at your target heart rate. Warmups and cooldowns are important, but they don't count toward your total.

PART TWO FEAST
AND THRIVE

MUST READS

The Busy-Man's Nutrition Plan

An aisle-by-aisle guide to improving your whole life
at the mini-mart

By Duane Swierczynski

If you live in one of the suburban enclaves of our great nation, you have likely observed this retail phenomenon: giant, mall-like, one-stop grocery stores from which you can purchase everything from sushi to diapers to $100-a-pound imported truffles, all while waiting for your clothes to be dry-cleaned.

That's nice, if you want to spend the afternoon wandering miles of aisles instead of hitting the links.

The time has come to celebrate one of our country's unsung suppliers of food and sundries: the mini-mart. Where else can you buy a cup of hot coffee, a cache of condoms, and a load of lottery tickets in a kwik 5 minutes?

Here's how the convenience store can simplify your life. After all, who needs sushi when all you want is a sandwich?

IN THE DAIRY SECTION

- Grab a plain 8-ounce low-fat yogurt and dump in half of a generic bag of nuts and dried fruit. You'll get less sugar, fewer calories, and more protein (3 extra grams) than in one of those yogurts with fruit already added. Note: This trick does not work with a raw egg, a bottle of beer, and a Slim Jim.
- Convenience stores tend to overcharge on every item except for the staples: milk, bread, and eggs. Stock up on those when you duck in.

AT THE HOT DOG COUNTER

- One of the original 15 Commandments (even God needed an editor): Thou shalt not eat pork by-products that spin. If you simply must have a rotisserie dog, make it one that's a bit shriveled. According to processed-food expert Barry Swanson, Ph.D., of Washington State University in Pullman, wrinkled wieners look terrible but usually have had more heart-strangling saturated fat cooked out of them.

- While you're at it, dress that dog to the nines: Spicy relish contains capsaicin, which can speed your metabolism and in turn help burn fat. Ketchup will baste your prostate gland with lycopene and your stomach with flavonoids—both potent cancer fighters. And onions contain allicin, to lower cholesterol and make your breath stink.

AT THE DELI COUNTER

- If there's a poster in the window advertising THE EMPIRE STRIKES BACK: COMING SOON, stick with ham sandwiches. Meats that have been cured are better able to resist the organisms that lead to spoiling, says meat-safety expert John Forrest, Ph.D., of Purdue University in West Lafayette, Indiana. Salami is another meat that's been cured . . . of everything except its high fat content.
- Before you take the leap, wait until the clerk isn't looking and then—quick—touch the sandwich case. The glass should feel cool and even have a bit of frost, says Forrest. Not sure? When in doubt, avoid anything green that moans when you touch it.

IN THE CHIP ZONE

- Your Dorito decision: Cooler Ranch or Nacho Cheesier? Neither. 3D's Jalapeno Cheddar have 10 fewer calories and 3 grams less fat per serving.

IN THE CANDY AISLE

- Not only is the Oh Henry! the healthiest candy bar around—lowest in saturated fat, and high in protein and carbohydrates—it is also the only one named for a major literary figure. The Alexandre Dumas–inspired 3 Musketeers bar doesn't even come close.

IN THE CAKE CORRIDOR

- The healthiest snack cake? Low-Fat Cream-Filled Chocolate Tastykakes. Eat the two in the pack and take in 200 calories, 3 grams of total fat, 1 gram of saturated fat, 42 grams of carbohydrates, 3 grams of protein, and 1 gram of fiber. That's right—fiber in cupcakes!

AMOUNT OF MONEY THE AVERAGE GUY SPENDS AT THE GROCERY STORE PER YEAR: $2,964

AMOUNT OF MONEY THE AVERAGE GUY SPENDS ON FAST FOOD AND PIZZA PER YEAR: $2,157

QUIK SEDUCTION

We asked chef David Goldberg, spokesman for the American Personal Chefs Association, to create the impossible: a romantic, five-course gourmet meal using only convenience store items. Not only did he do it but, amazingly, no part of the meal involves beef jerky.

What to Buy

- 4 ounces of spreadable cream cheese
- Small box of crackers (anything but saltines—"they're too salty and not particularly attractive," says Goldberg)
- Vacuum-sealed bag of sliced pepperoni
- Small jar of Spanish olives
- Prepared bag of salad with Caesar dressing (or lettuce, tomato, and dressing)
- 4 ounces of Parmesan cheese
- 2 pints of half-and-half
- Can of tomato soup
- Box of shaped pasta (and we don't mean "spaghetti-shaped")
- Can of mushroom soup
- 5-ounce can of chicken (look near the tuna; it's there)
- Bottle of your favorite white wine (if you live in a state where mini-marts can't sell liquor, move)
- Hershey's chocolate syrup
- Frozen pound cake
- Can of fruit cocktail
- Can of whipped cream (because every romantic meal should end with whipped cream)

What to Stuff in Your Pock . . . Er, Take Complimentary Samples Of

- Packages of croutons (look near the soup—get as many as you can before people begin to stare)

What to Make

Appetizer: H'ors de Gas 'n' Go: Slather cream cheese on a cracker. Add a slice of pepperoni and an olive—"with a red pimiento, for color," adds Goldberg. Make a dozen or so.

Salad: The Caesar-Eleven. Divide the bagged salad between two plates. Cover each with a little dressing, the free croutons, and a dash of Parmesan cheese. "Parm" the rim of the plate, too. "These garnishes will make it look gourmet, even though it's not," says Goldberg.

Soup: Quik-Tomato Surprise. Use the half-and-half, not water or whole milk, to make the soup. "It gives it a different consistency and a much sweeter flavor," says Goldberg. Then float more croutons on top, and sprinkle on some Parmesan. And yes, Parm the rim of the soup bowl.

Entrée: A-Plus Chicken-Mushroom Alfredo. Cook the pasta according to the package directions; drain. Throw the cream of mushroom soup into a pot and stir in a cup of half-and-half. Heat—but don't bring to a boil—then simmer and stir. Stir in the chicken, which is precooked, and add 2 tablespoons of wine. Cook for 2 to 3 minutes and remove from the heat. Dump some of the pasta on a plate, top with the sauce, add a dash of Parmesan—on the sauce part only, not the rest of the pasta—and sprinkle on some parsley flakes, if you have them handy. Parm the rim of the plate, and you're finished.

Dessert: Pump 'n' Pantry Delight. On a small plate, make a fancy-pants squiggle design with the Hershey's syrup. (Avoid satanic pentagrams.) Add a slice of pound cake, followed by fruit cocktail, followed by whipped cream, followed by hot sex right there on the Parmesan-dusted table.

Nutrition disclaimer: This meal is for occasional seduction purposes only. It is not a healthy dinner. (Read: Don't dine à la mini-mart every day.)

IN BEVERAGE ALLEY

- Drink apple juice to wash down all of your questionable mini-mart meals. University of California researchers found that it helps prevent the clogging of arteries that results from the LDL ("bad") cholesterol in saturated fat.
- Or grab a bottle of iced tea—the green kind. It has less sugar and caffeine than soda, and it packs phytochemicals that may help lower cholesterol and prevent prostate cancer. It may also help you lose weight: Research has shown that men who take green-tea supplements burn more calories and fat.
- Partial to trendy drinks with stuff like kava kava and ginseng? Choose them only if you like the taste, not because they look like they should be good for you. These beverages will have virtually no effect on your health.

AT THE CHECKOUT

- Skip the new "dental" gums: They're no better than regular gum, and they cost more. Chewing any sugar-free gum produces saliva, which in turn neutralizes the acids that cause plaque and cavities. But research has shown that gums with natural peppermint oil, such as Dentyne Ice or Extra, are best for hiding onion and garlic odors.

Food Fixes

You could just eat. Or you could beat stress, build muscle, protect your prostate, save your heart, and survive a hangover. Here's your menu

By Brian Good

THE PERFECT FOODS FOR PREVENTING PROSTATE CANCER

Tangerines. They turn margaritas into medicine, thanks to tangeretin and nobiletin—flavonoids that inhibited the growth of prostate cancer in the lab—

NUMBER OF TIMES PER WEEK THE AVERAGE GUY COOKS AT HOME: 2

NUMBER OF TIMES PER WEEK THE AVERAGE GUY EATS IN A RESTAURANT: 5

and vitamin C. Researchers found that a high-C diet may cut prostate-cancer risk by 23 percent.

Tequila. We don't know if the worm has anything to do with it, but Harvard researchers found that downing two alcoholic drinks a day may reduce your risk of an enlarged prostate.

Broccoli. It tastes better when you realize that a study of 1,200 men showed that those who regularly ate the most broccoli and other cruciferous vegetables reduced their prostate-cancer risk by 41 percent.

Sweet potatoes and carrots. Count it: 4,250 milligrams of beta-carotene. That's enough of the antioxidant to help reduce your risk of prostate cancer by 32 percent.

Chicken. Grab a breast; you'll get more than half of your Daily Value of selenium. According to one study, men taking a selenium supplement for $4\frac{1}{2}$ years were 63 percent less likely to die of prostate cancer than those who took a placebo.

Whole wheat tortilla and beans. Both contain selenium and a heavy dose of fiber. Canadian researchers found that a diet high in soluble fiber lowered levels of prostate-specific antigen, the body's marker for the presence of prostate cancer.

Wheat germ. A study at the Fred Hutchinson Cancer Research Center showed that men who took supplemental vitamin E had a 20 percent lower risk of prostate cancer, while those who took zinc daily had 45 percent less risk. Wheat germ is high in both.

Watermelon. It's red for a reason: Watermelon contains lycopene, a phytochemical that may reduce your prostate-cancer risk by as much as 40 percent.

Make 'Em into a Meal
Tangerine Margaritas

1	ounce tequila
$\frac{1}{2}$	ounce lime juice
$\frac{1}{2}$	ounce triple sec
2	ounces tangerine juice

Mix the tequila, lime juice, triple sec, and tangerine juice and serve over crushed ice.

Makes 1 serving.
Per serving: 125 calories, 0 grams (g) protein, 7 g carbohydrates, 0 g fat (0% of calories)

Spicy Mexican Vegetables

2 teaspoons canola oil
1 sweet potato, diced
1 large carrot, cubed
1 cup broccoli florets
1 chile pepper, diced
2 tomatoes, diced
1 cup corn
1 tablespoon cumin

Heat the oil in a nonstick skillet and fry the sweet potato, carrot, broccoli, and pepper for 5 to 7 minutes, or until tender. Stir in the tomatoes, corn, and cumin. Cook until the corn and tomatoes are hot. Salt and pepper to taste.

Makes 4 servings.
Per serving: 121 calories, 3 g protein, 23 g carbohydrates, 3 g fat (22% of calories)

Chicken Enchiladas

1   pound chicken breast, cubed
1   green bell pepper, chopped
½   teaspoon cumin
½   teaspoon chili powder
1   can (16 ounces) fat-free refried beans
1   cup wheat germ
6   whole wheat flour tortillas
1   can (10 ounces) spicy salsa
3   ounces shredded reduced-fat Cheddar cheese
    Salsa
    Sour cream

In a nonstick skillet over medium-high heat, cook the chicken, pepper, cumin, and chili powder for 4 minutes. Remove from the heat and add the beans and wheat germ. Add ¾ cup of the chicken filling to each tortilla, roll up, and place seam side down in a nonstick baking dish. Top with the salsa. Cover and bake at 350°F for 40 minutes. Garnish with salsa, sour cream, and cheese.

Makes 4 servings.
Per serving: 536 calories, 49 g protein, 65 g carbohydrates, 14 g fat (24% of calories)

THE PERFECT FOODS FOR MAKING MUSCLE

Iced tea sweetened with honey. University of Memphis researchers found that those subjects who ate the sticky stuff had higher and longer-lasting levels of glucose, which may help restore the muscle fuel glycogen after exercise.

Steak. Meat builds twice as much muscle fiber as other protein sources, such as tofu and tuna. Make your meat beef and you'll also get testosterone-boosting amino acids. Testosterone helps you lift more weight and build more muscle.

Almonds. You need your nuts; they're high in magnesium. In a Western Washington University study, people taking extra magnesium were able to lift 20 percent more weight than those taking a placebo.

Broccoli. Athletes in one study suffered less postworkout muscle damage when they took a vitamin-C supplement than when they took a placebo. Consider broccoli your vitamin-C supplement; a half-cup has 60 milligrams, more than any other vegetable.

Brown rice. It has more of the amino acids arginine and lysine than the white stuff you throw at the bride and groom. University of Houston researchers found that men who took arginine and lysine supplements had 2½ times more muscle-building growth hormone than the saps who got the placebo.

Low-fat ice cream. Scoop out some chocolate for more magnesium. Plus, just a half-cup contains 63 milligrams of calcium, the mineral your biceps, your triceps, and all your other 'ceps need to contract properly.

Make 'Em into a Meal
Almond Beef Stir-Fry with Oriental Brown Rice

Stir-Fry

> 1 teaspoon canola oil
> ½ pound lean boneless top round, cut into thin strips
> 1 teaspoon peeled, finely chopped fresh ginger
> 3 tablespoons slivered almonds
> 2 cups frozen broccoli florets, thawed
> ½ cup beef stock
> 2 tablespoons soy sauce

Rice

> 1 cup instant brown rice
> 2 teaspoons peeled, finely chopped fresh ginger
> 1½ tablespoons soy sauce

To make the stir-fry: Heat the oil in a heavy, nonstick skillet over medium heat. Sauté the beef. Stir in the ginger, almonds, and broccoli, and stir-fry for another 3 to 4 minutes. Stir in the stock and soy sauce. Cook until bubbling.

To make the rice: Cook the rice according to the package directions. While the rice is simmering, stir in the ginger. When the rice is done, fluff it with a fork and drizzle with soy sauce.

Top ½ cup of the rice with half of the stir-fry and serve immediately.

Makes 2 servings.
Per serving: 484 calories, 33 g protein, 55 g carbohydrates, 13 g fat (24% of calories)

THE PERFECT FOODS FOR SURVIVING A HANGOVER

Apricot juice. It's the best fruit-juice source of vitamin C, an antioxidant that prevents alcohol from damaging your cells. Bonus: It'll help relieve your dehydration-induced headache.

Scrambled eggs. Binges drive away dates and vitamin B_6, causing you to wake up alone and feeling "out of it." Good thing eggs are one of the top sources of B_6 as well as sodium and protein to help your dehydrated body retain water.

Hot sauce. Just a dash will turn your eggs into ibuprofen. That's because the red peppers in hot sauce are the top source of capsicum, a natural painkiller. In one small study, it eliminated the headaches of nearly half of the subjects.

Whole wheat cinnamon-raisin bagel. Despite the hole, bagels are good at soaking stuff up, like all the extra acid in your churning stomach. And the whole wheat kind is even better. Cinnamon may add more antioxidant protection from postbinge free radicals.

Honey-date yogurt spread. Sounds like trail food, we know. But honey and dates are the best sources of fructose, which has been shown to boost alcohol metabolism by 25 percent. The yogurt? It has bacteria that will help calm your stomach.

Kiwifruit. Truly first-aid fruit, thanks to proteolytics, enzymes that may help break down the proteins behind indigestion. Kiwis are also the most vitamin- and mineral-dense fruit around.

Strawberries. More vitamin C to help clear the martinis out of your blood. One half-cup has roughly 50 percent of your recommended daily intake of C.

Mint tea. Make it with two teabags—regular and mint. Mint is packed with the pain-relieving ingredient methyl salicylate. Caffeine heals your head by shrinking swollen blood vessels.

Make 'Em into a Meal
Hot Pepper Eggs

  ¼ cup diced onion
  ¼ cup diced red bell pepper
  1 egg
  2 egg whites
  1 tablespoon chopped parsley
     Hot sauce

In a nonstick skillet, fry the onion and pepper with 1 teaspoon water. Add the egg, egg whites, and parsley. Stir until the eggs thicken and set. Remove from the heat and top with hot sauce.

Makes 1 serving.
Per serving: 132 calories, 14 g protein, 6 g carbohydrates, 5 g fat (36% of calories)

Kiwifruit and Strawberries

  4 kiwifruit, sliced
  2 cups sliced strawberries
  2 tablespoons orange-juice concentrate

In a large bowl, mix the kiwifruit, strawberries, and orange-juice concentrate. Chill until ready to serve.

Makes 2 servings.
Per serving: 160 calories, 3 g protein, 39 g carbohydrates, 1 g fat (1% of calories)

THE PERFECT FOODS FOR PREVENTING A HEART ATTACK

Grape juice. The Concord kind is loaded with flavonoids, compounds that one early study showed could reduce risk of heart disease by up to 25 percent.

Orange juice. We knew Canada was good for something: A University of Western Ontario study showed that drinking OJ daily may help raise your "good" HDL cholesterol.

Salmon. This bear bait is high in omega-3's—good fats that can reduce your risk of heart disease—and the amino acid arginine. Research shows that extra arginine may improve circulation by 30 percent.

AMOUNT OF BEEF IN POUNDS
THAT THE AVERAGE GUY EATS IN A YEAR: **26**

AMOUNT OF CHICKEN IN POUNDS
THAT THE AVERAGE GUY EATS IN A YEAR: **57**

Spinach. Nothing you can pull out of the ground and put on your plate has more calcium and potassium, minerals that can lower your blood pressure. Spinach is also high in folate, which may cut homocysteine (a compound linked to heart disease) by up to 25 percent.

Kidney beans. Ignore the name; this is heart food. Researchers at Tulane University found that eating beans four times a week can lower the risk of heart disease by 19 percent.

Onions. They come with two compounds—quercetin and kaempferol—that inhibit LDL oxidation, the process that leads to heart disease.

Green apples. Or red, or yellow. All apples are high in pectin, a gelatin-like substance that helps keep cholesterol out of your blood.

Make 'Em into a Meal
Grape-Juice Cocktail

$\frac{1}{2}$ cup orange juice
$\frac{1}{2}$ cup grape juice
$\frac{1}{2}$ cup carbonated water
1   tablespoon sugar

In a blender, combine the orange juice, grape juice, water, and sugar.

Makes 2 servings.
Per serving: 89 calories, 1 g protein, 22 g carbohydrates, 0 g fat (0% of calories)

Poached Salmon and Spinach

$1\frac{1}{2}$ cups water
$\frac{1}{2}$ cup white wine
2   cloves garlic, minced
2   scallions, sliced
2   salmon steaks (4 to 6 ounces each)
1   cup frozen spinach
     Pinch of nutmeg
     Chili powder to taste
$\frac{1}{4}$ cup shredded part-skim mozzarella cheese

Preheat the broiler. In a skillet, boil the water, wine, garlic, and scallions. Add the salmon and return to a boil. Reduce the heat, cover, and simmer until the fish flakes easily with a fork. In a medium saucepan, cook the spinach, drain, and stir in the nutmeg. Place the fish on a pan coated with nonstick spray, top with the spinach and chili powder, and sprinkle with cheese. Broil until the cheese melts.

Makes 4 servings.
Per serving: 100 calories, 13 g protein, 4 g carbohydrates, 4 g fat (36% of calories)

Southwest Salad

    1   can (14½ ounces) red kidney beans, drained
    1   can (15 ounces) corn, drained
    ½   cup diced scallions
    1   can (14½ ounces) diced tomatoes with green chiles
    ⅛   cup lime juice
        Pinch of chili powder

In a large bowl, combine the beans, corn, scallions, tomatoes, lime juice, and chili powder. Chill for several hours before serving.

Makes 4 servings.
Per serving: 163 calories, 8 g protein, 34 g carbohydrates, 2 g fat (9% of calories)

Caramel Apple Wedges

    6   ounces fat-free caramel sauce
    4   apples, cored and quartered

Warm the sauce in the microwave. Dip the apple pieces in the sauce and serve.

Makes 4 servings.
Per serving: 219 calories, 0 g protein, 54 g carbohydrates, 0.5 g fat (2% of calories)

THE PERFECT FOODS FOR BEATING STRESS

Papaya. Stress sucks potassium, vitamin C, and manganese out of your body, resulting in fatigue, sore muscles, difficulty concentrating, and a rise in blood pressure. Get those nutrients back with one papaya, the best fruit source of all three.

Ricotta cheese. Researchers found that people who ate a daily 2.8 grams of whey (the liquid in the cheese) produced fewer stress hormones. They also had 48 percent more tryptophan, the substance that tells your body to release more of the feel-good chemical serotonin.

Whole wheat pasta. It'll give you extra tryptophan and the steady supply of energy you need to fight off stress-induced fatigue.

Turkey sausage. Turkey is a good source of tryptophan and pantothenic acid—a B vitamin vital to the production of stress-fighting hormones. Plus, the zinc in turkey may help keep you from being worried and weak. One study found that zinc supplements increased muscle strength and endurance.

Whole wheat bread sticks. Whole grains are rich in folate and other B vitamins that help supply your brain with the fuel it needs to keep you sharp when you're stressed.

Dark chocolate. Want a runner's high without the annoying running part? Eat a little dark chocolate; it will give you a shot of endorphins, a natural morphine.

Milk. Even the low-fat kind has protein that will elevate your levels of the stress-fighting hormones dopamine and norepinephrine.

Make 'Em into a Meal
Papaya Soda

    1   cup papaya nectar
    1   cup orange juice
    1   cup lemon-lime soda
        Ice

In a blender, combine the papaya nectar, orange juice, soda, and ice. Blend well and drink.

Makes 2 servings.
Per serving: 176 calories, 1 g protein, 44 g carbohydrates, 0 g fat (0% of calories)

Turkey Lasagna

    ½   pound turkey sausage, casings removed
    2   large yellow onions, chopped
    2   teaspoons oregano
    2   cans (14 ounces each) diced tomatoes
    3   cups nonfat ricotta cheese
    1   cup grated Parmesan cheese
    9   whole wheat lasagna noodles, cooked

Preheat the oven to 350°F. In a large skillet, quickly fry the sausage, onions, and oregano. Stir in the tomatoes. In a bowl, combine the ricotta and half the Parmesan. Spread a third of the tomato/meat mixture in a lightly oiled 9" × 13" baking dish. Arrange three noodles in the dish and spread half the cheese mixture over them. Repeat these layers. Top with the last layer of noodles and Parmesan. Cover with aluminum foil and bake for 45 minutes. Remove foil and bake for 15 minutes more. Let stand for 15 to 20 minutes before serving.

Makes 6 servings.
Per serving: 372 calories, 29 g protein, 40 g carbohydrates, 12 g fat (29% of calories)

PERCENTAGE OF MEN WHO SAY THAT WHEN THEY COOK THEY LEAVE THE KITCHEN UNTIL THE FOOD IS DONE: 14

PERCENTAGE OF WOMEN WHO LEAVE: 9

Italian Hot Chocolate

$\frac{1}{2}$ cup unsweetened dark cocoa
$\frac{1}{3}$ cup sugar
$\frac{1}{2}$ cup boiling water
$\frac{1}{2}$ cup water
1 cup fat-free milk

In a medium bowl, mix together the cocoa, sugar, and boiling water. Stir in the water and milk; microwave until hot.

Makes 4 half-cup servings.
Per serving: 103 calories, 4 g protein, 25 g carbohydrates, 1 g fat (9% of calories)

What's Missing from Your Diet?

Hint: It's on this list

By Katrin McDonald

What in the world is wrong with you? What's missing from your life? You've got your karma and you've got your chi. But you're still feeling so lousy that you joined Oprah's Book Club.

Maybe it's time to try looking for your missing nutrient: copper, folic acid, iron, magnesium, phosphorus, omega-3 fatty acids, or zinc. If one of these is absent from your diet—and chances are, one is—you'll get sick, you'll get sore, and you'll get stupid.

Once you know what's missing, where are you going to look? Forget journaling and meditating. Try shopping. Here's your list.

YOUR SYMPTOMS: Runny Nose, Coughing, Fever
What may be missing: Copper

Who says it isn't a precious metal? When University of North Carolina at Greensboro researchers infected human cells with bacteria, they found that the cells with normal copper levels killed two to three times more bacteria than did cells with low copper levels. They also produced up to 60 percent more cytokines—chemicals that trigger the body's immune response. "The fact that

**POUNDS OF BUTTER
THE AVERAGE AMERICAN EATS PER YEAR:** 4

these were otherwise healthy cells shows just how sensitive our immune system is to a lack of copper," notes study author Mark Failla, Ph.D.

Where to find it: In your breakfast. One bowl of raisin bran, a slice of buttered whole wheat toast, and a cup of hot chocolate will give you more than a third of what you need each day. Copper has also been spotted in lobster, cashews, and salmon.

YOUR SYMPTOMS: Huffing and Puffing, Even without a Cigarette; Lack of Stamina during Aerobic Exercise

What may be missing: Zinc

Zinc is the fitness mineral for men. A USDA study recently found that men on a low-zinc diet had a 40 percent decrease in red-blood-cell activity. "The longer it takes red blood cells to transfer carbon dioxide to your lungs, the harder it is to breathe," says study author Henry Lukaski, Ph.D. Plus, without enough zinc, your body can't clear the lactic acid out of your muscles, and that makes them very heavy. In fact, simply trying to get out of your own way will send your heart racing and make your breathing labored.

Where to find it: In a lean hamburger on a whole wheat bun; it has three times the zinc of that chicken sandwich you think is a healthier choice. You'll also find zinc in baked beans, peanut-butter-and-jelly sandwiches, and scrambled eggs.

YOUR SYMPTOMS: Headaches, Sleepless Nights

What may be missing: Magnesium

Think of magnesium as your body's bouncer; without enough of it, uninvited calcium will rush into your cells and wreak havoc on key hormones and neurotransmitters. After a little while, blood vessels become constricted and your head starts hurting, says Burton M. Altura, Ph.D., professor of physiology and pharmacology at the State University of New York at Brooklyn. "Too little magnesium may also result in increased brain activity, making it difficult for you to fall asleep."

Where to find it: In a baked potato topped with broccoli and a slice of melted cheese, plus a glass of milk. Magnesium is also found in almonds, frozen fish fillets, bananas, and whole grain breads and cereals.

YOUR SYMPTOMS: Brittle Bones, Frequent Stress Fractures, Teeth That Crack when Opening Beer Bottles

What may be missing: Phosphorus

You'd think that guzzling calcium-fortified orange juice would buy you a set of unbreakable bones. We used to think that, too. But it turns out that adding extra calcium to your diet without an equal amount of phosphorus will actually increase the odds that sticks, stones, and just about anything else will break your bones. "Extra calcium can make the composition of the bones unbalanced," says Joseph Spence, Ph.D., director of the USDA's Human Nutrition Research Center. "Your body will continue to build bone, but without enough phosphorus, the composition will be fragile."

Where to find it: In a Canadian-bacon-and-egg sandwich on a whole wheat English muffin. This modified McMuffin has 348 milligrams of phosphorus, exactly what you need to balance the 350 milligrams of calcium in a glass of fortified orange juice. You can also find phosphorus in pizza, macaroni and cheese, and chicken vegetable soup.

YOUR SYMPTOMS: Constantly Sore Muscles, Aching Joints, Difficulty Picking Up Gym Bag without a Spotter

What may be missing: Omega-3 fatty acids

If you've stopped trying to show off by bench-pressing the stairclimber and you still feel sore all the time, you may need more omega-3's in your diet. Researchers from Down Under recently found that men who ate the most omega-3 fatty acids had 26 percent lower levels of prostaglandins—fatty acids that cause muscle soreness. Taking in more omega-3's can counterbalance prostaglandin production and may decrease recovery time and diminish muscle pain, says William Lands, Ph.D., a senior science advisor at the National Institutes of Health.

Where to find it: In pizza with anchovies. A shrimp cocktail or a tuna sandwich (made with white tuna) on whole wheat bread is also high in omega-3's.

YOUR SYMPTOMS: You're Getting Dumber, You Can't Concentrate, and You Laugh at Your Own Stupid Jokes

What may be missing: Iron

That's right, iron, also known as kryptonite to men. Studies have linked high levels of iron, in excess of 10 milligrams a day, to an increased risk of heart disease in men. But if you're too good about watching your iron intake and

WHY NOT JUST TAKE A MULTIVITAMIN?

We thought you'd ask that. Sure, taking a multivitamin is an option; it's just not the best option. Not every multi has these nutrients or has them in adequate or safe amounts. You also miss out on a ton of phytochemicals, plant compounds that have health benefits such as cancer prevention and lower risk of heart disease.

Downing a handful of individual supplements is no answer, either. "Separating nutrients into individual supplements such that they can't interact with other nutrients isn't as effective as eating food," says Gary Miller, Ph.D., a professor of health at Wake Forest University in Winston-Salem, North Carolina. Besides, food tastes better.

you're on a low-fat diet that's light on meat, you could be coming up short. Without enough iron, your body has trouble ferrying oxygen through your bloodstream and dropping it off where you need it most: your brain. "When oxygen isn't reaching the brain, you feel light-headed and tired. Cognitive performance can suffer, too," says Gary Miller, Ph.D., a professor of health at Wake Forest University in Winston-Salem, North Carolina.

Where to find it: In a Caesar salad. Just make sure it's a big bowl, add some chicken, and go heavy on the lemon juice. Eating foods high in vitamin C, like lemons, along with an iron-rich meal improves your body's absorption of the mineral, says Miller. Iron also turns up in lean beef, dried fruit, and raisin bran.

YOUR SYMPTOMS: Forgetfulness. For Example, You Forgot You Read This Already. This, Too

What may be missing: Folic acid

... And your keys. Sure, there are a lot of reasons your memory could be going, but why not eliminate the easiest one first? (Okay, the second easiest, if you're Woody Harrelson.) According to a recent Swedish study, those people who bombed on a series of memory tests also had the lowest blood levels of folic acid. Researchers speculate that a shortage of folic acid may cause a spike in levels of homocysteine, an amino acid that damages blood vessels in the heart and the brain.

Where to find it: In a bowl of three-bean chili. One serving contains more than half of your daily requirement of folic acid. It's also present in orange juice, corn on the cob, and guacamole.

The Lard Is Your Savior

Want to lose your belly, gain hard muscle, and build an athlete's heart? Eat more fat

By Adam Campbell

Really big, life-changing advancements in food science don't come very often. Take sliced bread. It's been 73 years since that little feat made headlines. Come to think of it, there hasn't been a real blockbuster since 1974—the year edible underwear was invented.

But one of the latest nutritional paradigm shifts could be an even greater boon to mankind than apricot-flavored panties. A growing pile of research proves that one of the healthiest things you can eat is the very evil you've supposedly been trying to avoid: pure fat.

Pure monounsaturated fat, to be specific. That's the variety of grease found in nuts, olives, and avocados. It tastes just as good and satisfies your hunger just as well as its killer cousins, saturated fat (the type found in beef and butter) and trans fat (the "partially hydrogenated vegetable oil" found in chips and cookies), but it doesn't carry the health risks those fats do. Instead, it actually reverses those health risks.

Molecularly, saturated fat and trans fat are loaded with hydrogen atoms, which make both solid at body temperature. When you eat fats, they become part of the liver membrane, and solid fats make it more difficult for your liver to absorb and filter out harmful LDL cholesterol—sludge that eventually clogs every artery it touches. So a diet high in saturated fat (more than 30 grams a day) can lead to impotence, heart attacks, and strokes.

In contrast, the monounsaturated-fat molecule is missing two hydrogen atoms and is liquid at body temperature. Eat the stuff and it'll make the liver membrane more "fluid" and allow LDL cholesterol to pass more easily into your liver and out of your body. That little trick pays enormous dividends. In fact, eating a diet rich in monounsaturated fat can give you . . .

A stronger heart. Pennsylvania State University researchers found that diets high in monounsaturated fat and low in saturated fat lowered LDL cholesterol and triglycerides (both big factors in heart attacks) by 14 percent and 13 percent, respectively, after about 3 weeks. "These results show that eating more monounsaturated fat can reduce your heart-disease risk by 25 percent," says study author Penny Kris-Etherton, Ph.D.

Bigger muscles. Research has shown that men who eat more monounsaturated fat have higher testosterone levels, although researchers don't yet know why. The more natural testosterone you produce, the more easily you'll gain muscle.

Harder erections. Testosterone doesn't just build biceps.

Greater endurance. Runners in a State University of New York study maintained a vigorous pace for 10 minutes longer after snacking on peanuts for a month. "Gram for gram, a high-monounsaturated-fat diet provides more energy than the extra carbohydrates you're eating on a low-fat diet," explains Peter Horvath, Ph.D., lead author of the study. "And more energy means better performance."

Quicker thinking. Italian men whose daily diets included about 75 grams of monounsaturated fat scored better on cognitive tests than men who ate less than that. In fact, those who consumed the least were the stupidest of the bunch. "As we age, the neuronal cells in the brain require more monounsaturated fatty acids to keep their membranes strong," says Antonio Capurso, M.D., the study author.

Looser pants. Brigham and Women's Hospital nutritionists found that among two groups of people who had lost an average of 11 pounds, those who had eaten a diet high in monounsaturated fat were still slim 18 months later, while their cohorts on a low-saturated-fat diet quickly regained weight. "Participants on the high-mono diet reported they didn't feel as if they were dieting," says Kathy McManus, R.D., one of the study authors.

Eating five handfuls of pecans will provide your daily quota of 60 grams of monounsaturated fat, but it's easier to eat regular meals that are rich in the good fat. Here are four easy-to-prepare meals that contain at least 10 grams of monounsaturated fat but have no more than 600 calories.

Guacamole and Tuna Pitas

1	can (9 ounces) light tuna, packed in oil (canola or olive)
¾	cup store-bought guacamole
¼	cup chopped tomatoes
1	teaspoon lemon juice
1	tablespoon light mayonnaise
2	6" whole wheat pitas

Combine the tuna, guacamole, tomatoes, lemon juice, and mayonnaise in a bowl and blend thoroughly with a fork. Split the pitas in half and fill each half with ¼ cup of the mixture.

Makes 2 servings.
Per serving: 556 calories, 45 grams (g) protein, 43 g carbohydrates, 24 g total fat, 10 g monounsaturated fat

Garlic-Pesto Chicken

2	cups rotini pasta
1	tablespoon extra-virgin olive oil
1	pound chicken breast, cubed
1	package (16 ounces) Birds Eye frozen mixed vegetables
½	tablespoon minced garlic
1	teaspoon salt
3	ounces pesto sauce
2	tablespoons grated Parmesan cheese

Cook the pasta according to the package directions. Heat the oil in a large nonstick skillet over medium-high heat. Add the chicken and cook thoroughly. Add the vegetables, garlic, and salt, and cook for 5 minutes. Reduce the heat and simmer for 5 minutes. Add the pesto sauce. Serve over the pasta and sprinkle with the cheese.

Makes 4 servings.
Per serving: 593 calories, 37 g protein, 52 g carbohydrates, 27 g total fat, 15 g monounsaturated fat

Sausage and Sun-Dried-Tomato Pizza

    1   8" refrigerated pizza crust
    1   jar (13 ounces) sun-dried tomatoes in olive oil
    3   ounces pesto sauce
    1   package (6 ounces) shredded part-skim mozzarella
    1/4 pound smoked turkey sausage, sliced thin

Preheat the oven to 450°F. Cover the crust with half of the tomatoes. Top with the pesto sauce. Sprinkle with cheese, and add the sausage. Bake for 6 to 10 minutes.

Makes 4 servings.
Per serving: 600 calories, 26 g protein, 50 g carbohydrates, 35 g total fat, 18 g monounsaturated fat

Mexican Cheese Omelette

    3   eggs
    1   tablespoon water
    1   teaspoon taco seasoning
    1/2 cup canned diced tomatoes and green chiles, drained
    1   tablespoon canola oil
    1/4 cup shredded reduced-fat Cheddar cheese
    3/4 cup store-bought guacamole

Whisk together the eggs, water, seasoning, and tomatoes. Heat the oil in a 7" nonstick skillet over medium heat. Pour in the egg mixture and cook until

FATS AND FIGURES
The top 10 sources of monounsaturated fat

1. Extra-virgin olive oil	20 grams per ounce (g/oz)	7. Peanuts	7 g/oz
2. Canola oil	16 g/oz	8. Black walnuts	4 g/oz
3. Pecans	12 g/oz	9. Avocados	3 g/oz
4. Almonds	10 g/oz	10. Guacamole**	2 g/oz
5. Cashews	8 g/oz		
6. Peanut butter*	7 g/oz		

* Reduced-fat varieties have less monounsaturated fat.
** Make sure that avocados are the first ingredient listed and that the guacamole contains no partially hydrogenated oils.

it begins to solidify. Add the cheese. Fold the omelette; cook for 2 minutes. Top with guacamole.

Makes 1 serving.
Per serving: 441 calories, 25 g protein, 15 g carbohydrates, 30 g total fat, 14 g monounsaturated fat

Good Carb, Bad Carb

Finally, an easy way to eat better and stay well

By Janis Jibrin, R.D.

The glycemic index is coming. Sounds complicated, but it isn't. What it is, some health experts believe, is the most exciting nutrition breakthrough on the horizon.

Invented in the early 1980s by University of Toronto researchers as a tool to help control diabetes, the glycemic index ranks carbohydrate foods by their effect on your blood-sugar levels. Today, it's an accepted diabetes-control strategy in Canada, Australia, England, and elsewhere. And for that reason alone, it deserves more attention here.

The biggest surprise of all seems to be that the glycemic index may offer dramatic health benefits not just for diabetics but for almost everyone.

"We're learning that the type of carbs you eat really makes a difference in your health," says glycemic-index researcher Christine L. Pelkman, Ph.D., of Pennsylvania State University in State College. And the glycemic index helps you choose the best carbs for you.

With our easy cutout pocket guide to 118 foods on pages 59 and 60, you can use the glycemic index to choose meals and snacks that give you an edge against diabetes, heart attacks, and possibly even cancer. And don't be surprised if you find yourself losing weight to boot.

THE GOOD . . . AND THE NOT-SO-GOOD

The glycemic index (or GI, for short) assigns carbohydrate-containing foods a number based on how they affect your blood sugar, or blood glucose, after you eat them. Foods with a GI under 55 cause only a little blip in blood sugar; those in the 55 to 70 range raise it a little higher; and carbs with GIs above 70 send blood sugar soaring. We're learning that low-GI carbs are healthy; high-GI carbs, in excess, are not.

What explains the difference in numbers? No matter what form the carb initially takes—the lactose in milk, the starch in a bagel, the sucrose in table sugar—eventually, your body breaks it down to glucose. Glucose winds up in your bloodstream, fueling your cells. What makes a GI number high or low is how quickly the food breaks down during digestion. The longer your body has to wrestle with the carb to break it down into glucose, the slower the rise in blood glucose and the lower the GI.

It's not always easy to predict a food's GI. Often, fiber-rich foods have lower GIs. Fiber, especially the soluble type in oats and beans, creates a web in the intestines that traps carb particles. Not surprisingly, beans have low GI numbers.

But when fiber is ground finely, as it often is in whole wheat flour, it doesn't present enough of a digestive challenge to lower the GI value. That explains why whole wheat bread has a GI number nearly identical to white bread. (But whole wheat bread is still a healthier choice than white bread because of its extra fiber and other nutrients.)

Surprisingly, table sugar has a lower GI than potatoes. That's because it's made of two sugars, glucose and fructose; the glucose half sails right into the bloodstream, while the fructose segment has to detour through the liver, where it slowly gets converted into glucose. But the starch molecules in potatoes are strings of glucose. Boiling, baking, or mashing a potato causes the starch molecules to burst, making it easy for glucose to enter the bloodstream.

HIGH GI = HIGH RISK

The problem with eating lots of high-GI foods is this: When your blood sugar soars, so does the hormone insulin. Insulin's main duty is to scoop up excess blood sugar and store it safely in muscle tissue. In moderation, insulin is a good guy, but it becomes a killer when its levels spike repeatedly, triggering diabetes, heart disease, and possibly cancer.

Unfortunately, insulin is spiking all the time in the millions of guys who feast on high-GI fare such as bagels, doughnuts, french fries, and other quickly absorbed starchy carbohydrates. Experts point out that modern diets offer lots more opportunity to eat starchy high-GI foods than the diets on which human beings evolved.

THE VINEGAR TRICK

Glycemic index experts say that the acid in vinegar or lemon juice can substantially blunt the effect of a food on your blood sugar. That means that adding vinegar to your french fries or making potato salad with a vinaigrette dressing are two smart, tasty ways to lower the GI of potatoes.

MAKE THE GLYCEMIC INDEX WORK FOR YOU

I. One per meal. Try to choose one-third to one-half of your daily starches from the low-GI list. You're well on your way if you include one low-GI starch—for instance, a bowl of old-fashioned oatmeal, ½ cup beans, or some lentil soup—per meal.

2. Go whole grain. With a few exceptions, whole grain–based foods such as barley and bulgur have a low GI, mainly because their high fiber content slows digestion.

3. Rough it up. The least processed and rougher the grain or flour, the lower the GI. That's why pasta, which is made from a coarse-milled wheat, has a low GI even if it's not whole grain.

4. Bring it down low. Only have time to make instant rice? Just add some beans. Throwing in a low-GI food brings down the GI

rating of the entire meal. Adding some fat or protein also lowers the GI level.

5. Be savvy about snacks. When you snack, you tend to have just one food, all by itself. That's fine if you're having a low-calorie snack, whether the GI is high or not. But if you're having a high-GI bagel or doughnut with hundreds of calories, the glucose won't get blunted by other foods. So avoid starchy, high-GI foods as snacks.

6. Load up on fruits, vegetables, and legumes. Most have a low GI, and you would have to eat pounds of the ones that don't to affect blood sugar. By the same token, don't binge on low-GI foods that are high in calories, such as Snickers candy bars. Gaining weight will raise your blood sugar, too.

TAME THE KILLERS

The good news is, switching to a low-GI diet results in a minimum outpouring of insulin, and that has healthy ramifications all over your body. Here's what a low-GI diet appears to help you do.

Stop diabetes. Diabetes, which is characterized by higher than normal blood sugar, has reached epidemic proportions in the United States, afflicting 7.5 million American men. Most have type 2, prompted by two very American conditions: excess weight and a sedentary lifestyle. And millions more are walking around with a degree of insulin resistance just shy of diabetes.

"The beauty of the glycemic index for diabetics is that it not only helps control blood sugar and insulin, but its appetite-suppressing effects help them lose weight. And weight loss alone can reverse type-2 diabetes," says Marc Rendell, M.D., director of the Creighton Diabetes Center at Creighton University in Omaha, Nebraska, and medical director of the Rose Salter Medical Research Foundation in Baltimore. Although he believes it's entirely possible to induce remission of many cases of type-2 diabetes using the glycemic index, he urges patients with diabetes to continue their current therapies and add low-GI foods only in consultation with a physician or registered dietitian.

So far, research testing low- versus high-GI diets for diabetics is promising. A 1999 Swedish study of type-2 diabetics found that 4 weeks on a low-GI diet

EASY LOW-GI SUBSTITUTES

High-GI Favorite	Lower-GI Choice
French bread, 95	100% stone-ground whole wheat bread, 53
Jelly beans, 80	Dried apricots, 31
Mashed or baked potato, 73 or 85	Roasted sweet potato, 54
Pretzels, 83	Popcorn, 55
Side of bread-stuffing mix, 74	Side of canned baked beans, 48
Vanilla wafers, 77	Oatmeal cookies, 55

lowered blood glucose and insulin by 30 percent compared to a high-GI diet. In a recent 4-month study led by the University of Toronto's Thomas Wolever, M.D., a low-GI diet markedly improved insulin sensitivity in a group of pre-diabetic insulin-resistant people. "If these trends were sustained—and I'm trying to get money to extend the study—these people could probably avoid getting diabetes," predicts Dr. Wolever.

Which is exactly the implication of several large-scale diet surveys. In a 6-year study of male health professionals, men eating the lowest-GI diets were 25 percent less likely to get diabetes. In the Nurses' Health Study, the most powerful diabetes protection—a drop in risk of one-third or more—came from eating a low-GI diet and getting lots of fiber from cereal (7.5 grams daily).

Drop pounds. Ever feel hungry just an hour or two after a meal? It could be because the meal had a high GI. Ironically, high-GI meals cause such a flood of insulin to cope with all the glucose that blood-sugar levels wind up lower than if you had never eaten. And low blood sugar may send out hunger alarms, according to Susan Roberts, Ph.D., nutrition professor at Tufts University in Boston and author of *Feeding Your Child for Lifelong Health*. In one study, overweight children (average age 10) at Children's Hospital in Boston spent 4 months on either a low-GI diet or a low-fat diet of equal calories. The clear winner: the low-GI diet, with an average weight loss of 4.5 pounds compared to 2.8 pounds on the low-fat diet.

Roberts suspects that high-GI carbs are partly behind America's epidemic levels of obesity. "GI is not the complete answer to everyone's weight problem," she says. "But aside from the research, I am personally convinced that low-GI diets help people lose weight, myself included. My husband and I were eating a relatively high-GI instant oatmeal or low-GI Irish oatmeal for breakfast, and I'd call and ask how he felt 2 hours later. Both of us noticed a big decrease in hunger with the low-GI oatmeal. Now I've become very aware of the GI of what I eat and quite consistently find myself hungrier after very high GI foods such as bagels, mashed potatoes, and the like."

YOUR POCKET GUIDE TO THE GLYCEMIC INDEX

Eat sparingly foods in *italics*; these are high in empty calories.

Low-Glycemic-Index Foods (Under 55)

Low-fat yogurt, artificially sweetened	14
Peanuts	14
Fructose	23
Plum	24
Grapefruit	25
Pearled barley	25
Peach	28
Canned peaches in natural juice	30
Soy milk	31
Baby lima beans, frozen	32
Fat-free milk	32
Fettuccine	32
Low-fat yogurt, sugar sweetened	33
M&M's Chocolate Candies, Peanut	*33*
Apple	36
Pear	36
Whole wheat spaghetti	37
Tomato soup	38
Apple juice	41
Snickers bar	*41*
Spaghetti	41
All-Bran	42
Canned chickpeas	42
Custard	43
Grapes	43
Orange	43
Canned lentil soup	44
Canned pinto beans	45
Macaroni	45
Pineapple juice	46
Banana bread	47
Long-grain rice	47

Parboiled rice	47
Bulgur	48
Canned baked beans	48
Grapefruit juice	48
Green peas	48
Chocolate bar	*49*
Old-fashioned oatmeal	49
Cheese tortellini	50
Low-fat ice cream	*50*
Canned kidney beans	52
Kiwifruit	52
Banana	53
Potato chips	*54*
Pound cake	*54*
Special K cereal	54
Sweet potato	54

Intermediate-Glycemic-Index Foods (55 to 70)

Brown rice	55
Linguine	55
Oatmeal cookies	55
Popcorn	55
Sweet corn	55
White rice	56
Orange juice from frozen concentrate	57
Canned peaches in heavy syrup	58
Mini-shredded-wheat cereal	58
Multi-Bran Chex cereal	58
Blueberry muffin	59
Bran muffin	60
Cheese pizza	60

(continued)

YOUR POCKET GUIDE TO THE GLYCEMIC INDEX (CONT.)

Intermediate-Glycemic-Index Foods (55 to 70) (cont.)

Hamburger bun	61
Ice cream	*61*
Quaker Chewy Granola Bar	61
Coca-Cola	*63*
Beets	64
Canned apricots in light syrup	64
Canned black bean soup	64
Macaroni and cheese	64
Raisins	64
Couscous	64
Rye crispbread	65
Table sugar (sucrose)	*65*
Instant oatmeal	66
Pineapple	66
Angel food cake	67
Grape-Nuts	67
Stoned Wheat Thins	67
American rye bread	68
Taco shells	68
Whole wheat bread	69
Life Savers	70
Melba toast	70
White bread	70

High-Glycemic-Index Foods (Above 70)

Don't avoid or limit foods in **bold**; these are low-calorie and very nutritious.

Carrots	**71**
Bagel	72
Corn chips	72
Watermelon	**72**
Honey	73
Kaiser roll	73
Mashed potatoes	73
Bran flakes	**74**
Bread-stuffing mix	74
Cheerios cereal	**74**
Cream of Wheat, instant	74
Graham crackers	74
Saltine crackers	74
Doughnut	75
French fries	76
Frozen waffles	76
Total cereal	**76**
Vanilla wafers	77
Grape-Nuts Flakes cereal	80
Jelly beans	80
Rice cakes	**82**
Rice Krispies cereal	82
Corn Chex cereal	83
Mashed potatoes, instant	83
Pretzels	83
Cornflakes	84
Baked potato	**85**
Rice Chex cereal	89
Rice, instant	91
French bread	95
Parsnips	**97**
Tofu frozen dessert	115

Keep your heart strong. High levels of insulin wreak havoc on the heart. "Elevated insulin triggers a bevy of heart-disease risk factors," says Michael Zemel, Ph.D., director of the Nutrition Institute at the University of Tennessee in Knoxville. Zemel reviewed the connections between the glycemic index and heart disease for a scientific journal and found that they include high blood pressure, increased fat storage, high triglycerides (a type of blood fat), and lower levels of HDL (the good cholesterol carrier).

Once again, low-GI foods appear to be the remedy. In the Nurses' Health Study, women eating diets with the most carbohydrates from high-GI foods were nearly twice as likely to develop heart disease.

Thwart cancer. A high-glycemic-index diet may even be linked to colon cancer. The hypothesis: The flood of insulin, glucose, and blood fats that stem from a high-GI diet fuels colon-cancer cells. Both human and animal research support this theory. For instance, colon-cancer patients are prone to insulin resistance, and giving insulin speeds up the development of colon cancer in rats.

Stay energetic and alert. Want more stamina? You have greater endurance when you exercise after a low-GI meal compared to a high-GI meal, most studies show. And low-GI meals might also give you a mental edge, hints Australian research. People who ate a low-GI breakfast (based on All-Bran) scored higher in a test of alertness than those who ate a high-GI breakfast (based on cornflakes).

"I think the low-GI breakfast increased alertness for two reasons: by fueling the brain with a slow, steady supply of glucose and by staving off hunger. People eating this breakfast didn't get hungry before lunch, while those eating cornflakes did. It's easier to be alert and focused when you're not hungry," speculates study leader Susanna Holt, Ph.D., R.D., of Sydney University's Human Nutrition Unit.

THE GI: NOT PC

While organizations in other countries—such as the Canadian Diabetes Association, Australia's International Diabetes Institute, and the World Health Organization—all recommend including low-GI foods as part of managing diabetes, the glycemic index gets only a brief mention in the most recent practice guidelines from the American Diabetes Association (ADA).

"At this point, we don't recommend the glycemic index because not enough is known, and there's no evidence that this method is better than the standard approach of counting carbohydrates," explains Marian Parrot, M.D., vice president of clinical affairs for the ADA. Although Dr. Parrot agrees that the GI is "not harmful" and that "nothing is wrong with the science," her main objection is that it's too complicated—people just can't be expected to remember and deal with all those numbers. And in fact, a substantial group of health experts agree that although the glycemic index may prove useful someday, it is "not ready for prime time."

In response, Creighton Diabetes Center's Dr. Rendell, who wrote a recent *New England Journal of Medicine* editorial backing the glycemic index, believes there's a bias against publishing research in this area. "It's just not politically correct. I've seen excellent research papers on the GI get put aside by medical journals; unfortunately, the best studies haven't been published," he asserts.

"The authorities in the field are too hung up on arithmetic," he says. "For instance, they bring up the fact that carrots have a high GI, so they're afraid people will stop eating carrots." But GI experts never advise avoiding high-GI foods that are low-calorie salad vegetables or fruits. "If high-GI foods such as carrots are also low in calories, you'd have to eat pounds of them to make much of an impact on blood sugar," says the University of Toronto's Dr. Wolever, coauthor of *The Glucose Revolution.*

He recommends targeting those high-GI foods that are also high in calories, such as baked goods, highly refined breakfast cereals, and potatoes. Start to replace them with lower-GI foods, such as trading in bagels for 100 percent stone-ground whole wheat bread, instant rice for barley, or cornflakes for All-Bran. "Switching to these low-GI starches," says Dr. Wolever, "can make a tremendous difference in your health."

KNOW THIS

Headline Confusion

At *Men's Health*, we're sometimes baffled over health news—and heck, we report the stuff! Lately, it seems more and more newspaper headlines are telling us to watch out for the things that are good for us. As a rule, when long-standing health advice comes under fire, we start asking questions.

HEADLINE: FIBER DOESN'T CUT CANCER RISK, TWO STUDIES FIND

The research: Two studies, published in the *New England Journal of Medicine*, examined 3,200 people with a history of colorectal polyps—benign tumors that are precursors to colon cancer. Researchers said a high-fiber diet didn't reduce the risk of recurrent polyps.

Yeah, but . . . both studies looked at polyps, not colon cancer. Though all colon cancer starts out as a polyp, not every polyp develops into cancer. And since the study subjects had histories of polyps, they may have been at a higher risk of developing more. So they may have needed extra protection beyond the 30 grams of daily fiber they ate, says David Klurfeld, Ph.D., chairman of the department of nutrition at Wayne State University in Detroit.

What you should do: Try to eat at least 25 grams of fiber daily. Though studies haven't isolated fiber as the single ingredient that prevents colon cancer, it's still believed to be an important element in a diet that does. Plus, fiber reduces your risk of diabetes and heart disease.

HEADLINE: RESEARCHERS DOUBT BENEFITS OF ANTIOXIDANTS

The research: After reviewing research on vitamins C and E and selenium, a panel commissioned by the U.S. Food and Nutrition Board said that megadoses of these antioxidants didn't necessarily have disease-fighting abilities.

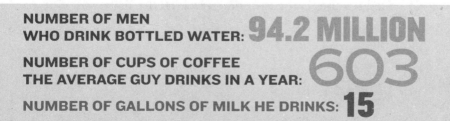

NUMBER OF MEN WHO DRINK BOTTLED WATER: 94.2 MILLION

NUMBER OF CUPS OF COFFEE THE AVERAGE GUY DRINKS IN A YEAR: 603

NUMBER OF GALLONS OF MILK HE DRINKS: 15

Yeah, but . . . the panel examined only the value and safety of taking antioxidants in extremely high doses—not what their impact was in a normal, healthy diet. In fact, the panel recommended that people get more C and E than they do now.

What you should do: Eat more foods that are rich in C, E, and selenium. Jeffrey Blumberg, Ph.D., chief of the antioxidants research lab at Tufts University in Boston, also recommends supplementing your diet with 100 to 400 milligrams of vitamin E to help prevent prostate cancer and heart disease, as well as 200 micrograms of selenium for extra prostate-cancer protection.

HEADLINE: TROUBLE FOR THE TITAN TOFU

The research: A study of 3,734 men by the Hawaii Center of Health Research concluded that those who consumed two or more servings of tofu a week were twice as likely to suffer from dementia.

Yeah, but . . . the researchers surmised that phytoestrogens—plant estrogens that mimic human estrogens—in soy may have interfered with brain function. But the men who ate the most tofu lived the longest, which could have put them at greater risk for old-age dementia anyway. And many of the study subjects may have had childhood nutritional deficiencies, which might have influenced their long-term brain function, says Harvard nutrition professor Meir Stampfer, Ph.D.

What you should do: Keep eating soy; it's been shown to lower cholesterol levels and possibly lower the risks of prostate cancer and osteoporosis. But until further research is completed on soy and brain function, try to limit your weekly intake to 190 milligrams of isoflavones—the main phytoestrogens in soy. A soy-protein shake has about 60 milligrams, and an 8-ounce glass of soy milk has 16 milligrams.

Three Good Reasons to Keep Drinking Beer

1. It's heart-healthy. Many studies suggest that moderate drinking—one, maybe two drinks a day—may help prevent heart disease. But before you choose your dinner cocktail, consider which aspect of your particular blood chemistry puts you at risk. If you need to raise your good cholesterol (HDL), make red wine your medicinal alcohol. But if your blood tests show elevated levels of homo-cysteine, substitute a cold frosty one for the merlot. Scientists at the Nutri-tion and Food Research Institute in the Netherlands gave a group of men wine, beer, gin, or water with dinner, switching beverages every 3 weeks. The wine and gin raised homocysteine levels a bit; the beer didn't. The beer bumped up the level of heart-protective vitamin B_6 by 30 percent—twice the increase that wine and gin caused. Just remember that we're talking about suds in moderation—downing an entire six-pack can actually deplete B_6.

2. It's bone-healthy, too. You thought it was clean living that's kept Gramps spry all these years? Turns out it's the alcohol. In a study of 445 people, re-searchers at Creighton University in Omaha, Nebraska, found that moderate alcohol consumption leads to stronger bones when you're older. "Alcohol re-duces the factors that cause bone loss," says Prema Rapuri, Ph.D., the study author. Rapuri found that seniors with the highest bone density drank two to four servings of beer or wine each week.

3. It calms an upset stomach. Sipping on a highly carbonated beer can settle a stomach just as Seven-Up or Sprite can. Plus, the alcohol helps buffer pain. "I've never seen a true medical study supporting this," says Larry L. Alexander, M.D., medical director of Central Florida Regional Hospital's emergency de-partment, "but I have patients who tell me it works. The only time you have to be careful is if you have an ulcer or gastritis. Alcohol can inflame that."

DOWN THE PIKE

Chocolate That Heals?

Coming soon: Chocolate that's less fattening, cholesterol-fighting, and delicious. Well, maybe.

For two periods of 2 weeks each, Swiss scientists plied 10 men with either regular chocolate or calcium-enriched chocolate. Those who ate the latter absorbed 13 percent less cocoa butter, a fattening ingredient commonly added to chocolate bars to extend their storage life.

The men who ate the calcium-fortified chocolate also showed a 15 percent reduction in LDL cholesterol, the "bad" cholesterol that clogs arteries. Best of all, they reported no taste difference between the two types of chocolate.

Now, if those scientists could only find an antidote for chocolate addiction. . . .

DOES IT WORK?

Don't Drink the Grass

Wheat-grass juice

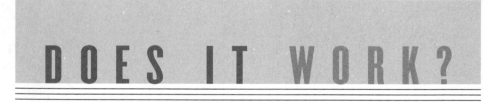

Time was, you would drink anything your buddies offered—you even have the college transcripts to prove it. Now that you're older and smarter, you take your drinking cues from more reliable sources. Here's what Jacqueline Berning, Ph.D., R.D., a sports nutritionist who works with the Denver Broncos and Colorado Rockies, says about this AstroTurf-colored health drink.

People drink it for the minerals, vitamins, and amino acids that the wheat grass supposedly has sucked out of the soil. But you're not a plant. Your body doesn't need chlorophyll. Plus, as you would expect, the stuff tastes like a mowed lawn.

COOL STUFF

Blend In

TailGator

When it comes to outdoor alcohol-delivery systems, a beer cooler is as high-tech as most men get. But there are times when a sophisticated blended beverage is called for and your extension cord won't reach—like on the boat, or in solitary. Pull out the TailGator, a gasoline-powered blender with a 25 cc, $2\frac{1}{4}$-horsepower engine and variable speed control. Fire up this sucker at your mother-in-law's garden party and charm the ladies with a 64-ounce pitcher of strawberry daiquiris in 15 seconds. The TailGator weighs 10 pounds and costs $295 (888-874-7677). Smaller and less rowdy is Black & Decker's single-speed PartyMate ($40, 800-231-9786), which runs on the same rechargeable batteries as your cordless drill.

Drink Your Vegetables

Omega 1000 Fruit-and-Vegetable Juicer

Juicers make us think of guys who get weekly colonics. But the fact is, juicing is great for any man who wants his fruits and vegetables without having to actually sit down and eat them. Of the machines we tried, the Omega 1000 ($249, 800-633-3401) pulverized fastest, left the most juice, and was the easiest to clean. For a day's worth of vegetables that's easy to swallow, Barbara Gollman, R.D., suggests combining three carrots, 1 cup of raw spinach, $1\frac{1}{2}$ teaspoons of fresh ginger, and $\frac{1}{2}$ cup of water.

**PERCENTAGE OF MEN
WHO REPORT HAVING CHOCOLATE CRAVINGS:** 15

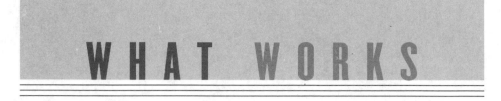

WHAT WORKS

We face a literal smorgasbord of food choices every day. Wheat bread or rye. Butter or margarine. Lager or stout. Most guys let their taste buds decide. We suggest you also use your head to determine what's best for your body. After all, what you eat has a major impact on your health and well-being. Anyone who's had one too many helpings of baked beans knows that. Here's how to truly drink to your health and eat to your heart's content.

I. **Shake on cinnamon, shake off diabetes.** According to the USDA, cinnamon helps control blood-sugar levels. Ground cinnamon—the spice, not the flavoring—stimulates the production of glucose-burning enzymes and boosts insulin's effectiveness. In one study, cinnamon made insulin 20 times more capable of breaking down blood sugars. "Adding a teaspoon of cinnamon to your diet each day will give you the same benefit," says the USDA's Richard A. Anderson, Ph.D.

2. **Eat rye bread to lower your cholesterol.** According to a small study done at the University of Kuopio in Finland, delicatessens have one menu item that may actually lower your lipid level: rye bread. Researchers took blood samples from 18 men who had consumed rye and wheat breads as part of their diets for 4 weeks. Men who ate large amounts of rye bread had a 14 percent reduction in their total-cholesterol levels and a 12 percent drop in LDL ("bad") cholesterol. "We assume the benefit comes from the high fiber content of rye bread," says Hannu Mykkanen, professor of clinical nutrition and coauthor of the study.

3. **Protect yourself from gum disease and cancer with OJ.** We already know that orange juice is good for fighting colds and heart disease, but two new reports show that as little as one glass of orange juice a day may help ward off both gum disease and cancer. In the first study, researchers analyzed vitamin-C intake and gum-disease levels in 12,400 adults. They found that getting less than 60 milligrams a day of vitamin C increases the risk of periodontal disease by more than 150 percent. In the second study, scientists found that bioflavonoids in orange juice counteract and destroy many of the enzymes that help tumors develop.

4. **Fight heart disease with cranberries.** A study from the University of Wis-

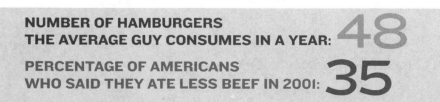

NUMBER OF HAMBURGERS
THE AVERAGE GUY CONSUMES IN A YEAR: 48

PERCENTAGE OF AMERICANS
WHO SAID THEY ATE LESS BEEF IN 2001: 35

consin found that cranberry juice contains just as many heart-healthy flavonoids as grape juice and red wine. "The antioxidants in cranberry juice can prevent arterial clogging," says Ted Wilson, Ph.D., the study coauthor. Wilson recommends drinking two 8-ounce glasses of cranberry juice each day, or alternating between grape and cranberry juice for maximum protection.

5. Grill a safer burger. Having burgers for supper? Flip them frequently while cooking them over low heat. A study in the *Journal of the National Cancer Institute* found that this is the most effective way to kill E. coli and limit formation of carcinogens in the meat as it cooks.

6. And make it healthy—without turkey. If you're going to eat a burger or hot dog, order one with everything. Bad foods can turn healthy when you add toppings like these:

Mustard: Curcumin, which makes mustard yellow, has been shown to reduce inflammation as well as half-strength cortisone does (when you eat the mustard, not when you smear it on your legs).

Spicy relish: Capsaicin, the stuff that makes red peppers hot, may help you lose weight by speeding up your metabolism and suppressing your appetite. Other ingredients may slow the formation and spread of cancer cells.

Mayonnaise: Linoleic acid is the good fat in low-fat mayo. According to one study of 650 men, linoleic acid lowered the risk of developing prostate cancer by 30 percent.

Ketchup: Lycopene, the red substance in tomatoes, may reduce the risk of prostate cancer by 25 to 40 percent. The flavonoids may reduce the risk of stomach cancer by as much as 56 percent.

Onions: The allium in onions lowers cholesterol levels and blood pressure and may also help prevent ulcers as well as stomach cancer.

7. Know what drinks go with your food. Lose the "red with beef, white with fish" mantra. These drinks will raise your meal to the next level.

If You Eat . . .	Have a Drink That's . . .
Barbecue	Cold and crisp. Like a Bud. Anything lighter will taste watered down against fiery sauces. Anything darker will cover the flavor
Chinese	Slightly bitter. A Heineken or a whiskey drink will go best with the garlic and ginger, says Dale DeGroff, former head bartender at New York's Rainbow Room
Indian	Strong or fizzy. DeGroff suggests a gimlet (gin and lime juice), a heavily hopped beer, or a pale ale like Bass Ale to neutralize the hot curries
Italian	Red. A rich, full-bodied red wine is the best thing to accompany a traditional Italian meal—besides a rich, full-bodied Italian girl. Try an Australian Shiraz
Mexican	Citrus-flavored. Why else do you think so many people order margaritas or lime-plugged Coronas? The fruits cut through the oils and grease
Seafood	Mild and citrus-flavored. It'll mimic a squirt of lemon on fresh fish. Try a sauvignon blanc. For beer, go for a Michelob or a wheat microbrew

8. Turn canned salmon into quesadillas. Eating salmon from a can seems wrong somehow, like wearing a suit to your softball game. But it's one of the easiest ways to get protein and heart-healthy omega-3 fatty acids. So we taste-tested a bunch. The winner: Bumble Bee. Now try this 5-minute recipe.

¾ cup (about 6 ounces) tub-style light cream cheese with chives and onions
8 8" fat-free flour tortillas
1 can (8 ounces) salmon
1 cup chopped green bell peppers
1 cup chopped onions
¼ teaspoon ground black pepper

Spread the cream cheese over the tortillas. Divide the salmon, peppers, and onions evenly among four of them. Press another tortilla on top of each. Heat a nonstick skillet coated with cooking spray over medium-high heat. Cook the quesadillas for 2 minutes on each side. Cut into wedges.

Makes 4 servings.
Per serving: 358 calories, 22 grams (g) protein, 39 g carbohydrates, 12 g fat (30% of calories), 6 g saturated fat

9. Know your spreads. Is the real stuff healthier than the artificial? Use this handy reference.

Butter versus margarine. If you must have either, butter is the smarter choice because margarine is loaded with trans fats, says Sue Saunders, R.D., director of nutrition at dietsmart.com. Use "lite" whipped butter, which is lower in saturated fat. Or use soft tub margarine, which has fewer trans fats than the stick kind.

Whipped cream versus Cool Whip. Calorie-wise, they're about the same, says Saunders. So take your pick: More fat? Or more chemicals? Or you could just put a can of evaporated nonfat milk in the freezer, along with a metal bowl and a beater. Take them out in 30 minutes and whip the milk. "No fat, calories, or artificial ingredients," says Saunders.

Real crab versus imitation crab. Imitation crab is surimi, or pressed white fish, along with some artificial flavoring and coloring. Nutritionally, both foods are about the same. But there is a difference in flavor. "If you're eating crab alone, use real crab," says Saunders. "If you're eating crab as part of a salad or other dish, surimi is fine."

Eggs versus egg substitutes. If you're scrambling them or throwing them at cars, use the real thing. But in recipes where the flavor is masked, use the fake ones.

10. Look for hidden sources of sodium. Sometimes it's easy to spot the extra salt in your diet; that ain't fairy dust on the rim of your margarita, amigo.

Other times, it's not so apparent. This could be a problem if you're overweight, diabetic, or "salt-sensitive," meaning you have a higher risk for developing high blood pressure. Heavy men are at particular risk. Researchers at Tulane University recently found that heavy guys with the highest salt intake were 89 percent more likely to die of a stroke than low-salt guys. Some stealth foods can quickly push you past your daily allotment of 2,400 milligrams of sodium.

Food	Mg of Sodium
I can Campbell's chicken-noodle soup	2,225
8 oz Campbell's tomato juice	750
2 cups Kellogg's raisin bran	700
2 slices Velveeta cheese	660
3 or 4 pancakes (6" diameter)	590
2 slices whole wheat bread	300
I medium chocolate shake	300

II. Fight fatigue with peanut butter. To keep from tiring out during endurance events like, say, marriage, nutritionists suggest you eat energy bars. But Ohio State University researchers found that blood-sugar levels actually crashed a half-hour after people ate energy bars high in carbohydrates and fat— meaning the subjects felt more tired than when they started. Our advice: Eat a tablespoon of peanut butter on a piece of bread. That has close to the perfect fatigue-fighting ratio of nutrients (40 percent carbohydrates, 30 percent protein, and 30 percent fat) needed to keep your energy up.

12. Protect your heart with walnuts. Spanish researchers fed people with high cholesterol a heart-healthy diet (vegetables, fish, very little red meat or eggs, olive oil as the only cooking fat) for 12 weeks. For half of the time, the researchers cut the amount of olive oil by 25 percent and made up the fat calories with walnuts. Though LDL-cholesterol levels dropped during both halves of the 12 weeks, they dropped significantly more during the walnut weeks. "These results came from only 8 to 11 walnuts a day," says study author Joan Sabatè, M.D., Dr. P.H., from Loma Linda University in California. It's possible that a combo of monounsaturated fats (olive oil) and polyunsaturated fats (walnuts) whacks cholesterol.

13. Drink wine to beat cold sores. According to a study published in *Antiviral Research,* resveratrol—a compound found in grapes—stopped the cold sore–causing herpes simplex-1 virus from multiplying. Researchers aren't sure if this works in humans, but red wine isn't exactly castor oil, so give it a try.

14. Drink dark beer and dodge kidney stones. Don't want to know what the labor of childbirth feels like? Another good reason to have a beer. Dark beers like stouts and porters are high in hops, a beer ingredient that's believed to keep stone-forming calcium from accumulating in your kidneys. Finnish researchers studied approximately 27,000 men and estimated that each glass of beer they drank in a day lowered their kidney-stone risk by 40 percent. Just don't binge; what's good for your kidneys isn't necessarily good for your liver.

15. Or drink coffee. If your doctor tells you to cut back on coffee because it contains compounds that may bind with calcium to form stones, he isn't up on his research. A study review published in the *American Journal of Kidney Disease* found that those who drank coffee had a lower risk of kidney stones. "A few doctors will still say to avoid it, but the best data we have suggest it has a protective effect," says David S. Goldfarb, M.D., of New York University's medical center. But since caffeine is a diuretic and dehydration is known to increase your risk of stones, drink plenty of water.

16. Protect your prostate with pineapples. Or guavas. Or cantaloupes. It doesn't matter. Increased intake of fructose, the sugar found in fruit, may combat benign prostatic hyperplasia (an enlarged prostate—BPH, for short). Here's the theory: Fructose helps reduce phosphate levels in your body, and too much phosphate may raise your levels of 1,25-(OH)2D, a chemical that's been linked to both BPH and prostate cancer.

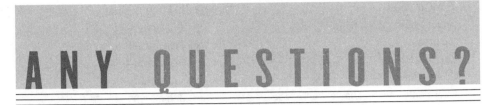

ANY QUESTIONS?

Rubber Stopper

How can I keep microwaved food from tasting rubbery?

—J. S., Tulsa, Okla.

The microwave oven is an amazing device that can make an ordinary piece of food taste as if the British cooked it . . . in a fraction of the time! If you're tired of eating rubber sole, try these suggestions from Mary Ellen Camire, Ph.D., a professor of food science and human nutrition at the University of Maine at Orono.

Turn it down. Use lower power (70 to 80 percent) and wait an extra minute or two. (Fine foods such as bean-and-bacon burritos must be allowed to breathe a little.)

Break it apart. Foods heat more evenly in smaller pieces, reducing mushy spots.

Throw in the towel. To reheat pizza, put a paper towel underneath to absorb moisture. This keeps the crust from turning into a doggie chew toy.

Spin it around. A micro with a carousel gives the best results.

"Some foods are going to turn rubbery no matter what you do," says Camire. For example, without much fat to soften it, the protein in low-fat cheese often turns to leather in the microwave. Try melting it in a low-tech toaster oven instead.

Frosty Fragrance

How long can you keep stuff in the freezer before it gets that "freezer smell"?

—N. T., Salt Lake City

Modern freezers go through a warming cycle to prevent frost buildup, says Carolyn Manning, R.D., associate professor of nutrition and dietetics at the University of Delaware in Newark. This means your food is partially thawed and refrozen over and over again. While not dangerous—the food remains cold enough to prevent bacterial growth—this isn't any way to treat a slab of porterhouse. To beat the funk, stick to the following guidelines.

Type of Food	Freeze No Longer Than . . .
Soups, stews, casseroles	1–2 months
Ice cream	1 month; less if ice crystals have formed
Lunch meat, hot dogs	1 month
Cooked meat	1–2 months
Raw steaks, chops, roasts	2–6 months
Raw ground meat	2–3 months
Raw poultry	4–6 months
Raw seafood	2–4 months
Cooked or smoked seafood	Do not freeze
Former mob boss	Indefinitely

Stomach Safety

I bring my lunch from home and leave it in a plastic container on my desk. My co-workers tell me that I'm going to get sick. How long can food sit at room temperature before it spoils?

—C. Z., Galveston, Tex.

Bacteria thrive above 60°F, so your leftover Chinese could be a real petri dish by noon. Food left at room temperature may look and smell okay, but it could contain high levels of the bacteria that cause food poisoning, says food-science professor Linda Harris, Ph.D., of the University of California at Davis.

If you don't have an office fridge or just don't feel like walking to it, pack your lunch with a reusable frozen gel pack. Or use a frozen juice box. It'll give you two benefits: The juice will be thawed by lunch, and your food will last a few extra hours out in the open. The following chart shows how long typical lunch foods will survive a morning on your desk at room temperature.

Food	Hrs Safe at Room Temperature
Tuna-salad sandwiches	1
Beef, bologna, leftovers with meat	2
Macaroni salad, pudding	2
Soup	3
Yogurt	4
Hard cheeses such as Cheddar	5
Salad, oil-based dressing	6
Fruit pies	7
Peanut-butter-and-jelly sandwiches, cake	8
Bread, raw vegetables, cookies, dried fruits, dried meats	All day

Omega Man

I despise fish, but my kids' frozen fish sticks aren't too bad. Do they have any of those omega-3 oils that are supposed to be so good for you?

—M. N., Midland, Tex.

Fish sticks may be great because you can dip them in beer, but they're hardly the nutritional equivalent of salmon or tuna. Six fish sticks have only half a gram of cholesterol-lowering omega-3's, compared with nearly 2 grams in a 4-ounce piece of salmon, says nutrition professor Gail Frank, R.D., of California State University at Long Beach. If you can't stomach fish, you can still find omega-3's in canola oil, which has 3 grams of omega-3's per 2 tablespoons. But don't eat more than a tablespoon a day; each tablespoon has 14 grams of fat.

Peanut Gallery

My girlfriend buys all-natural peanut butter because she thinks it's healthier, but I'd rather eat the smooth stuff you don't have to mix first. Is the peanut butter I like really less healthy?

—P. K., Redmond, Wash.

Natural peanut butters are like the latest ab machines: They look inviting but do little to trim your gut. While creamy peanut butters have a bit more sugar than the all-naturals, both types have 180 to 190 calories and 16 to 17 grams of fat per 2 tablespoon serving, says Cindy Moore, R.D., director of nutrition therapy at the Cleveland Clinic Foundation. The main difference is that the smoother kinds look and taste better. That's because brands like Skippy, Jif, and Peter Pan contain minute amounts of partially hydrogenated vegetable oil, which keeps their oils from separating during storage the way those in natural peanut butters do.

PART THREE
TURBOCHARGE YOUR SEX LIFE

MUST READS

Prostate Strategies

Three ways to get a better prostate-cancer screening

Let's face it: If you want a sex life, you need a healthy prostate. Heck, if you want a life at all, you need a cancer-free prostate. You've probably heard that it's a good idea to get your gland an annual checkup. What you may not know is that a yearly exam is not always enough.

We asked some of the country's top urologists what they'd insist on if their prostates were on the line. Their advice: Go beyond the standard routines the average doc is likely to suggest. Here's what you should know about when it comes to getting tested for prostate cancer.

The standard routine: Once you turn 50, you undergo a digital rectal exam (the finger) and a PSA (prostate-specific antigen) test each year. If your total PSA reading is 4 nanograms per milliliter (ng/ml) of blood or greater—a high count that suggests that cancerous cells may be producing PSA—your doctor may refer you to a specialist for a prostate biopsy.

A better strategy: Start getting PSA tests at age 40 if you have a family history of prostate cancer. Be certain your doctor performs a percent-free PSA test that measures both free-floating PSA and those bound to other molecules, known as complex PSA. The test has been around for several years, but not all urologists use it. Cancerous prostate cells seem to produce more complex PSA. Your doctor should send your blood sample to a university medical center that performs the percent-free test.

Also, ask your doctor if your PSA reading is normal for your age and race. Asian men produce the least PSA, white men produce slightly more, and black men have the highest natural PSA counts. Most urologists would ignore a PSA reading of 3.3 ng/ml in a 52-year-old black man, but if you're Japanese, that's high enough to suggest cancer.

The standard routine: Your prostate biopsy takes six tissue samples.

A better strategy: Double the take. "The standard six-sample prostate biopsy can miss cancer," says urologist Jonathan Epstein, M.D., of Johns Hopkins University in Baltimore. "That's why we take 12 core samples and include more outer regions of the prostate." This is called an extended-sextant biopsy, and it scans a wider field to spot malignant cells. It won't cause any more pain than the usual biopsy, says Dr. Epstein.

The standard routine: Your doctor sends your biopsy to a nearby hospital for analysis.

A better strategy: Cut the error margin. "If it were me, I'd have it sent to one of the best prostate-cancer centers for analysis. It doesn't cost a penny more," says Dr. Epstein. Your urologist should know the leading institutions. Most important, demand that at least two pathologists review the results and, if a tumor is present, agree on exactly how aggressive it is (its grade). "At least 15 percent of prostate-cancer cases are graded wrong, and grading determines what kind of treatment you get," says Dr. Epstein. A combination of tests, such as CAT scans, bone scans, and MRIs, can help determine the grade of your cancer.

Sex Snacks

An A-to-Z guide to the 24 best foods for erections, orgasms, and just playing around

By Brian Good

The way we see it, one primal urge deserves another. That's why we've always felt that food and sex go together like strawberries and cream. Or milk and honey. Or whipped cream and chocolate sauce. You get the idea.

What you spread, lick, or eat during sex can be about more than just making a mess. Pick the right foods and you'll boost your sex drive, strengthen your erections, and increase the power of your orgasm. Brazil nuts, celery, liver, and sweet potatoes don't sound sexy? As far as your body's concerned, they are. Here's our guide to the best foods for sex.

APPLES AND BLUEBERRIES

Fruit helps improve the taste of your semen by making it sweeter and less salty. Plus, apples and blueberries are loaded with fiber that pushes excess cholesterol through your digestive system before it can be broken down, absorbed, and deposited along artery walls. Lower cholesterol means cleaner arteries and better bloodflow to your penis. Translation: stronger erections over the long term.

Eat them: Every day. For foreplay, try using pureed blueberries as fingerpaint on her face and body. Clean with tongue.

BRAZIL NUTS

No food packs more selenium than the brazil nut. Studies show that selenium may help prevent the growth and formation of prostate-cancer cells. It may also enhance fertility: In a British study, men with previously low levels of selenium who increased their intake of the nutrient improved the quality of their sperm cells.

In addition, "all types of nuts and grains are good sources of vitamin E," says vitamin expert and nutrition professor Paul Lachance, Ph.D., of Purdue University in West Lafayette, Indiana. "Vitamin E is essential for preventing damage from free radicals and may also help to reduce the signs of aging. Vitamin E also prevents the natural breakdown of testosterone in your body and helps keep your sex hormones at their proper level."

Eat them: Before dinner, at least one night a week.

CELERY

It may taste like little more than crunchy water, but celery contains androsterone, a hormone found in the male body. Researchers believe that androsterone acts like a pheromone and is at least partially responsible for enhancing a man's attractiveness to women.

Eat it: About 30 minutes before making your move. Androsterone is released through your sweat shortly after being eaten. As things begin to heat up, your partner may notice her attraction to you increasing.

CEREAL

Check the label and pick a brand loaded with thiamin and riboflavin, such as Bran Flakes or Grape-Nuts. Both nutrients help ensure that your body uses energy as efficiently as possible. They also enhance nerve function. Since sexual stimuli travel to and from your brain along nerves, better function translates to more intense stimulation.

Eat it: Every morning.

CHEESE

Eating foods high in protein naturally boosts levels of dopamine and norepinephrine, brain chemicals that heighten arousal during sex.

Eat it: Like the French do—as a snack to cleanse the palate after a meal.

CHICKEN

Chicken is a lean source of protein that helps to reduce levels of a naturally occurring compound called sex-hormone binding globulin (SHBG). As you might guess from the name, having too much of the stuff is bad since it bonds with sex hormones and prevents them from doing their job.

Eat it: About three times a week.

NUMBER OF MINUTES THE AVERAGE MAN MAINTAINS AN ERECTION DURING SEX: 14

CHILE PEPPERS

Spicy foods have a reputation as aphrodisiacs because they speed up your metabolism, causing an elevated heart rate and sweating. Eager lovers may have confused these symptoms with sexual attraction and arousal. The metabolic boost is provided by capsaicin, an oil found in chile peppers. Pretend you don't know that, though, and you'll get an added charge from south-of-the-border fare—at least until the heartburn sets in.

Eat it: In guacamole. Combine a ripe avocado with one clove of crushed garlic, half of a minced jalapeño pepper, a teaspoon of lemon juice, and 3 tablespoons of low-fat sour cream. Mash with a fork or blend with a food processor until creamy, then spread on tortilla chips, tacos, or enchiladas.

CHOCOLATE

The cocoa in chocolate contains methylxanthines, compounds that help carry nervous-system signals throughout your body. Having lots of methylxanthines in your body benefits you during sex because it increases stimulation, ensuring that your skin registers even the slightest movement against it. Chocolate also contains phenylethylamine, the same chemical your brain produces when you fall in love.

Eat it: With your tongue. Melt dark chocolate (the cocoa is more concentrated than in milk chocolate) in the microwave until lukewarm, then dribble it onto the places your partner most likes you to lick.

COFFEE

Besides helping you stay awake and alert in the evening, the caffeine in coffee acts as a stimulant, speeding up your metabolism and enhancing your circulation. Improved circulation leads to increased arousal.

Drink it: After dinner.

EGGS

Eggs are an excellent of B vitamins, your body's natural stress-reducers. Bs improve your sex life by helping to lower elevated levels of stress hormones that may contribute to performance anxiety or premature ejaculation. "B vitamins are also involved in the breakdown of cholesterol into other substances," says Lachance. "Without B vitamins, your body wouldn't be able to produce either sex hormone or sperm cells." You also need plenty of those B vitamins in your diet in order to have powerful orgasms, since the nutrients increase testosterone levels in the body and help to fuel the sex drive by keeping your thyroid, nervous system, and adrenal glands working at peak level.

Eat them: A couple times a week.

GINSENG

The herb first gained popularity as an aphrodisiac simply because ginseng roots look like penises. Today, however, researchers know the root acts as a mild stimulant.

Eat it: In Chinese stir-fry. Grate a small piece of the root and brown it with garlic and onion before adding vegetables and meat to the mixture.

GREEN TEA

It's not just good for calming your nerves before sex. Research shows that the antioxidants in green tea help to prevent the development of all forms of cancer, including prostate cancer. Prostate cancer isn't just deadly, it's also a major cause of impotence in men over 50. In one animal study, green tea reduced tumor growth by more than 50 percent.

Drink it: With the Chinese stir-fry, above.

HONEY

Honey is packed with boron, a mineral that helps your body produce vital sex hormones such as testosterone. It's also nature's very own sports drink, providing you with all the energy you need for a night of passion.

Eat it: Off her face; honey is also a natural skin moisturizer.

LIVER

It doesn't sound sexy, but there's no better source of vitamin A than liver. Studies show that men with the highest daily vitamin-A intakes also tend to have higher sperm counts and better sexual functioning. Vitamin A also helps prevent dry and itchy skin.

Eat it: Once or twice a month.

MILK

Besides providing protein for energy and for the repair of sore muscles after a long night of lovemaking, milk contains calcium and phosphorus, both of which help to build energy reserves within your muscles and boost your libido. Calcium also gives muscles the nutrients they need to contract properly and prevent cramps. That can help keep an unplanned charley horse from putting a damper on your spring-squeaking fun.

Drink it: Twice a day.

OATMEAL

Anything made with oats will help to increase the amount of testosterone available in your bloodstream. Testosterone can get stuck to other compounds in your body as it moves through your bloodstream—but oats produce a chemical that frees bound testosterone, allowing it to return to the blood supply. The higher your testosterone level, the greater your sex drive—and the more powerful your orgasms.

Eat it: Stealthily. Mix some into ground beef before grilling burgers or frying meatballs.

OLIVES

Olives are another traditional aphrodisiac, but they can also be a lot of fun.

Eat them: In bed. "Try having your partner suck the filling out of one while you hold it in your mouth," says *How to Give Her Absolute Pleasure* author Lou Paget.

ORANGES

Citrus fruit is high in vitamin C, a nutrient that has been linked to increased sperm production. In one study, patients taking over 200 milligrams a day of vitamin C increased their sperm counts by over 110 percent and improved their sperm motility. Vitamin C also helps keep skin strong and supple. Finally, according to Lachance, C helps revitalize other vitamins in your system, including vitamin E and selenium. "It makes them available to your body so that you have a second chance to use them," he says.

Eat them: Without using your hands. Break an orange into sections, than challenge her to feed them to you one by one, using any part of her body except her hands. Return the favor.

OYSTERS

Another case of appearance leading to reputation; oysters became known as an aphrodisiac simply because of their resemblance to female genitalia, according to Paget. Like steak and chicken, they're a good source of zinc—a mineral necessary for high fertility levels and good prostate health. In a study from Singapore, men with high levels of zinc in their systems had significantly better fertility than men with lower levels.

Eat them: In soup. Mix 2 tablespoons of butter, some grated onion, a pint of oysters, 2 cups of milk, and 1/2 cup of light cream. Cook over a double-boiler until hot. Add parsley, salt, pepper, and paprika.

PUMPKIN PIE

In a study conducted at Chicago's Smell and Taste Treatment and Research Foundation, researchers found that eating pumpkin pie caused an immediate increase in bloodflow to the penis.

Eat it: With vanilla ice cream. Additional research from the foundation shows that the scent of vanilla is one of women's top turn-ons.

STEAK

Lean red meat is another good source of zinc. Zinc boosts libido by reducing your body's production of prolactin, a hormone that can cause erection problems and interfere with arousal. Red meat also increases testosterone production. "Zinc is part of all the enzymes your body produces," says Lachance. "Every enzyme—including testosterone and semen—has zinc within its structure and won't function without it." If your body doesn't have enough zinc, it will even go so far as to simply halt enzyme production until its supply is replenished. That can leave you virtually unable to perform.

Eat it: With her. Zinc works in women, too, helping increase natural lubrication. Buy lean cuts.

SWEET POTATOES

Ancient civilizations used to consider the lowly yam to be an aphrodisiac. Beta-carotene, which is responsible for giving sweet potatoes their orange color, enhances libido by improving the function of hormone-producing glands. The more beta-carotene in your body, the better your ability to make the hormones that regulate sex drive.

Eat them: Instead of baked potatoes. Wrap them in foil and bake at 400°F for 45 minutes.

TOMATOES

When tomatoes were first discovered, people called them love apples because of their supposed ability to boost sex drive. While we're not sure about the effect on libido, researchers do know that tomatoes are the best source of a nutrient called lycopene that is one of the most potent prostate-cancer fighters ever discovered. Lycopene works by reducing damage within the body caused by virtually all types of carcinogens. In one study, men who ate 10 or more servings of tomatoes or tomato sauce each week reduced their prostate-cancer risk by 41 percent.

Eat them: In ketchup, spaghetti sauce, and pizza. Because lycopene is not damaged by cooking or processing, it's even more potent in concentrated tomato sauces than it is straight from the garden.

ZITI

Whether it's squiggly or straight, pasta is an important source of carbohydrates. According to a Belgian study, athletes on a high-carb diet had 77 percent more endurance than those who went light on carbs. You don't need us to tell you that the greater your endurance, the longer the fun can last.

Eat it: In salad. Mix 1 cup of cooked pasta with tomatoes, olives, kidney beans, cucumbers, and feta cheese. Garnish with olive oil, vinegar, salt, pepper, and dill.

Break Your Sexual Slump

Sex gotten boring? Predictable? Nonexistent? Here's how to get out of any bedroom rut and regain your all-star form

By Brian Good and Zachary Veilleux

Our favorite baseball player of all time is Clete Boyer. Not because his name is Clete (well, maybe partly because his name is Clete) but because of how he broke an ugly 1-for-17 slump on August 31, 1969. Clete was at the plate when Morganna—the ultra-buxom, blonde "kissing bandit"—ran onto the field and planted one on Clete's face. Clete's response: an RBI single, followed by a scorching eight hits in his next 15 at-bats. The lesson: To break out of a slump, you just need the right inspiration.

Is your sex life like Clete's dry spell? Lots of effort, but nothing to show for it? Maybe you haven't had sex in weeks, or maybe when you have it, it's uninspired. Or maybe your once-loyal fans are booing you before you even walk onto the field. Whatever your bedroom dilemma, you don't need to rely on buxom blondes to turn things around (though we do endorse them). You just need to keep swinging.

YOUR SLUMP: You've Played the Same Position for Your Whole Career

If you've been with the same woman for a long time, chances are good that even if you don't have sex routinely, you settle for routine sex. Maybe she prefers you on top, so that's what you do every time, because it's like the DH rule: easy and effective.

Break it: You need to change the way you play—or at least where you play. Try one of these techniques for a change of pace.

Slow and shallow. Be more disciplined with your thrusting. Ask her to lie facedown, flat on the bed, legs together. Lie on top of her, penetrating from behind. The curve of her butt will limit how far you're able to enter her. That benefits both of you: The first 2 inches of her vagina are not only the most sensitive but also the tightest, because they swell with blood during intercourse. Use slow, measured thrusts to put your most sensitive spot (the head of your penis) alongside hers. Do it right and she'll stop trying to trade you for a player to be named later.

Kneeling together. If she lacks the enthusiasm to take the lead, try this position, courtesy of the guys at www.sexandhealth.com: Sit on your knees,

PERCENTAGE OF MEN WHO WOULDN'T WANT TO STAND IN FOR A MALE MOVIE STAR DURING A SEX SCENE: 79

feet tucked under your rear. Have her sit the same way, positioning herself between your legs. You rock up and back using your thighs; she slides up and down by pushing on your knees with her hands. She'll be in control of your depth and speed, so she can have it exactly the way she wants it, but she won't feel as if she's the only one putting on a show.

YOUR SLUMP: You Swing at Low-And-Away Sliders Every Time

If you've had a lot of sex with your wife or girlfriend, she knows how you're going to try to excite her even before you do. That game plan isn't very exciting for anyone.

Break it: The key to outsmarting—and satisfying—your partner is to change your pattern constantly so she'll never know what's coming. That translates to better sex—and more of it.

Start with the backs of her knees. Men tend to be very linear about how things should happen, and women know this, says *How to Give Her Absolute Pleasure* author Lou Paget. "They know their men will go here for 15 seconds and there for 30 seconds, and then think everything is okay. It's like getting on the dance floor with someone who does the same step all the time."

Make trapezoids with your fingers. When you're stroking your partner, don't move up and down her body in straight lines. "When you use a straight stroke, the nerves in the skin aren't surprised when they're touched," says Paget. However, when you use wavy lines and the stroke is irregular, the nerves have no idea what's next, and they become that much more excited. Pick areas that aren't generally exposed to light. Parts like the back of her arms are only used to feeling the pressure of clothing, so they're much more sensitive—and easier to stimulate—than other parts of her body.

Hit the showers. Paget recommends the PulsaBath ($12)—a small, Nerf-like waterproof ball with a built-in vibrator. "You can use it to rub all over each other's bodies in the shower or bath," she says.

YOUR SLUMP: You Swing at the First Pitch

Think about it: An at-bat is much more exciting when the batter stretches the count to 3-2 and then fouls off a half-dozen pitches. When he flies out on the first pitch, it's hardly worth noticing. Same thing with

PERCENTAGE OF AMERICAN WOMEN
WHO OCCASIONALLY FAKE ORGASMS: **70**

PERCENTAGE OF BRAZILIAN WOMEN
WHO OCCASIONALLY FAKE ORGASMS: **44**

sex: Finish the job in 3.7 seconds and she won't remember why she was there in the first place.

Break it: Products that help with premature ejaculation may seem like a quick fix—desensitizing creams, antidepressants, and even household numbing products like Chloraseptic are all known to help you last longer. But in almost all cases, you're much better off doing a little extra work on your technique. "Products for premature ejaculation may work, but they reduce the quality of sex you're having, since they're making your penis less sensitive," says Aaron Pierce, a marriage therapist in Temple, Texas. Try these techniques to help curb premature ejaculation.

Change positions frequently. A University of New Brunswick study found that men who vary their sex techniques have greater ejaculatory control than men who generally stick with one position.

Exercise before you go to bed. You'll release a surge of hormones that your system then has to break down. That causes a mild lull throughout your entire body, including your penis.

Have sex in the morning. Your sensory system is mildly depressed when you first wake up, so it takes longer for you to reach complete arousal.

YOUR SLUMP: You're Embarrassed to Even Wear the Uniform

It's hard to believe, but sometimes men are the ones who hesitate to climb into bed. One common reason: Stripping off their shirts means showing off their beer guts.

Break it: To get rid of your gut, flip to the fitness section of this book. In the meantime, make the best of what you have. Sex journalist Susan Crain Bakos suggests positions—such as rear entry—in which you won't feel conscious of her staring at your fat.

YOUR SLUMP: You Hit Better in Batting Practice Than You Do in the Game

Some men have trouble ejaculating or climaxing during sex because they've become accustomed to masturbation, says urology professor Gregory Broderick, M.D., of the Mayo Clinic in Jacksonville, Florida. The problem: You can control the pressure and pacing of your hands, and you can't do the same with her body parts.

Break it: We're not suggesting less masturbation, but maybe you need to think about how you do it. Try this technique, which mimics intercourse: Apply lubricant to your hands and place them palm to palm. Curve your palms lengthwise to form a tube, with your fingertips pointed at your feet. Then use only your thighs to create motion. That will help retrain your penis to respond more to her body parts than to yours.

YOUR SLUMP: You Lost Your Bat (And It's Your Only One!)

While it's normal for occasional erection problems to keep you out of a few games, you don't want to be benched permanently.

Break it: Let your penis know who's boss. A new study of 776 men found that those who exhibited "dominant" traits—men who were able to influence others or express their opinions forcefully—were half as likely to develop erection problems as less dominant men. "Somebody who's inclined to negative self-evaluation may be less likely to perform when given the opportunity, as opposed to a man who's confident in his abilities," says urologist Laurence Levine, M.D., of Rush-Presbyterian–St. Luke's Medical Center in Chicago. In other words: Have confidence in your penis and it will serve you well.

YOUR SLUMP: You Have No Minor-League Prospects

If you're having sex in order to produce a whole new crop of rookies, not connecting with the pitch can make your sexual relations more frustrating than enjoyable. The scariest statistic: About 40 percent of infertility is caused by problems with the man's equipment.

Break it: Stop the pregame celebrations: Excessive alcohol and cigarettes have been connected to lower sperm counts. Some drugs and supplements are just as bad; steroids, muscle-building supplements like DHEA, and even common heart medications like calcium channel blockers can keep you from fatherhood. While you're at it . . .

Avoid certain health foods. Phytoestrogens in plant foods such as soy, tofu, and beans can damage your sperm. It's good to get a small amount of phytoestrogens for your prostate health, but eating them excessively may decrease sperm production, says Harry Fisch, M.D., director of the male-reproductive-health center at Columbia Presbyterian Medical Center. Limit your intake of phytoestrogens to 190 milligrams (mg) weekly (a soy-protein shake has 60 mg; 8 ounces of soy milk has 16 mg).

Pee freely. Men who urinate frequently or have to get up at night to urinate could have urinary infections that are damaging their sperm. "I get more pregnancies by prescribing antibiotics for urinary-tract infections than I do by prescribing fertility drugs," Dr. Fisch says.

Do plenty of off-season training. In a study from the University of Rochester Medical Center in New York, researchers found that men's fertility levels decrease by up to 40 percent as the weather turns warmer—meaning that you're at your most fertile during the winter months.

PERCENTAGE OF COHABITATING WOMEN WHO REPORT BEING DEPRESSED: 42

PERCENTAGE OF MARRIED WOMEN WHO REPORT BEING DEPRESSED: 18

Assess Your Marriage— And Your Sex Life

We'll walk you through it so you can enjoy a
fulfilling relationship—and a lifetime of great sex

**From *The* Men's Health *Longevity Program* (Rodale)
by the editors of *Men's Health* Books**

Go get yourself shaved and showered, big fella. You have a hot date tonight.
Do what you need to do to clear your schedule this evening. Call the
babysitter. Think of some impromptu options for you and your wife. This
should not be a preplanned event. Spontaneity is key.

If you're a bit rusty at this kind of thing, just relax and use your imagina-
tion. If it's a nice night, go buy a checkered tablecloth, a bottle of wine, some
crusty bread, and some cheese, and enjoy a faux-French evening under the
stars. If there's a local theater group putting on a production, go see that and
follow it with coffee and cheesecake. Or just walk along the river, holding hands
and swigging from a hip flask filled with a good 12-year-old scotch.

Above all, do not let your wife do anything to prepare for tonight except
get herself ready. If there are dishes in the sink and she's horrified that the
babysitter will see them, you load them into the dishwasher. If there are
snacks to pick up, you go get them. Reservations to be made? Tickets to be
purchased? Money to be withdrawn? You do it all. This evening is a gift to her.

Why are we so concerned with your love life? There are a whole slew of
reasons.

Consider first that happily married men live an average of 6 years longer
than single men. And when researchers at the Veterans Administration Medical Center in Miami checked the survival rates of 143,969 men with prostate
cancer, they found that those who were married lived almost 3 years longer
than those who were never married or were separated or divorced. A good
reason for that may be that women play a big role in men's choices to seek
medical care. University of California, San Diego, researchers found that
married men were 2.4 times more likely than bachelors to seek medical care.

Also, if you decide to chuck your marriage, you'll pay for it in more ways
than alimony. Researchers found that the trauma of divorce can be bad
enough to negate the health benefits of remarrying (unless some really serious
abuse went on in the previous marriage). Plus, other nasty things happen. The
suicide rate among divorced and separated men is $2\frac{1}{2}$ times higher than that
of married men. And your boy won't do so hot either. A 10-year study by the
National Institute of Mental Health found that, when a father leaves, it can
have a traumatic, long-lasting effect on his sons.

HOW ARE YOU DOING?

How is your marriage going? To help get a bead on the status of your relationship, ask yourself the following questions from the book *Fighting for Your Marriage* by Scott Stanley, Ph.D., Howard Markman, Ph.D., and Susan L. Blumberg, Ph.D. If you answer yes to one or two of these, that's fine. Everyone goes through rough patches. But if you consistently answer yes to a lot of these questions, it's a very good idea to start figuring out how you can improve your marriage. Life is too short to be miserable.

I. Do routine discussions often erupt into destructive arguments?

2. Do you or your partner often withdraw or refuse to talk about important issues?

3. Do you or your partner often disregard what the other says, or do you often use put-downs?

4. Does it seem that your partner interprets your remarks much more negatively than you intended?

5. Do you feel that there has to be a winner and a loser when you disagree?

6. Does your relationship often take a back-seat to other interests?

7. Do you often think about what it would be like to be with someone else?

8. Are you disturbed by the thought of still being with your partner a few years from now?

But enough scary stuff. It's not just that you'll live longer and healthier; most important, it's that your time here on Earth will be so much more pleasurable if you enjoy the woman next to you.

So for this one day, we want you to think a lot about your relationship with your wife. Is she your friend? Can you speak freely with her? Are you harboring lingering resentments? Are you bored with marriage or perfectly happy with it? Do you love your wife as she is today? Can you be sexually free and open with her? Be honest, and be willing to act. Nothing is more worth fighting for than a great marriage.

LOVE THE ONE YOU'RE WITH

The reason we told you to have an impromptu night out with your wife is that it smacks of something that may be missing in your relationship: romance.

Before you start cringing at the mention of that word, bear in mind that romance has gotten a bum rap. If you think it's all about cloying novels with Fabio on the covers, boring English movies where nothing ever blows up, or fat little cherubs bouncing around, think again. It's really all about sex and fun and keeping your marriage alive and strong.

So if the mere mention of the word *romance* creates an overwhelming urge to power up your buzz saw, it's time to change your attitude. And not just for her sake.

"For crying out loud, it's about being selfish," says *1,001 Ways to Be Romantic* author Gregory J. P. Godek. "You want to have more sex? Have more fun? Enjoy your days more? I'll tell you how to do it—be romantic." Here's a crash course in the art of romance.

Be spontaneous. "Many women, when they say they want romance, mean spontaneity," says Godek. That's why you need to surprise your wife tonight. It's the unexpected that shocks and delights. It proves to her that you've been thinking of her when she least expects it.

Work harder at uncovering the things that turn her on. One of women's biggest complaints is that men are stone-deaf when it comes to picking up cues, says *The Seven Dumbest Relationship Mistakes Smart People Make* author Carolyn Bushong. When your wife says, "Gosh, I love purple roses," take note, literally. Write it down and slip it into your wallet so you don't forget. Surprise her with the flowers later.

Turn off the television. Try it for just a week, says Godek. See how much time it frees up to spend with the woman you love. After a week, see if you want to make this a regular habit.

Be creative in the way you love her. Ultimately, you know your wife best. You have to tailor your acts of romance to best fit your relationship. You see, when it's all boiled down, the only way she knows that you love her is by the things you do. Keep at it, and you'll notice some amazing things taking place. "Do you remember how good you felt at the beginning of the relationship?" asks Godek. "That's what it can still be like."

SEX: IT'S WHAT'S FOR DINNER

Broccoli. Salmon. Carrots. These are some of the things that are incredibly good for you. Then there's sex. As far as we're concerned, sex is the most enjoyable longevity tool out there.

Researchers who studied sexual activity and mortality in a group of 918 men found that those who had the most sex had half the risk of death from heart disease compared to their less stimulated counterparts. Seeing that the average couple has sex 3,900 times during the course of their marriage, that's a lot of chances for sexual healing.

But do anything that many times, and you run the risk of your rutting becoming routine. Then it tapers off as one or both of you lose interest. Too bad, because you'll miss out on other bodily benefits, such as a healthier prostate,

FREQUENCY OF HIV TRANSMISSION IN THE UNITED STATES: EVERY 13 MINUTES

better quality sperm, less stress, and an expanded sense of well-being. Your penis even needs lots of erections to keep it standing at attention late in life. Here are some things you can do to keep your love life limber.

Look for the new in her. Here's the thought for the day: To know her is to never stop discovering her. Deep, eh? We picked that up from a commercial, but it's a wonderful idea that the person you've chosen to be with is, in fact, this vast, unexplored territory, replete with assets, qualities, virtues, and, yes, vices that you haven't even found yet. If you think you know her completely, think again.

"People are always changing. They're always going to surprise you if you give them the chance," says *Light Her Fire* author Ellen Kreidman, Ph.D. So make it a quest to find out new things about your wife. Ask her what she was doing when she heard that John Lennon had been shot. Find out what her favorite candy was as a child. Even seemingly stupid questions like this can spark discussions that will lead you to places you never knew existed.

Don't criticize; encourage. As time marches on, you may be surprised to notice how many imperfections your once-perfect partner is starting to develop. (Incidentally, she's noticing the same thing about you.) Time and gravity bash us all. But don't you ever let on. "It's surprising, the nasty things people can say to one another after they've been together for years. Most people don't even realize how cruel they can be to one another," says Kreidman.

START OFF THE NIGHT RIGHT

Want to increase your chances of a warm reception when you hit the hay? Want to enjoy the evening getting there? Here are some things you can do—or should not do—to secure her amorous interest in you this very night.

Do	Don't
Seek her out as soon as you walk through the door.	Root through the mail or roll around with the dog first.
Give her a kiss when you find her.	Ask, "Hey, when's dinner?"
Make dinner with her.	Go near the TV or sofa.
Ask her how her day went.	Get that glazed look when she actually starts to tell you.
Wash the dishes.	Forget to take out the trash.
Rub her feet while she reads.	Say her feet stink (even if they do).
Shower and shave before heading for bed.	Go near the bedroom at all without at least brushing your teeth.

Before you say something that will put your sex life in the deep freeze for months, ask yourself how it would have sounded coming out of your mouth during your dating years. This brings up another valuable point: You *are* still dating and courting her. You're trying to convince her to spend the rest of her life with you. Remember that.

Keep in shape. We all get older. Our bodies sprout more hair, our bellies threaten to burgeon, we "forget" to take showers every day. Just to clue you in: She still wants you to be physically attractive. "It's important to women that the men in their lives take care to look nice and to stay fit and healthy. This sends a message that you care about them enough to look good for them," says Columbus, Ohio, psychologist Robert Birch, Ph.D., who specializes in marriage and sex therapy.

That doesn't mean you can never wear your ratty gray sweatpants. Just keep it to a minimum. And don't let your belly hang out.

Be on the lookout for ruts. In any long-term undertaking, always remember that complacency is the killer of passion, the birth mother of boredom. Keep your eyes peeled for danger signs such as always having conversations about the same things and always spending your time together in similar ways. If you see the warning signs, act.

The world is full of happy couples celebrating 50th anniversaries and beyond. They don't have any special advantages over you; they have just chosen to work together to sustain a lifetime level of interest and wonderment about each other.

You can do it, too. We'd like to see the two of you on a park bench together years from now. Just don't hog all the pigeons.

What She's (Really) Thinking About in Bed

Here's how to find out—and how to turn her intimate thoughts to your advantage

By Janine Hazlewood, for the South Africa edition of *Men's Health*

Ever want to know what's going through her mind while you're going at it? A bit of mental wandering during sex is perfectly normal. According to a report by condom manufacturer Durex, almost one-third of adults fantasize about a celebrity during sex, 36 percent have flashbacks of someone in their past, and a sad 7 percent think about TV. Work worries or body-image anxiety could also be responsible for your partner's preoccupied look. "The

biggest sex organ is the brain. And, as emotional beings, women in particular need to be psychologically and emotionally prepared for sex," says sex
counselor Suzie Hayman, author of *Pandora's Book of Sexual Fantasies*.
"Men, on the other hand, can more easily be aroused by physical touch
alone." Read her body language and tune in to her thoughts and you're
more likely to push all the right buttons and reap the rewards.

SHE'S (REALLY) THINKING ABOUT . . .
Her performance

How you know: "If she's sticking out her boobs and tossing back her hair as
though she's auditioning for a part in *Deep Throat*, she's probably anxious to
impress you," says *Bodytalk* author and body-language specialist Judy James.
James also warns that you should watch out for suspiciously loud squeals of
delight: They're probably fake.

Why? Just as men don't feel they've got a result unless they've given
their partners earth-shattering orgasms, so women feel the same pressure to
have those killer orgasms—and look like Pamela Anderson in the process.
"Women's magazines have a lot to answer for," says James. "Now that
women know multiple orgasms exist, they feel inadequate unless they have
them."

Do this: "The main thing is to bring honesty back into the relationship,"
says James. She suggests trying morning sex, when your partner is sleepy and
unkempt. That way, you'll have lazy natural-style lovemaking: The spoon position is a good no-pressure option.

Your benefit: She'll relax and become more uninhibited, and once she's
stopped play-acting you'll build up to good, honest sex.

SHE'S (REALLY) THINKING ABOUT . . .
Pornography

How you know: If she's swapped her mismatched, ancient underwear for a
leopard-skin G-string and thigh-high boots—or shouts "Screw me harder!"
along with any other lines you recognize from that porno flick you watched together a few weeks ago—she may be reliving the experience in her mind's eye.

Why? "Although some women genuinely find porn offensive, there are a
great many who are really turned on by it—but don't like to admit it," says
Rowan Pelling, editor of *The Erotic Review*. "The women I've spoken to aren't
interested in soft-focus subtle erotica, they want to see explicit sexual images,
just as men do." Women also get turned on by porn with an element of kink-
iness—such as spanking, bondage, or threesomes—because it's forbidden.

Do this: She may have more of a naughty streak than you realize, so stop
hiding your stash of porn under the bed and give her a peek. Read or watch

together to see what turns her on. Then try out a few scenarios the next time you have sex. Invest in some handcuffs or treat her to some saucy underwear.

Your benefit: Your sex life will never be the same again. And next time you go to bed, she could be wearing her spiky heels and be ready to chain you to the bedpost.

SHE'S (REALLY) THINKING ABOUT . . .
Food
How you know: The fact that she often brings snacks to bed might be a clue. That and her rumbling stomach.

Why? "Food, drink, and sex are all related because they're very oral, sensual, pleasurable activities. The image of someone greedily licking or sucking a juicy peach is very erotic because that's how you'd like them to hungrily devour you," says Hayman. Cosmetics giant Revlon surveyed 1,000 people and found the most sensual foods to be champagne or wine (34 percent), strawberries (29 percent), chocolate (23 percent), and whipped cream (19 percent). Apparently pork chops didn't make the cut.

Do this: Bring food into the bedroom, drip chocolate mousse onto your partner's breasts, dine naked, and eat off each other. Play with contrasting sensations by alternating ice cream or an ice cube with warm custard.

Your benefit: Food-themed sex games are a great way of thinking erotically and putting the fun back into sex.

SHE'S (REALLY) THINKING ABOUT . . .
Her body
How you know: No need for rocket science here. If she always likes the lights off, avoids undressing in front of you, and opts for the missionary position (where she's less on show), she's fretting about her body. "Other giveaways are moving your hand away from trouble spots, holding in her stomach, and general bodily tension," says clinical psychologist Sayal Bennett.

Why? Women are inundated with images of pert and perfect Heidi Klums and Elle Macphersons. So it's not surprising that few feel they make the grade. Many women say their weight makes them feel inhibited during sex. "Women tend to be incredibly self-critical and worried they'll disap-

DIVORCE RATE FOR COUPLES WHO LIVED TOGETHER BEFORE GETTING MARRIED: 85

ODDS THAT THE AVERAGE MAN WILL GET DIVORCED: 1 IN 2.5

point their partner," says Bennett, "yet they're forgiving of their men's imperfections."

Do this: You may be her biggest fan, but does she know that? Does she know that even her wobbly bits are sexy to you? If not, tell her. Become the master of compliments, touch her bottom and thighs and say how good they feel—celebrate her womanliness. It's also worth compromising on lighting. If you want the lights on and she wants them off, meet halfway and use candles or subtle lighting, or invest in a dimmer switch.

Your benefit: Self-confidence is the biggest turn-on. If her self-esteem is healthy, she's more likely to be adventurous in bed and opt for positions where you'll get a good view of her body, such as rear entry. Don't forget to tell her how sexy her butt looks.

SHE'S (REALLY) THINKING ABOUT . . .
Sex with another woman

How you know: She's likely to have her eyes firmly shut and avoid your manly hairy bits. It's tenderness she's thinking about, so she may be kissing you gently or caressing her breasts.

Why? "Same-gender sex is one of the most common fantasies, but it doesn't necessarily mean she's got lesbian tendencies," says Hayman. The attraction is more to do with tenderness. "Women like the idea of exploring nonpenetrative sex, because clitoral stimulation—as opposed to vaginal sex—is what usually brings them to climax. Also, being with someone who knows exactly what to do is pure self-indulgence, like a massive act of masturbation."

Do this: "It's a good idea to ban intercourse for a few sessions," says Hayman. "Let your fingers and tongue explore erogenous zones other than the genitals: Try the back of the neck, which is rich in nerve endings, or suck her earlobes, toes, or fingers." To encourage her to share her fantasies with you, tell her yours. Get her to describe where she is and who she's with, and touch her accordingly.

Your benefit: Evidence suggests that people who fantasize are more likely to have higher libidos—the more you think about sex, the more you want it. And as sharing fantasies is one of the most intimate things you can do, it'll bring you closer. Plus, girl-on-girl action is the ultimate male fantasy, so this is one you'll both enjoy.

SHE'S (REALLY) THINKING ABOUT . . .
Having a child (or not)

How you know: Ideally, this is something that needs to be discussed out of the bedroom. If she's telling you to throw away the condoms, or if she sticks her legs in the air after sex (helping to ensure that your sperm hit the spot), she may have babies on the brain. Equally, if she is hypercautious about contraception and seems tense toward your climax, she could be panicking about becoming pregnant.

Why? The most obvious reason is that her body clock is ticking away or your relationship has gotten to the baby-making stage. "This is not an exclusively female preoccupation, but women are conditioned to think love equals babies, particularly if sex is good and there's a real connection," says Hayman. "Procreation was, after all, the original function of sex; and when you both feel that this is why you're making love, it's the ultimate in sexual intensity." On the other hand, if her career is just taking off or it's early in your relationship, she could be terrified of an unwanted pregnancy, which will inhibit her performance.

Do this: If she wants your babies, take it as a compliment. Men often have a knee-jerk reaction to baby talk, but it's quite likely just a flight of fancy. All she may really be after is warm, intimate sex. Hayman suggests going for face-to-face positions where you can get close and look into her eyes. Likewise, if you sense she's anxious about getting pregnant, show her that you understand her concerns; and discuss contraception before madly thrusting away.

Your benefit: Once the baby/contraception issue has been thrashed out and you've agreed on what you both want, you can get down to some great, worry-free sex.

SHE'S (REALLY) THINKING ABOUT . . .
Other men

How you know: If she has repeatedly mentioned any new male colleagues or has surprisingly renewed sexual enthusiasm, she could be daydreaming about someone other than yours truly. And—just in case you weren't sure—yes, calling out another man's name at the point of orgasm is a pretty good (and less subtle) clue.

Why? This doesn't mean she's about to run off with Mr. Fantasy—fantasies are something forbidden, rarely what you would want in reality. They are also very common. "Most people at some stage imagine making love to someone else. It could be a person they know, a faceless stranger, or a celebrity," says Hayman. "This is an inevitable part of a long-term relationship and doesn't mean you need to rush into a new one—just bring the thrill back into yours."

COUNTRIES THAT HAVE THE MOST SEX PER YEAR: RUSSIA, FRANCE, GREECE

Do this: Crank up your sex life. Remember when you first met and you pulled out all the stops with your athleticism and knee tremblers? If you only know three of the estimated 500 sexual positions possible, buy a copy of the *Kama Sutra*. Break with routine: Forget the bed—try the sofa, the shower, the garden. "It isn't someone else she wants," says Hayman, "it's the old you she wants back."

Your benefit: She'll remember why she fell for you in the first place, and it'll drive all thoughts of that new work colleague—and Brad Pitt—right out of her head. And with all that renewed enthusiasm flying around, it should be just like those good old sex-filled days.

SHE'S (REALLY) THINKING ABOUT . . .
Her job

How you know: If she hunches up her shoulders and seems tense or withdrawn in bed, she may have work worries on her mind. Sudden changes in the frequency of sex are a good indicator that stress is killing her sex drive.

Why? According to a recent survey for Stress Awareness Day, two out of five people think about work during sex. If your partner is stressed about a meeting in the morning or tired from a long journey home, she won't switch off the minute you hit the sack. "Stress and overwork are among the most widespread causes of loss of libido for men and women—caused by a dip in testosterone and estrogen levels," says *Increase Your Sex Drive* author Sarah Brewer, M.D. "Think how much sexier you feel on holiday when you know you've got time to relax." It's not all doom and gloom, however: Research shows that job satisfaction can have the reverse effect. A University of Wisconsin survey of 500 couples suggested that women who are fulfilled at work have better sex lives than those who don't, because it increases their self-esteem and this makes them feel even sexier.

Do this: Concentrate on building intimacy. Dr. Brewer advises helping your partner switch off by giving her a massage (try using essential oils like rose or jasmine, renowned for their aphrodisiac properties). Or share a warm, relaxing bath together. The aim is to seduce her before you get to bed. Then move on to oral sex or mutual masturbation, and finally penetration when she's ready.

Your benefit: She's less likely to rebuff your sexual advances if you're sensitive to her stress. And hopefully, she'll discover how to get you in the mood for sex next time you come home from a nightmarish day.

KNOW THIS

That's *Your* Clock Ticking

Though men don't have a fertility cutoff event like menopause, the older you get, the longer it may take to become a father. Researchers in England studied 8,000 couples who were trying to conceive and found that it took longer when the man was 5 years older than the woman—no matter how old the woman was. The study, the first to suggest that the age of the man is a key factor in conception, showed that for every year past age 24, the odds of becoming a father within 6 months dropped by 2 percent. Women with younger partners got pregnant more quickly. "The chances of it taking more than a year to make your partner pregnant increase twofold from age 25 to age 35," according to Chris Ford, Ph.D., a senior research fellow at University Division of Obstetrics and Gynaecology at St. Michael's Hospital in Bristol, England.

Better Sex Leads to Babies

If you're trying to have a kid, change sex positions as much as possible, or at least break out the chocolate sauce and feathers. Japanese researchers have found that the hotter the sex, the better your sperm count. Researchers compared semen collected from 19 fertile men when they masturbated with and without erotic videos. When they used the videos (and reported sexual satisfaction averaging 7.5 on a 10-point scale), the men's sperm counts were 46 percent higher than when they didn't (and gauged their satisfaction at just 5.6). "The more aroused you are when you ejaculate, the better the contractile activity in the glands that produce semen," says urology professor Larry Lipshultz, M.D., of Baylor College of Medicine in Houston. And if you're getting better contraction, you generate more volume of ejaculate as well as draw from younger, healthier sperm.

PERCENTAGE OF PEOPLE WHO THINK SEX IS OVERRATED, ESPECIALLY COMPARED WITH WORK: 62

PERCENTAGE OF PARENTS WHO OWN VIBRATORS: 15

Here Comes a Son

Unless you have a son, you're going to be mowing the lawn for the next 30 years. Luckily, some research suggests that you just might be able to tilt the odds in your favor. If you want to add a boy to the group . . .

Start young. A study published in *Fertility and Sterility* suggests that older parents are more likely to have girls.

Conceive in the summer. A German researcher suspects that heat kills more X (female) chromosomes, leaving the Ys (male) free to dart for pay dirt.

Masturbate often. Researchers found that Y-chromosome sperm die after living in the testicles for more than a few days. If you don't release them regularly, more live X-chromosome sperm will be waiting in your arsenal.

Uncut and Uncensored

Here's a good argument against having your baby boy circumcised: By lopping off the nerve endings in his foreskin, circumcision limits the sensations he feels. But it's not just the fact that he'll have better sex; he'll probably have more of it. In a recent British study, women were 40 percent more likely to have multiple orgasms with uncut partners than with those who were circumcised. The authors concluded that because foreskin helps the penis glide in its own skin, there's less friction in her vagina, which keeps her lubricated longer. An added bonus: The uncircumcised men lasted an average of 4 minutes longer than their circumcised pals.

Nonoxynol-9 Warning

A recent study suggests that the spermicide nonoxynol-9, which had been shown to kill the HIV virus in test tubes, may actually increase the risk of HIV infection. Researchers studied prostitutes in Africa and Thailand and found that the rate of HIV infection was almost 50 percent higher among women who used N-9 than in those who used a placebo vaginal gel, according to Lut Van Damme, M.D., of the Institute of Tropical Medicine in Belgium. N-9 users also had higher rates of genital lesions that are often gateways for HIV. The study isn't definitive, but for now, don't depend on N-9 to help protect you from HIV. In fact, use condoms without N-9 until the Centers for Disease Control and Prevention completes its reevaluation of the spermicide.

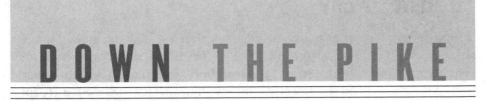

DOWN THE PIKE

New Erection Pill

A recent German study found that 75 percent of impotent men taking a drug called vardenafil were able to develop and maintain an erection long enough to reach orgasm.

The main difference between the new drug and Viagra (sildenafil) is that vardenafil works in much lower doses, says lead researcher Hartmut Porst, M.D. Lower doses translate into fewer side effects, such as headaches, flushed skin, and upset stomach, which are common with other treatments.

Vardenafil should be available in late 2002.

Yet Another Erection Drug

Researchers at the Medical College of Georgia are developing an alternative to the famous blue pill that will attack impotence in a whole new way.

"Viagra works by enhancing the relaxation of smooth muscles in the penis," says physiologist Thomas M. Mills, Ph.D., one of the lead researchers working on the new drug. "When those muscles relax, more blood can flow into them, creating a firmer erection." The new drug, which is still going by its experimental name—Y-27632—works on the opposite principle. Instead of relaxing muscles in the penis to increase bloodflow, Y-27632 increases blood-flow by blocking the body's ability to contract penile muscles in the first place.

So far, the research on Y-27632 is extremely promising, says Mills. Animals who are given the drug develop almost immediate erections that last for a sustained period of time. And while the drug has yet to be tested in humans, Mills expects clinical trials to be underway within a couple of years.

You can bet we'll be following up on this.

PERCENTAGE OF COLLEGE-AGE MEN WHO SAY THEY HAD SEX BEFORE AGE 18: 80

PERCENTAGE OF COLLEGE-AGE WOMEN WHO SAY THEY HAD SEX BEFORE AGE 18: 59

Tired of Latex?

There could be a better option on pharmacy shelves any day now. A recent study by the California Family Health Council has shown there's a new choice that's just as viable as the latex rubbers you grew up with. It's made from a material called styrene ethylene butylene strytene (SEBS). Fifty-four couples tested each type of condom—a latex Trojan Enz, the polyurethane Durex Avanti, and a SEBS condom—three times, rating them on acceptability, sensitivity, ease of use, appearance, and comfort. They also reported breakage rates: The latex condom broke once, the polyurethane condom broke three times, and the SEBS condom never broke.

The SEBS got high marks for being easy to unroll, fitting well, and allowing more sensitivity. It was also judged more attractive, quieter, and less smelly than latex. And the SEBS condom was the favorite among women.

SEBS condoms have been FDA-approved but are not yet being marketed to the public.

Invisible Condom

No, it's not a prank you play on a sorority girl. It's a colorless, odorless gel for use by women, and it'll prevent the transmission of sexually transmitted diseases—although it won't serve as an impromptu water balloon. Tests are just beginning, but it may be available in about a year.

DOES IT WORK?

Some At-Home HIV Tests

In theory, it sounds great: An at-home test you can use to make sure you're clean without the hassle and inconvenience of waiting rooms and appointments. But some kits may be unreliable.

The Federal Trade Commission evaluated five kits purchased through an Internet site, and all of them gave negative results when used on a known HIV-positive blood sample. The FTC has filed lawsuits against several companies who make or distribute the tests. One company, Medimax, recently settled out of court—and agreed to a permanent ban on the sale of their kit. "Only one home-testing kit currently has FDA approval," notes Brian Zack, M.D., director of sexual-health services at Princeton University. For reliable results, use the Home Access Express HIV-1 Test System, in which you send a blood sample to a lab by mail, then call a special toll-free number for results. Or simply see your physician.

Penis Enlargement

Your e-mail inbox probably overflows with junk from companies that want you to look at porn, buy Viagra, and increase the size of your penis. The latter is tempting, even for guys who are already average size or above. After all, if $40 a month and a couple of pills could really add extra bulge to your jeans, why wouldn't you do it?

Is there any science behind traction, vacuum pumps, supplements, penile exercises, hypnosis, and surgery being peddled from cyberspace? Not really. Surgery is "the only true way to guarantee a permanent enlargement of your penis," says E. Douglas Whitehead, M.D., director of New York Phalloplasty.

At a big cost. Aside from complications involved in any surgery, there's a chance your erection will no longer be able to stand up on its own or your penis will appear deformed.

Our advice? Make the most of what you've got. Learn positions and techniques that satisfy you and your lover. Heck, it's free.

COOL STUFF

Penile Numbing That Works

Prilocaine/Lidocaine Cream

We've always been a little skeptical of penile anesthetics. As far as we're concerned, numbing the penis—even to delay ejaculation—is like watching TV with the sound turned off: You can follow the plot, but you miss all the jokes. A new study from the Netherlands has caused us to reconsider. Researchers studied 15 men and found that those who used prilocaine/lidocaine cream—similar to the type prescribed by American doctors—were able to stay hard longer. Their times between penetration and ejaculation without the cream averaged about 2 minutes. With the cream, they averaged 8 minutes. The subjects' female partners also benefited from the cream: Only 29 percent of them experienced orgasm without the cream, while 69 percent did with the cream.

The subjects did report some unpleasant side effects such as numbness of the penis and a less than full erection, although they were still able to have intercourse. Although there is no research yet on the long-term effects of the cream, its efficacy may decrease over time, says lead researcher A. Koos Slob, Ph.D.

If you often ejaculate less than 2 minutes after penetration, talk to your doctor or urologist.

Count Sperm at Home

www.spermconfirm.com

Even with a good supply of porn magazines and an attractive nurse on the other side of the door, coming up with a sperm sample—on demand—can be a daunting task.

Fortunately, in the age of eBay, e-mail, and e-everything-else, fertility testing also has a presence on the Internet. A new service located at www.spermconfirm.com will test your sperm count and motility—and you never have to leave the house.

Just dial up the company's Web site and a few days later you'll receive your collection kit. Then go about your business in the privacy of your home, mix your specimen sample with a special preservative, and ship everything back to the company in the prepaid overnight package for next-day analysis. The company then mails the results back to you within 48 hours.

The procedure costs $75 and currently is not covered by most insurance companies.

PSA, ASAP

FastPack System

Nerve-wracking, week-long waits for the results of prostate-cancer screening tests could be a thing of the past thanks to a new blood-testing device called the FastPack System that works in about 15 minutes.

In fact, doctors who use the new equipment don't even need to send your sample to a lab. They simply fill a disposable syringe with a sample of your blood and let the machine do the rest. The equipment was recently approved by the FDA to measure levels of both free and total prostate-specific antigen (PSA)—blood chemicals doctors look for to indicate the possibility of early-stage prostate cancer.

Arousal Achiever

EROS Clitoral Therapy Device

The first FDA-approved device designed to treat female sexual-arousal disorder is now available. The EROS Clitoral Therapy Device, made by Uro-Metrics in St. Paul, Minnesota, is a pliable plastic cup attached to a palm-size, battery-powered vacuum pump. Before intercourse, a woman places it over her clitoris, and gentle suction enhances bloodflow to that area. The expanded arteries stimulate clitoral nerves, making arousal a better bet.

NUMBER OF ALCOHOLIC DRINKS THE AVERAGE MAN HAS PER DAY: 1.2

NUMBER OF DRINKS THAT LEAVE THE AVERAGE MAN UNABLE TO PERFORM SEXUALLY: 4

NUMBER OF SEXUAL ENCOUNTERS IN WHICH THE AVERAGE MAN OR HIS PARTNER HAS BEEN DRINKING: 3 OUT OF 5

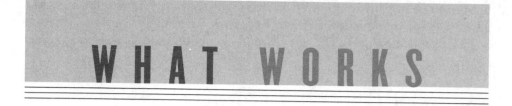

WHAT WORKS

Tons of things can douse the flames of her desire. Your beer gut. Stress. A squabble. Bedroom boredom. Your beer gut. Read on for the best ways to ignite a bonfire in your bedroom. We guarantee she'll replace her grumbling "Not tonight, honey" with purring delight.

1. To extend your manhood, lose your gut. You know extra weight is bad for your heart, but it also shortens your penis—you lose a half-inch for every 15 pounds you gain. Here's why: The fat pad that protects your pubic area creeps over the shaft's base as you get fatter, obscuring a perfectly good penis. A better diet and more exercise means more where it counts.

2. Fight better. Arguing isn't the most effective way to light the seduction fire. Here's how to shut off the tiff tap before it drowns your desire. First, you are both forbidden to use the word *why* during arguments, since it just spurs useless *because* replies. Second, you can't bring up any old news. Third, have cold drinks in your hands—preferably in plastic cups. Instead of screaming, you'll automatically pause and take a sip.

3. Get scared together. See scary movies, sleep in a haunted B&B, go skydiving, vote. It's a galvanizing crisis, which simply means that being terrified in each other's company may draw you closer emotionally—and erotically. You will synchronize your emotions and create physiological changes that mimic sexual arousal. It explains all the kissing in the streets at the end of World War II.

4. Appear sensitive. "One of the best ways for a man to seduce a woman he's just met is to reveal his vulnerable side," says David Givens, Ph.D., director of the Center for Non-Verbal Studies. "An easy and nonverbal way to do this is to display what's called your neck dimple, that V-shaped area just below your Adam's apple." Givens claims that open-collar shirts and V-neck sweaters that show off this area of the skin send the subconscious message that you're open and approachable—the opposite of what a tie expresses.

5. Put it simply. While research shows that men are attracted to women with larger vocabularies, the reverse doesn't hold true. (This explains the dating problems of our writing staff.) In an experiment involving 1,500 women, researchers found that the women's preferences for men remained the same whether the men talked like Dennis Miller or Dennis Rodman.

Since you won't score any points for reciting Shakespearean sonnets, feel free to continue answering with measured grunts.

6. Recall the best sex you had with her. Those kinds of fantasies are powerful motivators for you both. Talk about, and maybe relive, yours with her. Then give her the same courtesy. By reenacting the erotic fantasies you've carried, you can pump some pure energy back into your sex—and that's exactly what you need.

7. Read up. Women tend to be much more turned on by reading erotic words than by looking at dirty pictures—one reason she's not as excited as you are by your latest downloads. But you can turn this to your advantage by putting aside your laptop and picking up a paperback. Fifteen minutes of reading can replace 15 minutes of foreplay.

Have her put on something sexy and slide her some steamy passages from Henry Miller or her favorite romance novel before heading upstairs. She'll be primed.

8. Go along with her. In a recent survey, women admitted fantasizing about sex up to twice as often as men do. So how come she's not constantly jumping your bones? Because unlike your fantasies, hers are lengthy, interactive scenarios, says Karen Donahey, Ph.D., director of the sex- and marital-therapy program at Northwestern University in Evanston, Illinois.

You can get more action simply by giving her a scenario to spin. Toss her a line like this at lunch: "If anybody would look amazing in a French maid's outfit, it's you." You'll up your chances of her breaking out the feather duster after dinner.

9. Remember the kiss. "Women love to kiss, and I've heard a lot of them complain that guys just don't spend enough time on it," says *The New Male Sexuality* author Bernie Zilbergeld, Ph.D., a sex therapist in Oakland, California. But don't just do it more, do it better. Try varying the intensity (kiss her softly, then more passionately, then slow it down again). When you're done with her lips, move on to her cheeks, eyelids, forehead, nose, neck, or earlobes. Bonus points if you kiss her for several minutes without letting your hands roam—let her indicate when she's ready to move on.

10. Play head games. Notice how a lot of women play with their hair? It's not just a nervous habit—it feels good. Chances are she's wishing you would play with it, too. The scalp can be very sensitive to stimulation, and since she's probably not expecting you to lavish any attention on it, surprise her. "Having her hair brushed can be a very sensual experience," say Zilbergeld. Or run your fingers through it as you're kissing her; or simply caress her scalp gently with your hand.

11. Find her soft spots. Here's where you can get really creative. Try tenderly kissing the backs of her knees, the insides of her arms, her inner thighs, or the hollow of her neck. Women love to have these areas gently stroked, kissed, licked, or blown upon. Warning: These areas are all also made of very soft tissue, so tread lightly. "Gentle stimulation is going to be much more arousing than pressure that's hard or rough," says *Seductions* editor Lonnie Barbach, Ph.D., a San Francisco psychologist and sex therapist.

12. Go digital. Try sucking on her fingers or toes during foreplay or intercourse. (Granted, unless you're a contortionist, the toe thing may be a bit tough during intercourse, but you can usually find her fingers.) They're a lot more sensitive than you might think, and for whatever reason, a relatively large area in the brain receives sensation for them. "Lightly kissing or passionately sucking them, especially combined with the sensations you're causing in her genitals, can be incredibly erotic," says Barbach. We've heard that some women can even reach orgasm just by having their feet massaged.

13. Find true north. Austrian researchers have found that an oft-neglected region of the breast, the northern part from roughly 10 o'clock to 2 o'clock, provides even more arousal than her nipples. Investigate with light kissing and a gentle massage using the heel of your hand, not the fingers. The palm gives even sensation without causing pain.

14. Draw her in. Next time you're, you know, yodeling in the gully, don't just lick, the way most guys do. "Sucking on her clitoris and labia creates a unique feeling, and when contrasted with the usual friction can lead to more and better orgasms," says *The One-Hour Orgasm* author Bob Schwartz, Ph.D. This technique is better for you, too: You'll get fewer tongue cramps.

15. Taste the sensation. You love it when she gives you oral sex with a breath mint in her mouth. The mucous membranes that line your penis let mint pass through, giving you a cool thrill. But did you know that popping a curiously strong mint while you're giving her oral sex can lead to a curiously strong orgasm? Note to the wise: Peppermint oil can sting her. (One of our staffers found this out the hard way.) Stick to the original wintergreen flavor.

16. Press here for oral sex. Dentists aren't usually known for their passionate manner. But a recent study has some pretty interesting news for men and the women who want to love them—but don't enjoy performing oral sex because of that horrible gag reflex. In the study, the tooth-torturers gathered their most "orally sensitive" (read: "hurrallagggh!") patients and, using acupuncture or acupressure, stimulated their P-6 regions while simultaneously poking around in their mouths. In the majority of patients, the gag reflex diminished considerably.

Where's the P-6 region? No place too exciting: To find it, put the first three fingers of your right hand together and place them on the inside of her wrist. You press there while she pleasures you, and everybody ought to be happy.

17. Hypnotize her with your eyes. Want to drive her wild with desire? Look her straight in the eye during sex instead of burying your head in the goose down. Add in a little play-by-play of the action and solicit her opinion, too. The combination of eye contact and dialogue—that direct connection during sex—is an incredible turn-on for women.

18. Don't whisper. There is a biological connection between loud noise and sex. How else can you explain the way even bass players and drummers attract groupies? It turns out that a small part of your ear called the sacculus is stimulated by loud noises and sends a signal to your brain's pleasure center. Instead of whispering your dirty thoughts in her ear, say them out loud. Let your lips brush against her ear while you talk dirty—in a normal tone. This will sound loud to her because of the proximity, and she'll enjoy the movements of your mouth on her ear as well.

19. Have her give you a hand. Just before ejaculation, your testicles ascend like an aircraft's landing gear to provide more power to your takeoff. To give your equipment an even bigger boost, ask your partner to gently press upward on your testicles with the palm of her hand just before you ejaculate. This will heighten your arousal and add intensity to your orgasm, according to Schwartz.

ANY QUESTIONS?

Fastball

I got hit in the testicles with a baseball when I was a teenager, and one swelled and turned dark purple for a few weeks. Now I ejaculate too quickly. Is there a connection?

—T. L., New Castle, Del.

We doubt that anyone told you at the time, but you got a lucky bounce. Had the lob caused permanent damage, ejaculating would be painful or even impossible. Your rapid ejaculation probably stems from the fact that men are creatures of habit. "Most men masturbate to ejaculation as quickly as they can. So they're training themselves to ejaculate rapidly," says sex therapist Judith Seifer, Ph.D., R.N., a professor at the Institute for the Advanced Study of Human Sexuality in San Francisco. The best position for men who last less than 90 seconds during sex is with the woman on top. Being in the passive position helps you concentrate on delaying your orgasm. The missionary position can be counterproductive because it's harder for men to gear down when they're in charge of the thrusting.

Allergic to Women

After intercourse, I sometimes get a rash on my penis. I thought it might be a latex allergy, but it happens even when I don't wear a condom. Could I be allergic to my girlfriend?

—R. J., Tempe, Ariz.

Yes, you could be, but see a doctor first to make sure you don't have a sexually transmitted disease. Redness or a rash can be a symptom of genital herpes, gonorrhea, or something else just as delightful. If those are ruled out, then it could be that an allergy is being transmitted through sex. "Allergens like pollen, mold, dust, and pet dander can enter a person's system and make their way into her secretions," says immunologist Steven Witkin, Ph.D., of Cornell University medical center in Ithaca, New York. Washing up right after sex and using a condom both help. So does taking an over-the-counter antihistamine (such as Benadryl) an hour or so before sex.

'Fess Up

I had a herpes outbreak years ago and never had another. Do I still have to tell sex partners I have it?

—J. F., New York City

Yes, because even though you never have symptoms, it's still possible to infect someone else, says Felicia Stewart, M.D. If it's any consolation, you're far from alone. For adults who've had two to four sex partners, the odds of carrying the virus are 20 percent. That jumps to 25 percent if you've had five to nine partners, and 31 percent if you've had more than 10.

Once you have the virus, there isn't any way to get rid of it. In some cases, a doctor will prescribe an antiviral medication such as acyclovir to cut down on the frequency of herpes flare-ups. The best advice is to come clean with prospective partners and count yourself lucky; many people with herpes have it much worse than you do.

Pregnant Preference

My wife is 5 months pregnant, and I'm really attracted to her now. She thinks I'm nuts. Am I normal?

—P. L., Atlanta

No, you're not normal. You are a sick, sick man. Get counseling!

Actually, your body is probably just reacting to the increased levels of estrogen in your wife's body (and maybe her bigger breasts). When her estrogen levels soar during pregnancy, so will your testosterone, says sex therapist Judith Seifer, Ph.D., R.N., a professor at the Institute for the Advanced Study of Human Sexuality in San Francisco.

Even if both of you have an increased sex drive, you might worry that intercourse will be harmful. If she's having a normal pregnancy, it's perfectly safe. Seifer suggests trying the side-by-side rear-entry position if she's uncomfortable having sex. It's one of the easiest positions for expectant couples.

NUMBER OF AMERICANS INJURED BY THEIR BEDS AND BEDDING EACH YEAR: 437,980

PART FOUR
BLAST FAT

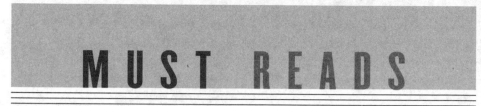

MUST READS

The Wet Diet

To lose your belly, just add water. Here's how to get more "wet foods" into your diet

By Kristyn Kusek

There's a secret ingredient in food. In the right amounts, it possesses a strange and awesome power—the power to help you lose weight as you eat!

"It" is water. Yep, take the same stuff you bathe in (well, not the same stuff), put it in food, and presto!—you have a bona-fide miracle weight-loss product on the end of your fork. According to *Volumetrics* author Barbara Rolls, Ph.D., no matter what you eat, you take in roughly the same amount of food, day in and day out. So while equal amounts of any food will fill you up, "wet food"—food with a high water content—will do it with fewer calories. The more water in a food, the less room there is for calories.

This doesn't mean you should go on a diet of watermelon, watercress, and water chestnuts. It means eating the right real food, the same food that Adam Drewnowski, Ph.D., director of the nutrition-sciences program at the University of Washington in Seattle, picked for the substitution list on the opposite page. Eat enough to save 500 calories a day, and you'll lose a pound a week. Eat more, and you'll lose more. In fact, you just may flush it away.

THE WET TEST

It's easy to tell whether a food is wet, dry, or just slightly damp: Simply pick up your grub, squeeze the heck out of it, and then measure how much water comes out. But that can get messy. Instead, try the more food-friendly method of dividing calories by weight in grams. Take the result, known as the energy density (ED), and see where it falls on this scale.

ED of 0 to 2.5 = Wet food (eat as much as you want)
ED of 2.6 to 6.0 = Dry food (eat sparingly)

Instead of Eating Dry . . .			Eat Wet . . .			Calories Saved
Breakfast	**Quantity**	**ED**	**Breakfast**	**Quantity**	**ED**	
Bacon	5 slices	5.0	Ham	I oz	1.8	131
Bagel with strawberry jam	I bagel	2.8	Low-fat yogurt with strawberries	6 oz	1.0	189
Burger King's French toast sticks	Approx. 5 sticks	3.9	McDonald's Egg McMuffin		2.1	150
Fruit toaster pastries	3 pastries	3.9	Pancakes with ¼ cup reduced-calorie maple syrup	2 pancakes	2.1	180
Lunch			**Lunch**			
Arby's Beef 'n Cheddar sandwich with fries	I sandwich	3.5	Subway's cold-cut trio with lettuce, tomatoes, onions, pickles, peppers, and olives on white bread	I 6" sub	1.5	359
Beef bologna with light mayo on whole wheat bread	3 oz of bologna	3.1	Tuna fish (packed in water) with light mayo on whole wheat bread	3 oz of tuna	1.1	175
Double cheeseburger	I burger	2.9	Steak wrap with vegetables	I wrap	2.1	264
Taco Bell's Santa Fe Beef Chalupa	I chalupa	2.8	Bean-and-cheese burritos	2 burrtios	2.0	62
Dinner			**Dinner**			
Cheese ravioli	2½ cups	3.2	Lasagna with meat	I serving (3½" × 4")	1.6	334
Hamburger	I medium-size burger	2.7	Meat loaf	3 oz	1.9	78
Hot dogs	2 dogs	3.2	Pork chop	3 oz	2.0	111
Pizza Hut's Pepperoni Lover's pizza	I slice	3.3	Homemade pizza	I slice	2.4	62
Roasted beef brisket	3½ oz	4.1	Beef pot roast with vegetables	3½ oz	2.3	177
Dessert			**Dessert**			
Brownies	2 brownies	4.0	Pumpkin pie	I slice	2.1	225
Cheesecake	I slice	3.2	Vanilla ice cream	6 oz (¾ cup)	2.0	58
Chocolate cake	4 oz	3.7	Chocolate pudding	4 oz	1.1	265
Chocolate-fudge cookies	3 cookies	3.5	Frozen fudge bar	I bar	1.4	128
Coffee cake	2 pieces	4.2	Apple pie	I slice	2.4	230
Snacks/Sides			**Snacks/Sides**			
French fries	I small order	3.0	Wendy's small chili	6 oz	0.9	305
Potato chips	3 oz	5.4	Potato salad	3 oz	1.3	340
Raisins	¼ cup	3.0	Grapes	½ cup	0.7	81
Salami, beef	3 slices	2.6	Shrimp	12 shrimp	1.0	115
Whole wheat fat-free tortilla quarters dipped in dressing	2 Tbsp	2.7	Whole wheat fat-free tortilla quarters dipped in salsa	2 Tbsp	0.3	166

Meals That Melt Fat

Our 2-week meal planner makes it easy

By *Men's Health* chef Vince Steinman

HOW TO USE THE PLANNER

1. Make a copy of the below lists and take it along for your Sunday grocery shopping. Buy everything on List A (we've kept the list to 12 items so you can breeze through the express lane).
2. Come home every weeknight and make a great-tasting meal—in just 15 minutes. Saturday and Sunday are potluck; you pick the two meals you want to make.
3. Eat like a king (okay, a duke) for a week, and lose a pound of fat. Here's how: Every meal serving weighs in at less than 500 calories, which is 500 calories less than the 1,000 that research shows the average guy eats for dinner. Multiply that calorie savings by seven, and you're 1 pound lighter.
4. Use List B for week 2. Swap in a few different ingredients, get five completely new recipes.

LIST A

2	pounds boneless, skinless chicken-breast tenders*
1½	pounds extra-lean sirloin strips*
2	packages (9 ounces each) Buitoni fresh angel-hair pasta
1	box (14 ounces) Uncle Ben's instant brown rice
1	bag (8 ounces) Kraft shredded reduced-fat Colby-jack cheese
1	dozen eggs
10	ounces ready-to-eat bagged spinach
1	jar (4½ ounces) minced garlic
4	onions
1	jar (26 ounces) Healthy Choice traditional spaghetti sauce
1	bottle (8 ounces) extra-virgin olive oil
1	bottle (5 ounces) A-1 steak sauce

LIST B

1½	pounds boneless, skinless chicken-breast tenders*
2	pounds extra-lean sirloin strips*
2	packages (9 ounces each) Buitoni fresh angel-hair pasta
1	box (14 ounces) Uncle Ben's instant brown rice
3	bell peppers
1	bag (16 ounces) carrots
4	onions
1	carton (16 ounces) Tropicana "No Pulp" orange juice
1	bottle (10 ounces) Kikkoman Lite soy sauce
1	jar (4½ ounces) minced garlic
1	jar (26 ounces) Healthy Choice traditional spaghetti sauce
1	jar (8 ounces) Dijon mustard

* Freeze half on the day you buy it. Cook frozen meat for an extra minute.

WEEK-I RECIPES
Monday
Colby-Jack Chicken

4½ ounces (half of a 9-ounce package) angel-hair pasta
1   egg
3   tablespoons beer (use St. Pauli Girl if you have it)
2   tablespoons shredded reduced-fat Colby-jack cheese
½   cup dried bread crumbs
½   pound chicken-breast tenders
1   tablespoon olive oil
¼   cup spaghetti sauce

Cook the pasta according to the package directions; drain. In a small bowl, beat together the egg and the beer. In another bowl, combine the cheese and the bread crumbs. Dip the chicken in the egg mixture, then in the bread-crumb mixture. Heat the oil in a nonstick skillet over medium heat. Add the chicken and fry for about 10 minutes, or until golden brown. Add the sauce and serve over the pasta.

Makes 2 servings.
Per serving: 461 calories, 36 grams (g) protein, 40 g carbohydrates, 16 g fat (31% of calories)

Tuesday
Tomato-Glazed Steak

½   cup brown rice
1   teaspoon olive oil
¼   cup thinly sliced onion
½   pound extra-lean sirloin strips
2   tablespoons spaghetti sauce
1   tablespoon steak sauce
½   cup spinach
¼   cup beer (got Sam Adams? pour him in)

Cook the rice according to the package directions. Heat the oil in a nonstick skillet over moderately high heat. Add the onion and the sirloin and brown for about 10 minutes. Add the spaghetti sauce, steak sauce, spinach, and beer. Cook for 5 minutes. Serve over the rice.

Makes 2 servings.
Per serving: 452 calories, 37 g protein, 41 g carbohydrates, 14 g fat (28% of calories)

Wednesday
Chicken Pasta Frittata

1   tablespoon olive oil
½   pound chicken-breast tenders
4½ ounces (half of a 9-ounce package) angel-hair pasta, cut into
     1" lengths
½   cup spinach
1   cup spaghetti sauce
2   eggs
⅓   cup shredded reduced-fat Colby jack cheese

Preheat the broiler. Heat the oil in a large nonstick skillet over medium heat. Add the chicken and brown for 7 minutes. In a large bowl, mix together the pasta, spinach, spaghetti sauce, eggs, and cheese. Pour the mixture into the skillet and cook for 5 minutes. Wrap the handle of the skillet with foil; broil for 3 minutes, or until browned.

Makes 2 servings.
Per serving: 474 calories, 41 g protein, 28 g carbohydrates, 22 g fat (42% of calories)

Thursday
Beer-Braised Beef with Onions

½   cup brown rice
½   cup flour
½   teaspoon salt
½   teaspoon pepper
½   pound extra-lean sirloin strips
2   teaspoons steak sauce
1   tablespoon olive oil
2   teaspoons minced garlic
½   cup thinly sliced onion
½   cup beer (best bet: Heineken)

Cook the rice according to the package directions. In a small bowl, combine the flour, salt, and pepper. Dip the beef in the steak sauce. Toss the beef in the seasoned flour, then shake off the excess. Heat the oil in a large nonstick skillet. Brown the meat, garlic, and onion for about 10 minutes. Add the beer and cook for 5 minutes. Serve over rice.

Makes 2 servings.
Per serving: 407 calories, 20 g protein, 34 g carbohydrates, 20 g fat (44% of calories)

Friday
Spicy Chicken and Pasta

$4\frac{1}{2}$ ounces (half of a 9-ounce package) angel-hair pasta
1   tablespoon olive oil
$\frac{1}{4}$ cup finely chopped onion
$\frac{1}{2}$ teaspoon flour
1   tablespoon water
$\frac{1}{2}$ pound chicken-breast tenders
2   teaspoons chili powder
$\frac{1}{2}$ cup spaghetti sauce

Cook the pasta according to the package directions; drain. Heat the olive oil in a nonstick skillet over medium-high heat. Add the onion and brown for about 1 minute. In a small bowl, mix together the flour and the water. Add the flour mixture, chicken, chili powder, and spaghetti sauce to the skillet. Simmer, uncovered, for 10 minutes. Serve over the pasta.

Makes 2 servings.
Per serving: 412 calories, 28 g protein, 30 g carbohydrates, 20 g fat (44% of calories)

WEEK-2 RECIPES
Monday
Sirloin Strips in Wine Sauce

$\frac{1}{2}$ cup brown rice
2   teaspoons olive oil (left over from List A)
1   teaspoon garlic
$\frac{1}{2}$ pound extra-lean sirloin strips
$\frac{1}{2}$ cup sliced onion
$\frac{1}{2}$ cup sliced bell pepper
$\frac{1}{2}$ cup dry red wine (check the cabinets; you've got to have a bottle somewhere)
2   teaspoons light soy sauce
$\frac{1}{2}$ teaspoon salt

Cook the rice according to the package directions. Heat the oil in a large nonstick skillet and sauté the garlic. Add the beef, onion, and pepper. Cook for about 10 minutes, or until tender. Add the wine, soy sauce, and salt; simmer for 5 minutes more. Serve over the rice.

Makes 2 servings.
Per serving: 505 calories, 37 g protein, 41 g carbohydrates, 16 g fat (29% of calories)

Tuesday
Skillet Steak with Mustard

$\frac{1}{2}$ cup brown rice
2 teaspoons olive oil
$\frac{1}{2}$ pound extra-lean sirloin strips
$\frac{1}{2}$ cup chopped onion
$\frac{1}{2}$ bell pepper, sliced into strips
1 tablespoon light soy sauce
1 tablespoon Dijon mustard

Cook the rice according to the package directions. While the rice is cooking, heat the oil in a nonstick skillet over medium-high heat. Add the beef, onion, and pepper. Cook for about 10 minutes. Mix in the soy sauce and mustard. Cook for 5 minutes, or until the meat is tender. Salt to taste. Serve over the rice.

Makes 2 servings.
Per serving: 478 calories, 37 g protein, 42 g carbohydrates, 16 g fat (30% of calories)

Wednesday
Chicken à l'Orange

$4\frac{1}{2}$ ounces (half of a 9-ounce package) angel-hair pasta
2 tablespoons olive oil
$\frac{1}{2}$ pound chicken-breast tenders
1 teaspoon minced garlic
$\frac{1}{2}$ cup orange juice
2 teaspoons light soy sauce
1 tablespoon flour
$\frac{1}{2}$ cup sliced carrot

Cook the pasta according to the package directions; drain. Heat the oil in a large nonstick skillet. Add the chicken and garlic and brown for about 10 minutes, or until tender. In a small bowl, mix the orange juice, soy sauce, and flour. Add the orange-juice mixture and the carrot to the skillet. Bring to a boil and simmer for 5 minutes. Serve over the pasta.

Makes 2 servings.
Per serving: 399 calories, 28 g protein, 31 g carbohydrates, 17 g fat (38% of calories)

Thursday
Green Peppers Stuffed with Beef and Rice

$\frac{1}{2}$ cup brown rice
$\frac{1}{4}$ cup sliced carrot
2   green bell peppers
$2\frac{1}{2}$ teaspoons olive oil
$\frac{1}{2}$ pound extra-lean sirloin strips
$\frac{1}{4}$ cup spaghetti sauce
$\frac{1}{2}$ teaspoon salt

Preheat the broiler. In a medium saucepan, combine the rice with the carrot. Cook according to the directions on the rice package. Cut off the tops of the peppers and scoop out the seeds. Rub the outsides of the peppers with $\frac{1}{2}$ teaspoon of the olive oil. Heat the remaining oil in a large nonstick skillet over medium heat. Add the beef and brown for about 5 minutes. Add the rice mixture, spaghetti sauce, and salt. Cook until heated through. Divide the beef-and-rice mixture between the peppers. Broil the peppers for about 5 minutes, or until browned.

Makes 2 servings.
Per serving: 507 calories, 38 g protein, 47 g carbohydrates, 18 g fat (32% of calories)

PERCENTAGE OF AMERICANS WHO SAY THEY ARE SATISFIED WITH THEIR WEIGHT: 68

PERCENTAGE OF AMERICAN MEN WHO ARE A HEALTHY WEIGHT: 39

PERCENTAGE OF AMERICANS WHO SAY THEY ALWAYS EAT WHENEVER THEY SEE FOOD: 39

NUMBER OF U.S. SOLDIERS DISCHARGED FOR OBESITY DURING THE 1990S: 41,799

Friday
Red-Wine Chicken with Garlic

4½ ounces (half of a 9-ounce package) angel-hair pasta
2 tablespoons olive oil
½ pound chicken-breast tenders
2 teaspoons minced garlic
¾ cup thinly sliced onion
½ cup dry red wine
½ cup orange juice

Cook the pasta according to the package directions; drain. Heat the olive oil in a large nonstick skillet. Add the chicken, garlic, and onion. Brown for about 10 minutes, or until tender. Add the wine and orange juice and simmer for 5 minutes. Serve over the pasta.

Makes 2 servings.
Per serving: 421 calories, 28 g protein, 29 g carbohydrates, 17 g fat (36% of calories)

Beat Fat for Good

Lose more fat in less time with this five-step metabolism-boosting plan

By Lou Schuler

Swear to God, this happened to me 3 years ago: I'm standing in front of a company urinal, taking a completely unmemorable whiz, when all of a sudden the button flies off my khakis and lands in the bowl. I leave work holding my pants closed, drive home, and put on another pair.

Up to this point, I'd ignored all the warning signs of my creeping corpulence. Sure, I'd gone up to 34-inch-waist pants after wearing 32s most of my adult life. But that had happened a couple of years before—ancient history by this time.

Then I started noticing the signs all day, every day. I saw an angry red ring

**ODDS THAT THE AVERAGE MAN
IS AT LEAST 30 POUNDS OVERWEIGHT:** 1 IN 5

around my waist when I undressed at night—a cry for help from the elastic in my Fruit of the Looms. I saw that the buckles on my belts no longer faced forward. They were starting to slope downward, pushed into submission by my expanding waistline.

The problem is easy to explain: My metabolism was slowing down. According to the Cooper Institute for Aerobics Research, the average person's metabolism slows 1 percent a year after age 30, as a result of lost muscle mass.

Metabolism is the speed at which your body burns calories. If you add muscle, no matter how old you are, your metabolism increases. But there's more to it than just adding muscle. What you eat and how you work out can also turn on your metabolic afterburners, taking inches off your waist almost as fast as you can put them on.

And I still haven't told you the best part of my story: I spend less time exercising now than I did 3 years ago, and the scale shows that I'm 10 pounds lighter.

Here's the fast and effective five-step plan that keeps the urinals of America safe from my buttons and can help keep your buttons dry, too.

STEP 1: HIT THE WEIGHTS

Aerobic exercise has many wonderful benefits: a longer life, a trimmer waist, a stronger heart, and fewer illnesses. But the way most of us do it—long, slow, and steady—doesn't increase 24-hour resting metabolism. In other words, you burn calories while you're exercising, but you don't get much fat-burning benefit when you're not.

To pump up your muscles as well as your resting metabolism, try the program on pages 124 to 125 for 4 weeks. A West Virginia University study showed that weight lifting can speed up your metabolism even while you're losing a lot of weight. In this study, weight lifters peeled off an average of 32 pounds but still saw their metabolisms increase 4 percent. The people in the study who were doing aerobics lost more weight—an average of 40 pounds—but that included 9 pounds of muscle. Consequently, their metabolisms slowed down an average of 14 percent.

What this means is that those with slower metabolisms will have more trouble keeping off the weight—a problem you avoid if you build muscle while dropping fat.

STEP 2: WHEN YOU DO AEROBICS, KEEP THEM SHORT AND FAST

There's a big difference between the slow, plodding aerobic exercise just impugned and harder, shorter sessions. Hard exercise signals your body to burn more calories of fat in the hours following your workout, according to research from the University of Virginia. The reason: The harder you go, the more growth hormone your body generates, and growth hormone is your number one fat fighter. The more you have during the day, the leaner you get.

A harder workout is also a shorter workout. You can't turn up the intensity without turning down the volume. Here are three ways to do that.

THE LAST FAT-BURNING WORKOUT YOU'LL EVER NEED

Workout A

Do three sets of 10 to 15 repetitions of each exercise in this lower-body workout. Rest a minute between sets. You can also do supersets: Do a set of squats followed by a set of deadlifts with no rest, rest 1 to 2 minutes, then repeat. When you've done three supersets, move on to the next pair of exercises.

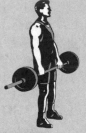

STIFF-LEGGED DEADLIFT

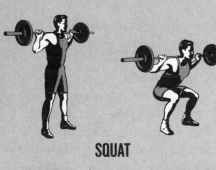

SQUAT

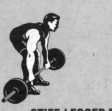
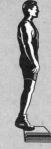
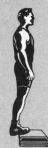

CALF RAISE

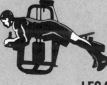

LEG CURL

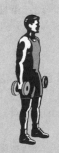
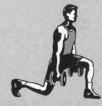

LUNGE

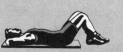

REVERSE CRUNCH
(or any abdominal exercise you choose)

I. Sprints

You can choose any aerobic exercise for this workout. Running is ideal, although you can also do sprints on a bike or in a swimming pool. Another option is to use a jump rope for your sprints, and jog in place in between.

Once you've picked your exercise, do this:

Workout B

Alternate this upper-body workout with Workout A, and do three or four workouts a week, total. Do three sets of 8 to 12 repetitions of each exercise in Workout B. You can also do supersets, as described in Workout A.

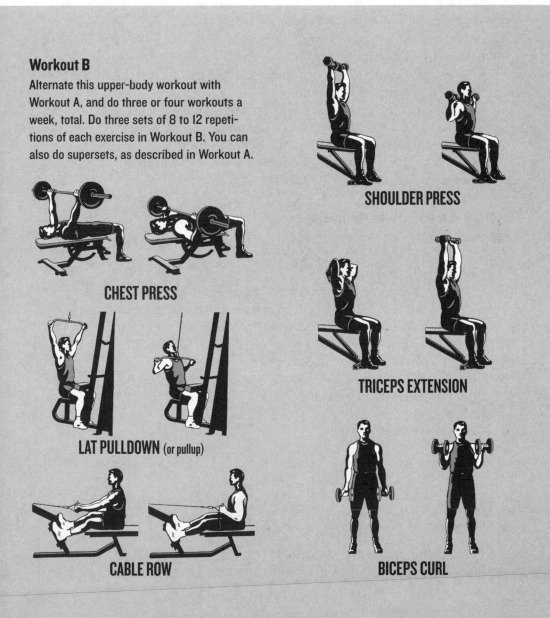

SHOULDER PRESS

CHEST PRESS

TRICEPS EXTENSION

LAT PULLDOWN (or pullup)

CABLE ROW

BICEPS CURL

- Warm up for 5 minutes (a brisk walk or light jog, if you're running).
- Go as hard as you can for 10 seconds.
- Go easy for 2 minutes (walk or jog, if you're running).
- Repeat for a total of 10 sprints and recovery periods.
- Cool down for 5 minutes by doing whatever you did to warm up. (The 2-minute recovery from your final sprint can count as part of the cooldown.)

2. Intervals
Choose any type of aerobic exercise you want, then . . .

- Warm up for 5 minutes.
- Go hard for 30 seconds—not all-out like the sprints but the best effort you can put out for 30 seconds.
- Go easy for 1 minute—just a brisk walk or light jog if you're running, or drop down a few levels if you're on a cardiovascular machine.
- Repeat for a total of 8 to 12 intervals and recovery periods.
- Cool down for 5 minutes (the 1-minute recovery from your final interval can count as part of the cooldown).

3. Hard, Steady-State Aerobics
Again, choose any exercise you want.

- Warm up for 5 minutes.
- Increase your pace until you're moving at 75 to 80 percent of your maximum heart rate. (Subtract your age from 220 to approximate your maximum.) If you don't have a heart-rate monitor and don't want to stop to check your pulse, just go at a pace that forces you to breathe deeply and rhythmically. You should be able to carry on short snatches of conversation but not deliver your entire conspiracy theory on how the president stole the Florida election.
- Maintain this pace for 20 minutes.
- Cool down for 5 minutes.

NUMBER OF POUNDS THE AVERAGE MAN GAINS IN A YEAR: 1.1

POUNDS A WEEK A TYPICAL MAN WILL LOSE BY EATING 300 TO 500 FEWER WEEKLY CALORIES: 1 TO 2

You should see great results from two or three of these workouts a week. You can mix and match them any way you choose. And you can use a different aerobic exercise each time you do any particular workout (for example, if you belong to a gym, you can do intervals on a stationary bike, treadmill, elliptical machine, or stairclimber).

STEP 3: SNEAK A SECOND WORKOUT INTO YOUR DAY

You can generate more growth-hormone release in a day with multiple exercise sessions, says *The Spark* coauthor Glenn Gaesser, Ph.D., an exercise scientist at the University of Virginia in Charlottesville. When Gaesser had a group of sedentary men and women exercise for 10 minutes two or three times a day, he found that they received all the health-and-fitness benefits normally seen in a conventional 3-month program—less body fat, improved cardiovascular and muscular fitness, greater flexibility, lower cholesterol. Except they achieved those benefits in 3 weeks.

Don't have time for a couple of trips to the gym per day? Don't worry. That's not the kind of second workout we're talking about. "The primary focus is to do exercises that don't necessarily build up a sweat. Three sessions that require showering afterward won't work," Gaesser says, since they're too time-consuming and energy-draining for men with busy lives. For beginning exercisers, 10-minute exercise sessions might include . . .

- A brisk walk at lunch or on your way to the train in the morning
- A quick weight routine with a pair of light dumbbells (You can keep them in your office and do this as a midafternoon break)
- A series of stretches when you wake up or before you go to bed

More advanced exercisers can try doing a short, intense aerobic session first thing in the morning before breakfast, then a weight-lifting session in the evening, after work. If that's impractical, you could simply do a hard workout whenever you normally would, with a session of your favorite stretches or abdominal exercises at another time of day. Keep it short—10 minutes is all you need.

STEP 4: FILL UP ON PROTEIN FIRST

A study in the *International Journal of Obesity* compared high-carbohydrate with high-protein diets for weight loss in extremely overweight men. Even though the calories were the same, the high-protein group lost 28 percent more weight in the 4-week study. More important, the metabolic rates of the men in the high-protein group were 14 percent faster than the others'.

Try eating 1 gram of protein per pound of body weight, suggests Thomas Incledon, Ph.D., C.S.C.S., president and director of sports nutrition at

Human Performance Specialists in Plantation, Florida. That's more than you need to build muscle, but the excess protein (order it up from "Protein Pluses," below) will help you burn fat.

Unfortunately, shopping for, preparing, and eating that much protein could turn into a part-time job. This explains the popularity of protein-based meal-replacement supplements. A single serving of Met-Rx, Myoplex, or Grow! contains between 37 and 42 grams of protein. All are sweetened with a sugar called maltodextrin, so you don't have to add anything but water and then mix them up in a shaker or blender. Two daily servings of any of the above gives you about 80 grams of protein.

Protein bars are another alternative, with one minor drawback: Many are made with chemicals called sugar alcohols, and too much of these can lead to serious flatulence. But you shouldn't experience this problem with one bar a day.

STEP 5: EAT THE RIGHT KIND OF CARBOHYDRATES

The best carbohydrates for your metabolism are those with a low glycemic index. The glycemic index measures how fast your body processes a food. Foods with a high index (such as white bread and highly processed breakfast

PROTEIN PLUSES

Here are some of the foods you can combine to hit your daily number of grams of protein.

Breakfast

I cup of fat-free milk (9 grams of protein)

2 whole eggs (13 grams of protein)

6 egg whites (21 grams of protein)

I cup of oatmeal (5 grams of protein)

2 slices of Canadian bacon (II grams of protein)

Lunch/Dinner

6-ounce can of tuna (41 grams of protein)

Arby's roast beef sandwich (22 grams of protein)

I cup of baked beans (12 grams of protein)

6-ounce chicken breast (53 grams of protein)

2 slices (6 ounces) of lean roast beef (49 grams of protein)

I cup of spaghetti (7 grams of protein)

Subway's 6-inch turkey sandwich on wheat (18 grams of protein)

Snacks

½ cup of cashews, or about 40 to 50 nuts (II grams of protein)

8-ounce container of low-fat yogurt (II grams of protein)

I ounce part-skim mozzarella cheese (7 grams of protein)

cereals) make you hungrier faster. In a study in *Pediatrics,* obese teenage boys ate 81 percent more after a high-glycemic meal than after one with a low glycemic index.

Unfortunately, there's nothing intuitive about the glycemic index. Many people consider pasta to be a fast-acting carbohydrate, but most pastas fall in the middle of the range. And a high-fiber cereal like Shredded Wheat is near the top.

In other words, if you want to use the glycemic index, you pretty much have to memorize it. Or use a cheat sheet like "Your Pocket Guide to the Glycemic Index" on pages 59 to 60.

The G.I. Joe Myth

Achieving a Perfect Body at Any Cost

By Donna Raskin

We have news for you: G.I. Joe may be harming today's generation of boys.

Don't believe it? Consider this. "G.I. Joe, who's been around for decades, is getting progressively more muscular," says *The Adonis Complex: The Secret Crisis of Male Body Obsession* coauthor Roberto Olivardia, Ph.D., clinical psychologist at McLean Hospital in Belmont, Massachusetts. If G.I. Joe Extreme, introduced in the mid-1990s, were a real man, he would have 27-inch biceps. Each biceps, in effect, would be nearly the size of his waist, not to mention that his arms would outsize those of most competitive bodybuilders. "His chest would also be 55 inches," says Olivardia. "But oddly," he adds, "his head would be tiny."

Okay, G.I. Joe is just a toy. But the body-over-brains world of men and eating disorders is very real. Experts estimate that men now constitute some 10 percent of those suffering from eating disorders of all kinds. That's between three million and five million men showing symptoms of bulimia, binge eating, anorexia, or exercise addiction. More precise numbers are hard to come by because it's an affliction that often goes unreported (and unrecognized, even by the afflicted themselves). "The most common thread among these guys is their secrecy," says Olivardia.

IT'S LIKE DRUG ADDICTION

"Most men with an eating disorder are bulimic," adds Olivardia. "They commonly throw up or use laxatives as part of their disease." Bulimia describes a cycle of bingeing and purging: You scarf down enormous amounts of food, then compensate for the indulgence by purging yourself of the calories in an effort to prevent weight gain. In contrast, anorexia, a disease in

DO YOU—OR DOES SOMEONE YOU KNOW— CROSS THE LINE?

If the phrase *eating disorders* conjures images of a young woman bent over a high school toilet, you might want to consider these others: The fat kid from your old gym class who's skinny today but only because he secretly purges after every meal; he still sees a fat kid when he looks in the mirror. Or how about the competitive runner who sits in the cube next to you? He eats only fat-free yogurt for lunch and goes ballistic any time the weather or a meeting forces him to miss an afternoon run.

For that matter, what about you? Do you work out for hours at a time even if you're hurt? Do you measure your biceps and lats after every workout? And even though the measuring tape says they're getting larger, do you still feel small?

If you or someone you know agrees with two or more of the following statements, seek help. To find a qualified professional, call the National Eating Disorders Association at (800) 931-2237.

1. People tell me I look good, but I don't agree and I don't believe them.

2. I used to enjoy sports and exercise, but now it feels like something I have to do no matter what.

3. I feel uneasy about food and eating, but I keep my feelings to myself because no one would understand.

4. I feel that the only part of my life I can control is my weight and how much I work out.

5. I can't go through a day without worrying about what I can or cannot eat.

6. I have had an out-of-control eating binge at least once during the past year.

7. I have done one of the following after a binge at least once during the past year: made myself vomit; used laxatives, enemas, colonics, or diuretics; fasted; exercised excessively.

8. If I got on the scale tomorrow and found out that I'd gained 2 pounds, I'd be very upset.

9. If I can't exercise to compensate for food I have eaten, I panic.

10. I don't believe I'll be able to find happiness until I'm in shape.

which sufferers starve themselves, is not as common among guys as the other eating disorders because it doesn't give them the physical results they're looking for. "They want the V-shape body," says Olivardia. Many men with eating disorders also have muscle dysmorphia, meaning that they see themselves as smaller than they actually are: Picture Lou Ferrigno looking in the mirror and seeing Woody Allen.

"We've also seen an increase in guys who use exercise as a form of purging," says Olivardia. "We describe them with the term *exercise bulimic*. So, they eat too much, then to get rid of the extra weight that might come on, they work out excessively." To understand these distinctions, see "Do You— Or Does Someone You Know—Cross the Line?"

Finally, there are those men who simply binge on food without purging. These are guys who eat enormous amounts of food for the psychological rush or feeling of comfort. As you might imagine, they're usually overweight. As you might *not* imagine, bulimic men also tend to be slightly overweight because their purging can't keep up with their bingeing.

Just as alcoholism isn't only about beer and drug addiction isn't simply about cocaine or heroin, eating disorders aren't solely about food. Typically, there are more deep-seated psychological roots to any addictive behavior. "Many psychological factors contribute to the development of eating disorders in men, including the pressure to succeed and to win at all costs, low self-esteem, poor body image, and strong feelings of inferiority or inadequacy," explains Olivardia.

THE DEALER IS YOU

Meet Dennis Henning, founder of the Freedom Institute in Santa Barbara, California, an organization that sponsors mind/body/spirit retreats—and a man who has suffered with eating disorders for 25 years. People with such disorders, says Henning, hear messages that "are special to them" and that act as triggers. He would know. Henning grew up being told he'd never amount to anything. He turned to food because it was "comforting—and it's easy to get." As he puts it, "No one knows there's a problem. It's not like there's a dealer coming to your house."

Ah, but the dealer is *you*. "At some point," says Olivardia, "bulimics and compulsive exercisers begin to feel like drug addicts. The habit isn't a choice [anymore]. Eating too much, throwing up, or exercising for hours actually makes the person feel good for a while—and maybe even euphoric." Emphasis on the "for a while."

Henning describes his first bulimic episode as "an amazing high. It just became that I wanted to eat so I could get that high. I could never control it. I was addicted to throwing up." Henning's diet eventually cost him hundreds of dollars a day and exacted a much higher price in friendships and lifestyle. Even once it was clear that he had a problem, asking for help was difficult, as it simply reinforced his negative feelings about himself: "I felt more shame and guilt. Pathetic. A loser."

In Olivardia's opinion, Henning typifies the syndrome. "Men are also usually at a worse stage once they do ask for help, because it takes them so long to seek someone out," says Olivardia—adding that by "worse," he means sui-

NUMBER OF POUNDS HEAVIER NONSMOKERS TEND TO BE COMPARED TO SMOKERS: 6 TO 10

PERCENTAGE OF MEN WHO WON'T STOP SMOKING, BECAUSE THEY'RE CONCERNED ABOUT WEIGHT GAIN: 16

cidal. "Their lives are consumed by food. They have no relationships. Their only relationship is with food and working out."

And too often, the downward spiral merely continues once they seek help. "They find themselves in a counseling group with all women, and that's not good," says Olivardia. "It's important for a man to know that he's not the only guy."

Henning agrees and adds, "There are so few counselors who understand men with eating disorders."

Not surprisingly, since as we've suggested, there are so many male sufferers who don't fully understand the problem. Help break that cycle. If you think you see some of the signs in close friends, pick a suitable guy-to-guy moment to ease into the subject. And don't neglect the most important guys in your life—your sons. Especially if they're into certain sports. Kids who participate in weight-restricted competition such as swimming, wrestling, bodybuilding, gymnastics, and running are at an increased risk of developing an eating disorder.

"We're going to see it more in the boys of today than ever before," says Olivardia. Especially if their squadron of toys includes unnaturally proportioned action figures like G.I. Joe.

KNOW THIS

Vanilla Rubs Out Chocolate

Sniffing a vanilla candle can fight a chocolate craving, according to scientists at St. George's Hospital in London. Among 160 volunteers, those given vanilla-scented skin patches lost an average of 4½ pounds, twice that of guys given dieting tips alone. "Vanilla may trigger the release of serotonin, making you less likely to crave sweets," says dietitian Catherine Collins, S.R.D. Collins says you can get the same benefit from sniffing any other natural vanilla scent.

Calcium Helps You Lose Weight

High-calcium foods help you shed fat quicker when mixed with a low calorie intake. A University of Tennessee study found that mice on a calcium-rich diet lost weight twice as fast as those on a low-calcium regime. Study author Michael B. Zemel, Ph.D., director of the university's Nutrition Institute in Knoxville, suggests four servings of low-fat dairy products daily.

Obesity: A Sickness?

Feeling pudgy? It might be a viral infection. According to a study published in the *International Journal of Obesity*, adenovirus-36 (Ad-36), a common virus that causes coldlike symptoms, could be one cause of obesity. Scientists at Wayne State University found that injecting animals with Ad-36 caused them to more than double their body fat.

In a separate study, 30 percent of obese subjects had been exposed to the virus—compared with just 5 percent of normal-weight people. "The

PERCENTAGE OF AMERICAN MEN
WHO ARE OVERWEIGHT (BODY-MASS INDEX 25 TO 29.9): **59.4**

PERCENTAGE OF AMERICAN MEN
WHO ARE OBESE (BODY-MASS INDEX OVER 30): **19.5**

number is high enough to suggest that Ad-36 is at least partially associated with obesity," says study leader Nikhil Dhurandhar, Ph.D.

More Good News about Fat

Fat might not be so bad after all. According to a University of Wisconsin study, a dietary fat called conjugated linoleic acid (CLA) may help increase your levels of lean muscle mass. Over a 6-month period, researchers gave CLA supplements or placebos to men and women starting an exercise program. Among those who gained weight, the CLA group gained almost twice as much lean muscle mass—45 percent compared with 26 percent. "CLA doesn't get rid of fat, but it can prevent new fat from attaching to your cells, and it may make results from exercise longer-lasting," says Michael Pariza, Ph.D. CLA is available as a supplement, but you probably already have some in your refrigerator. Beef and dairy products are both excellent sources of the stuff.

Ration Your Rations

Are the armies of chubbies you see nowadays evidence of mass inertia? Probably not. Researchers compared the body-mass indexes of more than 15,000 men and women in the armed forces over a 3-year period. The number classified as overweight rose significantly: from 50 to 54 percent.

The increase mirrors that among civilians, even though 67 percent of the military personnel engaged in vigorous physical activity 3 or more days a week, compared to 15 percent of civilians. The cause? Researchers say it could be food intake.

Don't chuck your lifting gloves just yet—the health benefits of exercise are well-established. Your best bet is to adjust your diet to your body. Use this formula as a guide.

1. Your weight in pounds: _____
2. Your basic calorie needs. Multiply line 1 by 11: _____ × 11 = _____
3. Your physical activity. Multiply line 2 by 20 percent if you currently get no exercise, by 30 percent for light exercise (2 hours a day on your feet), by 40 percent for moderate exercise every day, or by 50 percent for intense excrcise 3 or 4 days a week: _____ × _____ % = _____
4. Your daily calorie needs. Add line 2 and line 3: _____ + _____ = _____
5. Optional: If you want to lose weight, subtract 500 (so you can lose 1 pound a week). The result is your ideal daily calorie intake for weight loss: _____ − 500 = _____

DOWN THE PIKE

Anti-Fat Pill

A pill could soon be available to prevent you piling on the pounds. Professor Stephen Bloom from Hammersmith Hospital in London has discovered the area of the brain that controls calorie loss. He hopes to develop a drug that targets the area, in order to speed up metabolism.

Flip Your Fat Switch

Researchers have discovered a "fat switch" that determines whether cells turn into muscle or flab. Tests at the University of Michigan have revealed that the protein Wint-10b stops cells from turning into fat. It's hoped that anti-obesity drugs can be developed to control the protein.

DOES IT WORK?

Quick-Fix Diets

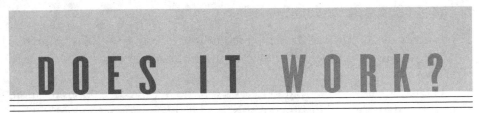 Putting yourself on starvation rations may send the scale nosediving by 6 pounds a week or even slightly more. But don't think it's all blubber that's been burned. It really is impossible to lose more than 2 pounds of fat per week. As for the rest, it's not just water: It's muscle and bone as well. Lose muscle, and your metabolic rate—the speed at which you burn calories—also plummets. For safe and sustained weight loss, cut your calorie intake by 500 a day and up your exercise to burn another 500. This way, you retain muscle and your metabolism while shedding over 7 pounds of fat per month.

COOL STUFF

Dieting in Cyberspace

Efit.com

We love going undercover, which is why we asked nutritionist Elizabeth Ward, R.D., to pretend she was a 5-foot-11, 225-pound man named Bob with high blood pressure and high cholesterol. Her mission (which she chose to accept): Find the best diet Web site to help Bob lose weight. The winner? Efit.com.

Efit.com charges more than some other sites, but it's well-worth its weight in benefits. Of all the sites, only this one offered Bob a truly personalized weight-loss plan: a 12-week low-fat, low-sodium program. Again Efit.com was unique—it was the only site to consider Bob's health issues and design the plan around them. And the program was realistic: 2,000 daily calories for a loss of 1 to 2 pounds per week. Efit.com costs less than sessions with a live dietician: $99 for 12 weeks of meal plans and professional advice from a cyberdietician.

Fast-Food Fat Finder

Eating Smart Restaurant Guide

If too many meals out have turned your gut into a flabby, uh, waist-land, this $5 tool from the Center for Science in the Public Interest may be easy to swallow.

The pamphlet-sized slide guide shows you the number of calories for more than 250 restaurant and fast-food meals. And it breaks down total fat, artery-clogging saturated fat, and trans fats (found in hydrogenated oils). You'll learn, for example, that an order of cheese fries packs more than 3,000 calories and 4 days' worth of artery-clogging fat. Now that's something to chew on.

Write: CSPI Restaurant Guide, 1875 Connecticut Ave. N.W., Suite 300, Washington, DC 20009-5728.

DIRECT AND INDIRECT U.S. HEALTH-CARE COSTS OF EXCESS WEIGHT AND OBESITY: $99.2 BILLION

AMOUNT AMERICANS SPEND ANNUALLY ON WEIGHT-LOSS PRODUCTS AND SERVICES: $33 BILLION

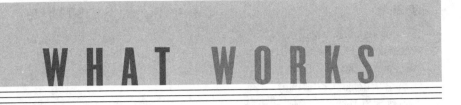

WHAT WORKS

Your abs versus your belly. If losing weight were no contest, we'd all be slim. Truth is, it's a battle. A battle of the belly, so to speak. As men, we know all about battles. We've fought and won them throughout history—on the frontier, in the trenches, at the office. Today we're at war with fat. And Americans are losing this fight in record numbers—more than half of us are overweight and some 20 percent of men are obese. So here's *your* battle plan: eating and exercise tactics that will make your belly fat surrender and clinch victory for your abs.

I. Combat restaurant sabotage. Restaurants are part of the global plot to make you fat. Secretly, unseen cooks in back rooms are thinking up ways of making sure that chubby men never disappear from the Earth. Foil their evil plot.

Order the steak—plain. Many chefs pour at least an ounce of butter (200 calories and 23 grams of fat) onto a steak—just so the meat will look juicier. Tell them to skip the glaze.

Make sure you can read the menu. One study found that people order more desserts when the foods are described with ethnic names.

Don't always order the salad dressing on the side. If you go to a restaurant that serves salads pretossed with the dressing, it's usually a much lighter coating than what most people end up dumping on, says Joey Abitabilo, a chef at the New England Culinary Institute in Montpelier, Vermont.

Toss the garnish. Those harmless-looking shredded carrots that dress up your beef are probably deep-fried; a half cup is 137 calories (four times the calories in raw carrots) and 12 grams of fat. Ask that they be grilled, or scrape them to the side.

2. Find hidden ways to lose weight. Maybe you hate running. If you need to justify that cheeseburger, figure out how many calories you can burn by doing other not-so-fun stuff. If it makes you feel better.

PERCENTAGE OF MEN TRYING TO LOSE WEIGHT USING DIET PILLS: 2

PERCENTAGE OF PEOPLE WITH EATING DISORDERS WHO ARE MEN: 10

Activity	Calories Burned by a 180-Lb Man
Making your bed (5 min)	13
Washing your hands (5 min)	16
Washing the dishes (10 min)	30
Calling your mother (30 min)	61
Foreplay (30 min)	61
Slow dancing (20 min)	81
Sitting in a meeting (1 hr)	122
Watching the kids (1 hr)	327
Cleaning the gutters (1 hr)	409

3. Be a double loser. Here's something to put smiles on the faces of the L.A. Clippers: Being bad at sports actually burns more calories than being good. Until you actually become good at something, your body has to work harder to stay in the game, especially in the following sports.

Sport	Calories a Good 180-Lb Player Burns	Calories a Bad 180-Lb Player Burns
Basketball (1 hr)	368, for a player who makes most of his shots	491, for a player who misses a shot, then runs in for his own rebound
Bowling	123, for a player who bowls 12 strikes a game for three games	245, for a player who bowls no strikes
Golf	1,473, shooting a 72 on an 18-hole course	2,227, shooting a 110
Running	785, finishing a 10-K race in 36 min	818, finishing in 1 hr
Tennis (1 match)	655, for a player who rarely hits the ball out of play	798, for a player who has to chase after stray balls

4. Prolong that full feeling. Here's the typical weight-loss formula: Eat less. It works for a while—2.4 days, to be exact—and then you're back on all fours, shoving Big Macs down your throat like a supermodel on her birthday. The key to weight loss isn't depriving yourself all the time; it's eating the foods that'll keep you full. Start here.

Add fat. Just make sure it's the monounsaturated type; it may help keep you from overdoing it at the taco bar later. Penn State University researchers recently found that men who ate mashed potatoes prepared with oil high in monounsaturated fat (such as olive oil) felt fuller longer than when they ate potatoes made with oils rich in polyunsaturates (such as vegetable oil). Use olive oil as salad dressing, or have a peanut-butter sandwich at lunch.

Add snacks. But they should be foods with a low glycemic index, meaning they won't cause your insulin levels to spike and your hunger to follow. Try low-fat chocolate milk, peanuts, or low-fat yogurt. For more low-glycemic snacks, see "Your Pocket Guide to the Glycemic Index" on pages 59 to 60.

Add carbohydrates. If you eat a lunch that's rich in carbohydrates, your body will release serotonin, a feel-good chemical. But in a couple of hours, those levels will drop—and you'll be more likely to binge. Try light popcorn to keep your serotonin levels even.

5. Ask for the wine list. In a study of more than 12,000 people, those who drank an average of six glasses of wine a week were significantly thinner than those who drank the same amount of beer. Beer has a lot of calories and may affect certain hormones that cause you to store more belly fat. For a good inexpensive wine, try Gossamer Merlot ($6). We're on our fourth bottle right now.

6. Lose your gut in intervals. One of the fastest ways to deflate your gut: interval running. Run for 300 feet (about one block) at half of your top speed, then rest 1 minute. Repeat this five times, going a little faster each time so you're in an all-out sprint for the last block (watch the applecart). Do this three times a week and you'll fit through turnstiles within a month.

7. Multitask your workout. Hunt for ways to make common exercises burn more fat; for example, swinging your arms on a stairclimber (instead of holding the railings) can burn an additional 300 calories in 30 minutes.

8. If you want to lose, lose the OJ. Despite its many health benefits, at roughly 115 calories from carbohydrates per 8-ounce serving, orange juice causes a quick sugar spike followed by a dip that makes you crave even more. Try eating your fruit instead; you'll get fewer calories, plus fiber to help you feel full.

9. Switch spreads. Margarine not only is high in heart attack–inducing trans fats but also contains 100 calories per tablespoon. A better spread is apple butter (37 calories and 0 grams of fat).

10. Ice your tea. Call it Miracle-Gro for your gut. If you can't stand unsweetened brew, just add extra ice to your regular tea; your body will burn about half the calories in a teaspoon of sugar as it warms the tea to 98.6°F.

11. Find your stuffed factor. Tighten your abs at the table after a meal, says weight-loss expert Mark Liponis, M.D. If this makes you feel queasy, you've

PERCENTAGE OF ADDITIONAL
CALORIES MEN BURN BECAUSE
THEY HAVE MORE MUSCLES THAN WOMEN: **10 TO 20**

PERCENT FEWER FOOD
CRAVINGS MEN EXPERIENCE: **15**

had too much. The added pressure your abdominal muscles put on your stomach clues you in on overeating long before indigestion does.

12. Eat as the Romans do. Eat supper with a family in Italy and you'll down six courses, each on a separate plate. So how do they stay so skinny? By eating one food at a time, they become satisfied with the food's flavor a little more quickly and eat less, says Sheah Rarback, R.D., of the University of Miami. Americans mix foods and tastes on one plate, so it takes longer—and more food—to feel satisfied.

13. Pinch away food cravings. In Oriental medicine, the little bud of cartilage directly above your ear canal (called the tragus) is the acupuncture spot that controls hunger. "Lightly pinching that area for 1 minute should cause food cravings to subside," says Joseph Carter, a spokesman for the Acupressure Institute of America.

14. Eat beans, lose weight. From black beans to kidney beans, all legumes are top sources of soluble fiber and lean protein—two things that satisfy your hunger, help burn fat, and stabilize your blood-sugar levels. Insert your own bean/fart joke here.

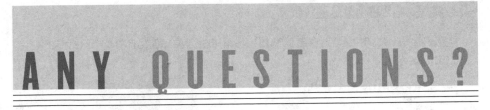

Have a Late Dinner

I often wind up eating dinner close to 10:00 P.M. My girlfriend says this habit will make me fat. Do I have to believe her?

—J. A., Houston

No. On the face of it, the idea that your body is less active at night and therefore unable to burn off the calories you shovel into it in the evening seems to make sense. But scientific research has shown that when you eat has no bearing on your weight. It's not when you eat that counts but what you eat—and how much of it—over a period of time.

Your body doesn't stop burning calories just because you go to sleep. In fact, if late-night eating suits your lifestyle, the best advice is simply to go with it. It probably means you'll be more likely to stick to your overall eating plan. Just try not to get crumbs in the bed.

Midnight Snack Attack

I stay up late and am always famished around midnight. Can you suggest something that'll satisfy my hunger and not turn to flab overnight?

—J. D., Tulsa, Okla.

A bowl of Wheaties. The best midnight snacks are high in carbohydrates and low in fat and protein, says Leslie Bonci, R.D., a spokeswoman for the American Dietetic Association. Meat and dairy products sit in your digestive tract for hours, while a bowl of cereal, a small bagel, or a whole grain English muffin will digest quickly. They may even help you fall asleep.

And stay off the late-night peanut butter. Protein foods are high in tyrosine, an amino acid that helps stimulate the production of dopamine, which in turn increases mental arousal and could keep you awake.

NUMBER OF ADULT DEATHS IN THE UNITED STATES ATTRIBUTED TO OBESITY EACH YEAR: 280,000

Chocolate Excuses

I can't break my chocolate habit. Is it any worse for me than other snacks?

—S. F., Springtown, Pa.

Don't believe all of chocolate's bad press. Okay, it is relatively high in sugar and fat, but it's by no means the worst snack you can scoff. Per helping, it supplies fewer calories than peanuts or French fries, coming in at 264 calories per 50 gram serving. The same weight of peanuts crams in 300 calories, and a small portion of fries has 280 calories.

Like any food, it will only guarantee your membership in the big-gut club if you eat too much of it. Go steady, and it can make up part of a balanced diet. More good news for chocoholics is that it doesn't cause acne, as you may have been told. And the tannins in cocoa can actually prevent tooth decay.

How Much Is Too Much?

What's the most weight I can safely lose in a month?

—C. J., Birmingham, Ala.

No more than 2 pounds a week, according to James O. Hill, Ph.D., director of the center for human nutrition at the University of Colorado in Denver. The biggest drawback of rapid weight loss? You're far more likely to regain the weight. People who drop pounds like Phish fans drop acid typically rely on extreme exercise programs or very low calorie diets, which are tough to maintain for more than a few weeks. Rapid weight loss also involves losing a lot of fluid, which can be dangerous, especially if you're engaged in serious exercise.

PART FIVE
PROTECT YOUR HEALTH

MUST READS

No Flu for You!

Seven easy steps to surviving the cold-and-flu season

By Rebecca Kleinwaks

The cold-and-flu bugs are swarming: This year, there will be 1 billion colds and 95 million cases of the flu in the United States alone. But while a billion colds is a statistic, 2 colds—the likely number you'll catch this winter—is a tragedy. Getting sick just twice can put you weeks behind at work and in the gym. It's also a leading cause of being quarantined in the spare room.

Sorry, science doesn't have a cure yet. But doctors have figured out how these viruses conspire to make you feel lousy. Thwart the bugs' insidious game plan and you'll not only get sick less often but also bounce back faster if you do catch something. So have a look at the sad, sniveling life of a common virus, then take the necessary steps to squash it like the bug that it is.

1. CONTACT

If your partner starts sneezing, the fellow in the next cubicle begins hacking like a coal miner, or the kids run a fever, heighten your alert. They might be packing a cold or flu virus, one of a horde of strains that plague people all winter. Those bugs want you next, but there are only three ways to get in: your nose, mouth, and eyes.

Your best defense: Keep your hands clean. Viruses are often passed from an infected person to a phone receiver or some other surface that other people then touch with their hands. In the case of the flu, they fly through the air and stick to things! To keep a virus from latching on to you, wash your paws every time you shake hands or wipe your kid's nose. Quick-drying antibacterial gel lets you clean up without leaving your office.

2. INVASION

Too bad you didn't duck when your kid coughed—or wash up before licking your fingers during that fried-chicken lunch. Within minutes, the virus you picked up or inhaled has settled into its spacious new home: you. Don't worry; it's not too late to ward off trouble.

Your best defense: First, get a flu shot. Second, from September through March—prime cold-and-flu season—drink even more water than usual. The mucous membranes that line the upper respiratory tract, one of your body's first defenses, work best when thoroughly moist, says Mary Hardy, M.D., director of integrative medicine at Cedars-Sinai Medical Center in Los Angeles. Eight 8-ounce glasses of water every day is the minimum; drink more and you're ahead of the game.

3. INCUBATION

Soon after entering, the virus has worked its way from your mouth or nose through the mucous membranes to your body's cells. The bug fools the special receptors that act as doorways, then walks on in and makes itself comfortable—and you miserable.

Your best defense: Start every day this cold season with a walk around the block. Contrary to what your mother told you, brief exposure to cold—after a good warmup—stimulates the immune system. Exercise can also help you feel better, as long as you don't overdo it. Although a study reports that working out neither lengthens nor shortens recovery time, the feel-good hormones you produce, called endorphins, will boost your mood.

4. INFECTION

After attacking a cell, the virus injects its genetic material inside and copies itself. This process takes about 12 hours, and you won't actually feel sick until two or three of these cycles are complete.

Your best defense: Within 24 to 48 hours of a flu strike, ask your doctor for amantadine—it'll cut the duration of your misery. Acetaminophen (Tylenol) will help aches and fever. As soon as you notice cold symptoms— runny nose, scratchy throat, fatigue—take a decongestant. But only one dose. The active ingredient, usually a pseudoephedrine combination, will open up the nasal passages and help your body flush away the invaders. Australian researchers found that taking a decongestant just once cut symptoms by 13 percent.

5. ILLNESS

All the copies the virus made now break out of the host cell and look for other cells to infect. This period, which lasts 3 to 5 days, is when you feel worst. Your nose starts running to wash away a cold virus, and you sneeze— another way the body tries to expel the infection. Your body tries to burn out the flu virus; that's why you have fever, chills, and fatigue.

Your best defense: If you feel really horrible, take a day off to rest. If you're still functional, just take it easy, cutting your usual workout in half and skipping after-work drinks. (Alcohol will make you feel worse.) Also: Wipe, don't blow. Blowing your nose can clog your sinuses with germ-laden mucus. You'll feel better faster if you let your body flush out the virus naturally.

6. GET BETTER—OR WORSE

All those symptoms that make you feel lousy—sore throat, headache, congestion—should be gone within a week, the average time it takes for the body's infection-fighting forces to eradicate a mild virus. But if you haven't been following our feel-good advice, an infection can move deeper into your upper respiratory tract to infiltrate your lungs and drag on for another week or more. If this happens, you'll be coughing—another attempt by your body to rid itself of the nasty virus.

Your best defense: See your doctor. He may prescribe medication that can help keep you from developing a secondary infection, such as bronchitis or pneumonia.

7. GET OUT AND STAY OUT

Since the initial contact, a whole army of cells within your body has been working to suppress and destroy the virus—one of countless viruses you could be exposed to this winter. Your body's cells then work feverishly to clean up the mess that's left behind. The only things that remain once the infection has been cleared out are memory cells. These will help protect you from that same virus for the rest of your life, making it much less likely you'll suffer from that strain again. Your collection of memory cells is the reason you now get fewer colds than you did as a kid.

Your best defense: Go back to your usual activities, as long as you feel better and your symptoms are under control.

The Ultimate Health Test

A revolutionary new $895 procedure allows you to see everything inside your body. Are you brave enough to peek?

By Joe Kita

I am staring at my potential killer. Given the chance, it could swiftly choke off my life. It's hiding deep within my circumflex artery, the blood vessel between my heart's left atrium and its right ventricle. It's a bright white speck of calcified plaque, cold and emotionless.

"This could kill me?" I ask, pointing it out on the computer screen.

ODDS THAT THE AVERAGE MAN WILL DEVELOP HEART DISEASE BEFORE AGE 60: 1 IN 3

ODDS THAT THE AVERAGE MAN WILL HAVE A HEART ATTACK: 1 IN 21

"This little dot right here could kill you, yes," says Harvey Eisenberg, M.D. I watch as he taps at his keyboard and electronically pulls the plaque out of the vessel, enlarges it, enhances it three-dimensionally, then measures its volume and density. The tiny deposit, which had been no bigger than a pinhead, is now looming in the middle of the computer screen, rotating under the doctor's inspection.

"Your job," he deadpans, "is to get rid of that."

FLASH BACK ONE HOUR

The waiting room at the HealthView Center for Preventive Medicine in Newport Beach, California, is serene. I sit facing a Japanese wall fountain, water trickling down across bromeliads. At its base is a pool, the bottom of which is spotted with pennies. Like the patients before me, I pitch in one for good luck.

I am about to undergo a new and potentially revolutionary procedure. For 15 minutes, a modified electron-beam computed-tomography scanner (EBCT) will take hundreds of picture-slices of my body, working methodically from neck to hips, just like a CAT scan. Special software will then transform this data into three-dimensional images of my heart, lungs, spine, stomach, prostate, colon, and every other internal organ. The result: a virtual tour of my insides projected on a computer screen.

I'm scared. I'm 40 years old, and although I'm lean and physically fit, my total cholesterol is a stubborn 230, and my father died at age 62 of a heart attack. I worry I may have only a couple of decades left.

And shortly, I will know for sure.

SO EASY IT'S SCARY

When it's time for my exam, a white-coated technician named Nancy shakes my hand. There is no nurse to take my blood pressure, check my weight, or press a cold stethoscope to my chest. No one even asks to examine the results of my last blood test. At HealthView, such things are obsolete.

Nancy ushers me into a beige, sterile-looking room and asks me to remove my belt and empty my pockets. There's no embarrassing open-backed gown to don. All my clothes stay on. The only prep work required is not eating or drinking for 6 hours prior, having three electrodes taped to my chest, and swallowing a cup of supercarbonated fluid to inflate my stomach.

Then I lie back on the scanner's tabletop surface and extend both arms above my head. Since small amounts of radiation will be emitted as the machine takes its snapshots, Nancy goes into another room and communicates via intercom. The tabletop slides slowly backward through a large ring. Unlike with some CAT scans or MRIs, there's no claustrophobic feeling. It's an open unit, with a perfect forest scene on the ceiling for me to gaze at. I feel as if I were looking up at heaven, which is not at all reassuring.

"Take a deep breath," says Nancy. "Blow it out. Now inhale again and hold."

The EBCT scanner screens my torso in three parts. I hold my breath for approximately 30 seconds during each. Then it takes two more, slightly longer scans, this time stuttering its way back up my body. And that's it. I sit up and put my belt back on, and then Nancy escorts me to the doctor's office for the typical hour-long consultation.

Dr. Eisenberg is the brain of this operation and, fittingly, his office looks like an air-traffic control center, only without the view. Computers clutter a wing-shaped desk, and behind them sits a wallful of video screens. The doctor himself is 60 years old but looks 10 years younger. That's a good sign.

A specialist in radiology, Dr. Eisenberg has been doing these physical exams/scans for 14 years. He's one of the largest providers, projecting 11,000 patients this year, or 30 to 40 per day. Tens of thousands of people have undergone the procedure, and many are alive today because it discovered a hidden problem. And it discovers something in everyone.

"I joke that I have a box of gold stars, and I'll put one on the forehead of the first person who gets through this without my finding something significant," he says. "I've yet to open the box."

Dr. Eisenberg insists, however, that this is as much a preventive procedure as it is a diagnostic one. Any symptomless abnormalities that are uncovered are likely to be in the formative stages, when they can be easily managed and eliminated. In fact, he claims that someone of my age who is scanned annually and follows recommendations could live into his 90s or 100s. That's 20 to 30 years longer than the average man's life span.

"The way medicine is practiced today is flat-out wrong," says Dr. Eisenberg. "Doctors are trained to wait for people to develop symptoms, and then react. Yet what person would conduct his business by sitting and waiting for catastrophes to happen? That's called crisis management, and everybody knows it doesn't work.

"Your body is not this wonderful machine with bells that go off the minute something is wrong. With major killers like heart attacks and strokes, in most people the first symptom of disease is the heart attack or the stroke, and more than a third of them die of it."

WHAT YOU DON'T KNOW CAN KILL YOU

Dr. Eisenberg recently scanned more than 350 physicians, and he says not a single one didn't become excited about the process. Those in the medical world who remain skeptical argue that too much knowledge can be dangerous, especially for younger patients like myself. For example, a small growth uncovered in the lung could remain small and asymptomatic for life, or even disappear on its own. Yet once you're aware of its existence, you'll risk life-threatening surgery in order to remove it.

That argument agitates the normally subdued Dr. Eisenberg. "You tell me what disease you don't want to know about," he says. "The answer to cancer isn't in the billions we spend on exotic surgeries. The answer to cancer is finding it very early, when you can effectively deal with it in any number of ways. Let me show you something."

And with that, he begins tapping at his keyboard, summoning to his computer screen a succession of virtual body parts. Each is an actual internal image, startling in its clarity, from a severely diseased patient who was supposedly perfectly healthy.

"This is a 53-year-old male who looks like Mr. America, in absolute top physical condition," he explains. "He had just come from Harvard's main teaching hospital, where he had a stress EKG, and a cardiologist gave him a clean bill of health. Yet look at all this plaque in his arteries. This is the kind of guy who just keels over, and everybody is amazed because he was so healthy."

"Now," says Dr. Eisenberg, shifting in his chair. "Let's take a look at you. . . ."

He begins with a survey of my body, a quick once-over to see if there are any obvious problems. It's difficult to accept that this image on the screen is me. I have become the frog in biology class. Dissected.

A window has been opened in my chest, and we peer into that. One of the doctor's first observations is that I have very little internal body fat (11 percent, to be exact). That's good for overall health, but it makes his job a bit more difficult. Fat appears as darkish areas on the scan, surrounding the organs and helping define them. "But it's still a good visualization," he assures me.

The doctor flips through the scanned images like pages in a book. Then he asks if I have any particular health concerns, and I mention my family history of heart disease. "We look at our parents and figure we're going down the same path," he says, "but that simply isn't true. No matter what we find, it can be readily dealt with, even if there's a bad genetic drive. So let's examine your cardiovascular system."

Dr. Eisenberg navigates the blood vessels of my body, steering through them like a veteran river guide. As he does so, he points out areas of interest while warning me of upcoming trouble spots. "At the undersurface of the aortic arch is an area of high turbulence, where the blood swirls around a corner; it's typically where we first see plaque formation." But I don't have any there, thank God.

He inspects my heart more closely, examining it now in 1 millimeter slices. And there, right at the origin of the circumflex artery, is a small white

PERCENTAGE OF CARDIOLOGISTS SURVEYED WHO TAKE DAILY VITAMIN-E SUPPLEMENTS: 39

PERCENTAGE OF CARDIOLOGISTS SURVEYED WHO TAKE ASPIRIN EVERY DAY: 42

dot. It's instantly visible against its black-and-gray backdrop. The white is calcified plaque, an actual bit of formative bone. It represents an artery that has begun to harden.

"Plaque is made up of fat, collagen, muscle fiber, and bone," explains Dr. Eisenberg. "Once the calcium gets into the plaque, it anchors it. And the anchoring, together with the mechanical stress of blood flowing against it, can cause a fissure. Blood then clots around this crack, rises up to plug the artery, and causes a heart attack."

At one time, it was thought that only large plaques have this effect. "But two-thirds of the time, the plaque causing a heart attack is less than a 50-percent blockage," he says. "So the real risk predictor is not how big your plaques are, but how many plaques you have. The more surface area they cover, the higher the probability that one will rupture."

Dr. Eisenberg scores each of his patients based on how much plaque he finds. I have two lesions: the one near my heart and another of similar size in an artery feeding my pelvis. (Thankfully, there is none in the vessels leading to my penis, which would signal impending impotence.) Their combined volume is 3.2 millimeters, giving me a score of 1.1 on a scale of 1,000. But before I can rejoice, he looks me squarely in the eye and says I am now carrying a disease that I have to take seriously.

At first, I find this difficult to accept. I mean, my score was pretty damn close to perfect. But the doctor explains that disease isn't something you measure by degrees. You either have it or you don't. What's present in me is the beginning of a deadly process. In fact, my score is exactly average for a 40-year-old guy. And while my risk of heart attack is low, Dr. Eisenberg stresses that I want to have a score of zero. "That's normal," he says.

RISK MANAGEMENT

The most striking part of this analysis for me is how crude and undependable it makes cholesterol testing seem. "Standard cholesterol testing has only a 7 percent to 10 percent predictor value," says Dr. Eisenberg. "It's not very good. Two-thirds of people with high cholesterol don't develop heart disease, and most heart attacks occur in people with normal-range cholesterol."

The second eye-opener is that despite all the time I spend exercising (10 hours per week), it doesn't completely protect me. I've entered the risk game at age 40, just like every other male. I have developed a disease. "That's the great male misconception," says Dr. Eisenberg. "Physical fitness does not completely protect you from this disease. While there's no question that going from sedentary to some reasonable level of activity changes your cardiovascular risk, it just takes you part of the way. Proper nutrition and stress control play even bigger roles. I've seen a lot of athletes in here, guys at the peak of fitness, who are loaded with plaque."

Now that mine has been quantified, my job is to either thwart its growth or eradicate it. Dr. Eisenberg suggests a multipronged attack: (1) Eat a low-fat, whole-food diet rich in antioxidants; (2) keep my immune system strong by managing stress more effectively; (3) take a baby aspirin every other day to thin my blood so additional platelets won't aggregate around my lesions; (4) have my blood examined by a lipidologist to determine exactly how my body metabolizes fat and whether I should consider taking medication; and (5) continue to exercise, but use it as a stress reducer rather than as disease armor.

"Untreated, plaques like yours grow at a rate of 20 percent to 250 percent per year," says Dr. Eisenberg. "But treated, they grow minimally or not at all, or even disappear. Now, let's take a look at your lungs."

I have never smoked a cigarette, and I am suddenly thankful for that. Dr. Eisenberg is scrolling through my lung field, one of the most complex structures in the body. The job is tedious, simply because there is so much lung structure. If you were to spread out the organs' entire anatomy, it would cover a tennis court. But what really makes this process painstaking, at least for me, is that he's searching for cancer. Yes, cancer inside me. "I'm looking for a little blip," he explains. "I can see it right down to a half-millimeter in size. On a chest x-ray, a tumor might have to be the size of my fist to produce a bulge in the border of the heart big enough to notice. So we're talking up to a 3,000-percent increase in sensitivity to lung cancer with this technology. The chest x-ray fundamentally belongs in the Smithsonian."

I can't help but hold my breath as he performs this virtual bronchoscopy. He inspects the individual branches of my airway tree, cuts them open, and even examines the surrounding air fields at the cellular level. This last component resembles a fresh, moist sponge. He terms it "beautiful," but to give me some perspective, he calls up the same section from a patient of similar age who smokes. The sponge is in black tatters.

"That's the result of inhaling 4,000 substances, including cyanide and carbon monoxide," he explains. "Secondary smoke can do that, too. If you want to help somebody stop smoking, this is how you do it. You show them their lungs. Well, you're doing pretty well so far. Want to move on?

"Now we're in the abdomen," says Dr. Eisenberg, continuing his play-by-play. "This is your liver, and this sac hanging off the bottom is the gallbladder. That looks okay, as does your spleen. These V-shaped structures are your adrenal glands. I can tell by their size and appearance that they're functioning normally. Now here is the pancreas, which is a deadly organ, . . ." he pauses to inspect it, as I pray silently, ". . . but I see no signs of tumors.

"In this area, I'm also searching for abdominal aneurysms," he goes on. "About 15 percent of men over 50 get them, and they can be lethal. None here, though. Now I'm looking at your prostate gland, which is a little enlarged. It's in the upper limits of normal, but it bears watching. I don't need to put my finger in your rectum to feel that. I can see it. You should start getting an annual PSA test.

"Moving on to the colon, you can see how difficult it becomes to trace the intestine through this area. That's because there's a lot of residue in your bowel—feces." He looks at me accusingly, but I swear I don't have to go. "If we had given you a cleansing prep, I'd be able to do a virtual colonoscopy."

Next, Dr. Eisenberg summons my stomach to the screen. Fortunately, it's emptier than other parts of me, and he is able to slice it in half and search for ulcers, cancer, and polyps. He finds nothing worrisome.

Finally, he zeroes in on my kidneys. They look good, except that toward the bottom of the left one, there's a white spot, similar to the plaque I saw near my heart. "That's a kidney stone," he says. "It's still small enough [less than a millimeter in diameter] that it should pass. But you'll need to drink a lot of fluid. If it grows larger and gets stuck, you'll think you've been kicked by a mule."

Without thinking, I reach for my cup of water on the desk, and swallow hard.

We're inside my spine now, the last leg of what's been a truly fantastic voyage. And the detail here is perhaps the most unbelievable. After examining my spinal column from the outside and pronouncing it "healthy," Dr. Eisenberg splits it and looks inside. He can not only measure the size of the spinal canal but also visually check for osteoporosis, a disease he says he finds just as often in men as in women.

"You're lucky," he says. "You were born with a really good spinal canal. These holes are gigantic, and there's nothing compromising the nerves. Your bones are solid blocks. There's no hollowing out. This is a healthy spine, and I don't see many of those."

But when he moves to a higher resolution and begins inspecting each vertebra, he detects some early signs of degeneration. Specifically, he notices a slight bulging in my bottom two disks.

"Despite the fact that your joints are normal, the ligaments around the joints are thickened," he explains. "This little bulging in here isn't normal. It's quite minor, and most people would say that's fine, but it isn't. The time to deal with it is right now."

Dr. Eisenberg guesses that I'm a runner, and he's right: usually 20 miles a week on pavement, for the past 6 years. That pounding is what's causing the compression. To alleviate it, he suggests I switch to power walking or trail running, or have my stride analyzed by an exercise physiologist.

"So that's it," he says, turning away from the computer. "We'll give you follow-up materials and send referrals. But before you leave, you need to understand one thing: The most important physician you'll ever have in your life is you. The actions you take on a daily basis will mean far more to how long or how well you live than anything any physician can ever do. Hopefully, this visual imagery will motivate you. What I've done is put you in charge of your disease."

4 WEEKS LATER

My desk is littered with empty water bottles, and every time I pee, I pay way too much attention to my stream. Any twinge in my chest reminds me of that piece of plaque, and my lower back has seemed a bit crankier lately, even though I've stopped running on hard surfaces. I fear that such intimate knowledge may turn me into a hypochondriac, a life not of ignorant bliss but in the constant shadow of death. It's going to be a long year before I go back, get rescanned, and see if I've made any progress.

Dr. Eisenberg isn't concerned. "It's important for you to be aware of your disease on a daily basis," he says, "because that's when you make decisions about diet, exercise, and stress control that ultimately affect it. I used to tell patients they needed to do X, or else Y would happen, but they rarely did it. With this technology, I supply a different kind of motivation. Yes, it can be disturbing, but that's what makes it effective."

And he's right. I just have to learn to keep it in better perspective. One unquestionable benefit, though, is the deep satisfaction that comes from knowing I won't be dying of natural causes anytime soon. I was right to buy extended warranties on all those appliances.

This experience has also colored my opinion of every facet of disease detection. Cholesterol screening, digital prostate exams, stress tests—they all suddenly remind me of a carpenter knocking on a wall to find a stud. But that's about to end. Next year, Dr. Eisenberg will unveil his latest technology, one beyond even the capabilities of this one, and he plans to license it everywhere. Soon, we won't be guessing anymore. You'll know, just as I do, what's going on inside you.

For more information about this procedure, call HealthView at (888) 724-8439. With a doctor's referral, your visit may even be covered by health insurance. It's recommended that men and women have a baseline scan at age 35. There is currently a 10-month waiting list.

How to Not Die

Fear the Reaper? We'd rather kick his black-robed butt. Here's how to beat Mr. Death at his own creepy little game

By Duane Swierczynski

Boil down the *Men's Health* philosophy to a few words and it's this: We don't want you to die.

And, as long as you're alive, we also want to you look good, have tons of sex, and be able to play folk songs using only your abs and a guitar pick.

That's why we've put together this encyclopedia of the misadventures that kill the men who didn't buy this book, along with the best ways to prevent every one of those mishaps. So if you want to live forever, here's a list of the things you have to avoid.

ANIMAL ATTACK
Deaths per Year: 107
Animals don't care who they kill. They're animals. They'll eat a cattle rancher and follow up with a PETA volunteer. It's all meat to them.

How to avoid dying: Dog (or wolf) coming after you? Don't run—you'll look like a steak with legs, says Luanne Freer, M.D., of Yellowstone Park Medical Services. Appear as threatening as possible; wave your arms to look bigger than you really are. Or call a lawyer. If the wolf starts to pounce, punch him square in the nose.

If a big cat is the problem, don't look him in the eye. Instead, do the threatening dance described above. But if that doesn't work, wrap your arms around your head and neck to protect the veins and arteries—this is where he'll bite first. Then kick the mother-loving crap out of him.

Bear? You can't outrun him, so drop into a ball and play dead. Or shoot pepper spray directly into his eyes—he'll run like Anna Nicole Smith from a prenup. Don't have pepper spray? Crouch down and make yourself as small a snack as possible.

BLACK DEATH
Deaths per Year: 2
According to the Centers for Disease Control and Prevention, there are still 10 to 15 cases of the plague reported each year in the United States alone (the hot spots: New Mexico, Colorado, California, Oregon, Nevada, and Arizona). In the Middle Ages, this was Death's greatest hit.

How to avoid dying: Rodent-borne fleas are the culprits, so if you live in the western part of the country and regularly play with roadkill, wear gloves and insect repellent.

CAR ACCIDENT
Deaths Per Year: 41,000
If the media treated the AAA like the NRA, you'd hear this little mantra more and more: Cars don't kill people. People with cars kill people.

How to avoid dying: You can cut your risk by wearing a seat belt (lowers your risk by 45 percent) and having an airbag (in conjunction with a seat belt, reduces your risk by 56 percent). Stay home on Saturday, when 18 percent of all deadly collisions happen—especially in Mississippi, Montana, and South Carolina, which have the highest rates of traffic deaths per vehicle mile. Tuesday is the safest day, hosting only 12 percent of fatal crashes.

One more thing: Let those people go. Eleven percent of fatal accidents occur when someone is too stubborn to yield.

CEREBRAL HEMORRHAGE
Deaths per Year: 26,230

Cerebral hemorrhages are often caused by aneurysms, weak vessels in your brain (the result of a birth defect, high blood pressure, or a head trauma).

How to avoid dying: If the problem is a birth defect or blood pressure, you need to avoid two head-splitting vices: smoking, which triples your risk of a rupture; and taking cocaine, amphetamines, or ecstasy, which can cause your blood pressure to spike and pop your top for good. The head-trauma problem is a bit easier to solve: Duck.

CHASING A FLY-AWAY HAT ONTO A SPEEDING HIGHWAY
Deaths per Year: 1

In 1992, a man was killed after he chased his cowboy hat into speeding traffic on Texas Highway 225. Don't let it happen to you.

How to avoid dying: Don't wear hats. That's one way. But if your propeller beanie blows onto the interstate and traffic is light enough, you might try this: Watch the cars. Count the seconds between the time you first see a car and the time it takes to pass you, judge carefully, then run for it. (Note: We assume no responsibility for what happens, since we already told you not to wear hats.)

CHRONIC LIVER DISEASE/CIRRHOSIS
Deaths per Year: 25,192

You want to live forever? We'll drink to that. But maybe you shouldn't.

How to avoid dying: Quitting your bottle-of-Chivas-a-day habit is a start. Can't do that? Then start drinking coffee. According to a recent Japanese study, 2 to 5 cups a day lowers the levels of gamma-glutamyltransferase (GGT) in your liver, thereby preventing some liver-cell damage. Kahlúa doesn't count.

CHRONIC OBSTRUCTIVE PULMONARY DISEASES
Deaths per Year: 112,584

They're the number five killer of men . . . but what the hell are they? A fancy-pants term for good old-fashioned emphysema and bronchitis.

How to avoid dying: You've stopped smoking. You've quit your coal-mining gig. You put away your Fun with Asbestos kit. So what else can you do to protect your lungs? Wear a dust mask when you're tearing apart your house—that'll prevent toxic junk from entering your chest.

COLON CANCER
Deaths per Year: 47,700

Death from down under. You knew about the importance of a checkup, but you were busy. Very, very busy.

How to avoid dying: Drink milk every day—or consider a 300-milligram calcium supplement. Calcium has been shown to decrease the recurrence of pre-cancerous polyps, says Robert Beart, M.D., chief of colorectal surgery at the University of Southern California in Los Angeles.

DIABETES
Deaths per Year: 64,751
The adult-onset kind can ambush you: One minute, you're in line at Baskin-Robbins; the next, you're facedown in the sherbet.

How to avoid dying: Eat more insoluble fiber (vegetables and wheat bran) and its dietary friend, soluble fiber (fruit, some beans, oats, barley, and rye). According to the *New England Journal of Medicine*, men who ate 50 grams a day of both kinds of fiber reduced their glucose by 10 percent and insulin by 12 percent.

DROWNING
Deaths per Year: 4,100
Every guy finds himself in over his head at some point in his life. Most guys just get fired. But some go under the hard way.

How to avoid dying: If you're floundering in warm water, the object is to stay afloat until you're rescued. To save energy, try the U.S. Coast Guard's "drown-proofing" technique: Float in the water, allowing your head to submerge between breaths.

In cold water? Screw drownproofing. Your goal is to maintain body heat by trying not to dunk your head—a source of tremendous heat (not to mention hot air). Unless there's a piece of driftwood nearby, don't try to swim any-where—that will only make you lose heat faster. Float with your legs together, elbows at your sides, and arms folded over your life jacket. No life jacket? Tread water—but just enough to keep your head above water.

DRUGS (ILLEGAL)
Deaths per Year: 10,123
Been using for years? Like, check this out, man. Before you check out, man.

How to avoid dying: If you insist on being a crackhead—and crack cocaine killed the most people in 1999, with heroin a close second—at least skip the booze. A recent study at Johns Hopkins University showed that cocaine actually makes your brain more vulnerable to alcohol-induced drain bramage.

PERCENTAGE BY WHICH TWO DRINKS A DAY LOWERS A MAN'S RISK OF HEART DISEASE: 50

PERCENTAGE BY WHICH THREE DRINKS A DAY INCREASES A MAN'S RISK OF LIVER DISEASE: 40

DRUGS (LEGAL)
Deaths per Year: 7,000
How to avoid dying: The nuns were right: Bad handwriting can be fatal. Ask your doctor to type or use capital letters on your prescription. If he balks, remind him of the Texas woman who in 1999 won $450,000 in damages from her dead-husband's doctor. The doc's penmanship was so atrocious, the pharmacist gave the husband the wrong meds, which killed him.

EARTHQUAKE
Deaths per Year: 12
Not even leaving L.A. will help you avoid a quake: They're a nationwide phenomenon with unseemly consequences. Like Eminem.

How to avoid dying: Forget standing in a doorway—it's not necessarily stronger than the rest of the house, says Carolyn Bell of the U.S. Geological Survey. Instead, take shelter under a sturdy table, and grab a cushion from the couch to place over your head and shoulders. This is also a great way to protect yourself during a frat party.

ELECTROCUTION BY A HOUSEHOLD APPLIANCE
Deaths per Year: 66
Step away from the toaster and put down the fork.

How to avoid dying: Remember everything Mommy told you about outlets and light sockets. Also, during a thunderstorm, stay off the phone. If you must make a call, stick to your cell phone, says Richard Kithil, president of the National Lightning Safety Institute. The bolt can't touch you there.

FALLING
Deaths per Year: 16,600
Life. It's nothing but ups—and downs. Same with death.

How to avoid dying: To prevent Gerald Ford-ing yourself into an early grave, practice standing on one leg with your eyes wide shut. "Your vision gives you stability," says Tim Hilden, a trainer at the Boulder (Colorado) Center for Sports Medicine. Removing visual input will only strengthen your other stabilizers. It also helps if you say "Ommmm . . ." a lot while you do this.

FIRES AND BURNS
Deaths per Year: 3,741
Tenth floor. Smell smoke coming from the apartment next door.

How to avoid dying: Fight that towering inferno with a roll of duct tape. If you're waiting for the fire department to rescue you, "seal the door with tape to prevent smoke from coming in," says Julie Reynolds, spokesperson for the National Fire Protection Association.

Or try blasting the blaze with a fire extinguisher. If that doesn't work, get the hell out.

Another option: For about $1 per square foot—or the price of a Jacuzzi—you can add a sprinkler system to your home. A sprinkler system essentially guarantees that you won't die in a fire.

GUNSHOT WOUND
Deaths per Year: 30,708 (26,189 of Whom Are Men)
Your risk of getting one escalates the moment an NFL player enters the room.

How to avoid dying: Immediately put direct pressure on the wound with your fingertips. This is more effective than using your palm, since the pressure will be focused on a tighter area. Shot in the arm or leg? Elevate it above your heart to reduce bleeding.

HEART DISEASE
Deaths per Year: 724,859
More than half of the 1.1 million coronary victims each year die on the way to the hospital. Why? Because they blow off their symptoms or delay calling 911 for help, says a study from Oregon Health Sciences University.

How to avoid dying: If you have even the slightest doubt, don't wait for your wife to get home from work to drive you to the hospital. Call an EMT pronto, Tonto.

And if you know you're at risk for a coronary, ask your doctor about other symptoms you may experience during an attack—including shortness of breath, nausea, and fainting. A study in the *Journal of the American Medical Association* revealed that one-third of heart-attack victims show up at the hospital with these symptoms rather than chest pain—making the patients twice as likely to die, since they aren't diagnosed as quickly as the complainers.

HYPOTHERMIA (EXCESSIVE COLD)
Deaths per Year: 685
You've locked yourself out of your igloo again—naked. Now what do you do?

How to avoid dying: Try some isometric exercises, which can produce heat: Press your hands together, palm to palm, then push down with one while pushing up with the other. This will develop heat energy without spiking your body's metabolism. Fingers frostbitten? Tuck them under your armpits to warm them up. Never use a heating pad to bring frostbitten skin back to life; the skin will burn—and that ruins the blanket.

INFLUENZA AND PNEUMONIA
Deaths per Year: 91,871
You, her, and 17 of her closest friends—all in one hot tub. The next day, you feel as though you're dying. What happened?

How to avoid dying: The tub was dirtier than your craven, wretched mind. Hot tubs that aren't working properly or that haven't been cleaned in the correct way have been known to carry an organism that leads to pneumonia. You jump in the tub, the germs jump in you.

So what do you do? How about the dishes? One study found that liquid dish soaps are really good at destroying the respiratory syncytial virus that can cause pneumonia; they do an even better job than so-called antibacterial soaps.

If it's flu, though, you can skip the dishes and go straight to the doc's office. Ask him about amantadine. The stuff has been shown to stop the flu dead in its tracks if taken at the earliest sign of symptoms.

INHALATION OF VOMIT
Bandleader Deaths: At Least 2
Everyone knows Jimi Hendrix choked on his own vomit. But you probably didn't know that swing-band leader Tommy Dorsey was the first musician to pull this stunt, way back in 1956, after eating a huge meal and taking too many sleeping pills. "This kind of choking occurs when someone has a severely diminished mental status," says Robert Norris, M.D., chief of the division of emergency medicine at Stanford University School of Medicine.

How to avoid dying: If you can't keep from severely diminishing your mental status, at least sleep on your side.

LIGHTNING
Deaths per Year: 63
In 1949, a bolt of lightning hit a Florida baseball field, electrifying the ground from first to second base. Three players were called out—permanently—because they didn't know the first thing about lightning survival.

How to avoid dying: Ironically, your best defense against lightning is a baseball-catcher's position: crouched, feet together, hands on ears, says Kithil. You might also consider wearing a skirt and pumps, since women are four times less likely to be struck by lightning than men are.

MENINGITIS
Deaths per Year: 768
How to avoid dying: Get a shot. Most people don't know there's a meningitis vaccine, but in fact it's been around for nearly 30 years. If your 18-year-old is headed off to Whatsamatta U. this fall, make sure your family doctor gives the kid the needle: College freshmen are more than six times as likely to contract meningitis as kids of the same age who aren't attending college.

NECROTIZING FASCIITIS (FLESH-EATING BACTERIA)
Deaths per Year: 160
The killer that stalks the hospital hallways is from the same family as ordinary strep throat. But the consequences can be far worse: Muscle, fat, and skin are

stripped away faster than you can say "Karen Carpenter." The early warning signs are fever, severe pain and swelling, and redness around a visibly infected area.

How to avoid dying: See your doctor quickly, and don't touch anything. The best prevention? Stay away from General Hospital—not that you wouldn't want to anyway. And wash your hands, especially if you're around someone with open sores and wounds. Or you could just break up with her.

OVERCONFIDENCE
Deaths per Year: Countless
F. M. Esfandiary was a noted futurist who claimed with utter certainty that modern science would enable him to reach his 100th birthday. He died at 69.

How to avoid dying: Don't tempt God.

POISONING (BY FOOD)
Deaths per Year: 5,000
There are more types of foodborne illnesses than there are Baldwins. The worst? Alec. Second worst? Salmonella, which kills about 585 people each year.

How to avoid dying: Pass on the Uncooked-Pork Swirl ice cream, and make sure you use a paper towel to dry your hands—especially if you're like most guys and use the same dish towel to dry the plates, wipe the counter, bathe the dog, and buff your chainsaw.

POISONING (BY UNSEEN GASES AND VAPORS)
Deaths per Year: 638
Carbon monoxide is the Steve Winwood of gases: odorless, tasteless, and colorless. And it can kill in minutes if you and a running car are locked in the same garage together, listening to "Back in the High Life Again."

How to avoid dying: Keep the garage door open until the song is over, Einstein. And if you're worried about leaks from your gas stove, buy a CO detector. Or check the flame on the top burners: Blue is good; yellow or orange means a slow leak.

PROSTATE CANCER
Deaths per Year: 31,900
How to avoid dying: Catch it early. If you do, you have a 70 percent greater chance of beating it. Have a prostate-specific antigen test and, after you turn 50, get a digital rectal poke once a year. For best results, ask a doctor to do it.

PERCENTAGE BY WHICH AFRICAN-AMERICAN MEN ARE MORE LIKELY THAN OTHER ETHNIC GROUPS TO DEVELOP PROSTATE CANCER: 50

PERCENTAGE BY WHICH DEATH FROM ALL CANCERS IS HIGHER FOR AFRICAN-AMERICAN MEN THAN WHITE MEN: 48

SEXED TO DEATH
Deaths per Year: Several (Though Few Complain)

You wake up surrounded by naked women, but somehow you just don't feel right.

How to avoid dying: Don't have sex between 6:00 A.M. and noon—at least if you've had heart surgery. One study found that sex can trigger a sudden cardiac episode, and it's more likely to happen first thing in the morning. To be sure, check with your doctor about your particular risks—and resume the horizontal mambo only after he's performed a few stress tests.

SEXUAL VOYEURISM
Deaths per Year: At Least I

According to the Darwin Awards, in 1999 a Mexican jailer who was spying on a prisoner's conjugal visit tripped over an air vent, smashed through a glass skylight, and fell 23 feet to his death. Could have happened to you, hombre.

How to avoid dying: Watch the Spice Channel.

STRANGULATION
Deaths per Year: 762

Attacked by a mugger who learned his trade during the Great Depression? You have only 3 to 4 seconds before you run out of oxygen.

How to avoid dying: Place your foot behind one of your attacker's legs, then twist violently and throw an arm in his face. With any luck, he'll trip over your leg and undo his grip on your throat, and you'll have time to catch your breath.

TESTICULAR CANCER
Deaths per Year: 300

If you've got 'em, check 'em. A bump on a nut could mean trouble.

How to avoid dying: Get treatment fast; if caught early, testicular cancer is a highly curable condition. Want to prevent it? Sever all ties to Ronald McDonald—if you're young and you have a high-fat diet, you're four times as likely to develop testicular cancer. Be especially careful if one of your boys never made the jump down. Cryptorchidism (an undescended testicle) can mean you have 2 to 11 times the average guy's risk of testicular cancer.

ZAMBONI MACHINE
Deaths per Year: None (Yet)

As far as we know, only one person has ever died in the maw of a Zamboni machine (and he's fictional—Carla's second husband on *Cheers*, who croaked at an ice show). But we needed a Z, so what the hell.

How to avoid dying: Don't date a figure skater.

What You Can Learn from My Heart Attack

15 men, 15 coronaries. Read what the survivors have to say

By Gavin Evans for the U.K. edition of *Men's Health*

Two years ago, my brother said to me, "The men in our family all died young, you know. Mainly heart attacks." Then he began to reel off a list of family members who'd succumbed. "Look at Uncle Rex: He was 38—your age."

His point struck home, so I cut out red meat, coffee, and salt, and took up running. One London Marathon down, several to go. My heart is fine, I think. I'm just more aware of it these days. Bdumm, bdumm, bdumm. . . . I've since met coronary survivors from all over the United Kingdom. Some were young, clean livers; others were older smokers, with poor diets and dodgy genes. All were taken by surprise. Let their stories be a lesson to every man. . . .

WHAT ARE THE WARNING SIGNS?

"The doctor said, 'You're having a heart attack,' and that made me mad. I actually told him, 'Don't talk shit to me.' I was 30, fit, ate no red meat, had low blood pressure, low cholesterol, and none of my family had had heart attacks, so I couldn't believe it. Later, I heard the cardiologist saying, 'He's had a really big heart attack, but because he's young and fit, he'll be okay.' He then turned to me and said, 'Brenton, you're an enigma.' They still don't know why the artery collapsed."

Brenton Joseph, lawyer; now 31

"I had heartburn, but my doctor said not to worry. Then one evening when I complained of the pain, my wife phoned the ambulance. I was irritated and told her, 'Don't be silly. You're wasting everyone's time. There are other really ill people who need it.' Without her, I would have died in my sleep. By the time the ambulance arrived, I'd suffered a massive attack and was technically dead."

Martin Beckwith, janitor; heart attack at 51, now 54

"I was 45, smoking two packs a day, eating loads of Mars bars, cheese, and butter; and at 5 feet 9 inches, I weighed 259 pounds, but I had no idea I was putting myself at risk. Fortunately, a nurse lived next door and recognized that I was having a heart attack—the ambulance rushed me to intensive care. Six weeks later, I felt the same symptoms, but this time I immediately knew what it was."

Graham Beeson, now 48, car dealer

PERCENTAGE INCREASE IN DIAGNOSED CASES OF DIABETES IN 30-YEAR-OLDS BETWEEN 1990 AND 1998: 70

"I WAS A STATISTIC THEY COULDN'T EXPLAIN"

Stephen Brown
Age 33
Bus Driver

Two years ago, Brown began to feel an odd discomfort in his chest as he was finishing his route. "It was a bit like trapped wind or indigestion at first, but as I continued driving it gradually got worse," he recalls.

Within a few hours, he was back to normal, the scare apparently over, and felt well enough to go grocery shopping. He returned home and sat down to watch the six-o'clock news, when suddenly the pain returned—only this time it kicked in without remorse. "It steadily got worse—at first like very severe indigestion and then this heavy pressure in the chest. You just can't get away from it." He staggered to his bed and collapsed. At 8:00 P.M., his wife called the doctor.

"He was unsure because of my age—I was so young—but he gave me an aspirin and rang for an ambulance." At the hospital, Stephen was wired to monitors and fed with drugs, and at 1:00 A.M., the doctor told him he'd just survived a heart attack.

"The morphine and other drugs they gave me took away the pain, and by the next day, I was feeling okay, but then the pain came back."

Eight days later, he was sent home with lots of advice about eating healthily. "My cholesterol level was low and my diet wasn't bad. I was exercising regularly, not smoking, not drinking too much. I was just one of those statistics they couldn't explain."

Four months on, he returned to work, but within a week the pain had returned. "The hospital said it was an angina attack. After that, I never went back to driving buses—too much stress."

Since then, Stephen has taken a job as a janitor at a local college. "I still feel it could happen—another heart attack—and I suppose this has changed my outlook on life. I don't really worry about money or anything like that. I just look at every day as an opportunity, and I take it."

"I recognize the signs only in hindsight. I realize now that I had a mild heart attack when I was younger, without knowing it; and I certainly had ample warning this time when I felt indigestion and chest pain. My parents said I looked awful, but I ignored it. The next day, I went to the office and felt more pain in the chest. My wife said, 'You don't look well,' and I said, 'I don't feel well.' It was only then that I realized I was in trouble."

Pat Allan, accountant; heart attack at 55, now 69

WHAT DOES IT FEEL LIKE?

"I finished batting, went to the showers, and began to feel weak. I started sweating heavily, got dizzy, and sat down. I thought I needed sugar, so I ate a chocolate bar. But when I got up, I fell over. I then felt a pain in my lower left arm and asked a friend to massage it. She knew the symptoms, so some of the guys carried me to her car and drove me to the hospital. When I was on the stretcher, it really hit me. I mean the pain was intense—unbearable. I was writhing in agony."

Brenton Joseph

"THIS CAN'T BE HAPPENING TO ME"

Ian Campbell
Age 31
Fireman

As a fireman and rugby player, Campbell gave no thought to the danger from within. Why should he? His diet was sound, his weight perfect, and he had no family history of heart problems. But one morning in 1991, while ventilating a building after fighting a fire, he felt unfamiliar indigestion pains. He ignored them for the rest of the day and night. But it was after he'd returned home from the pharmacy, having bought some indigestion tablets, that he was hit by a shock of chest pain. "It felt like a bricklayer's clamp was crunching my chest," he recalls.

Ian struggled to the phone and called for an ambulance. By the time it arrived, he was feeling better, but he was bundled off to the hospital. After an electrocardiogram and blood tests, it was confirmed that he'd suffered a heart attack. He had two more aftershocks over the next 3 days while in intensive care.

"My parents picked me up from the hospital after 11 days, and it was the first time I'd cried as an adult," he says. "I felt my life was gone. I'd overheard my commanding officer saying to my dad, 'That's the end of his career.' It really upset me."

Over the next year, Ian fought the battle of his life to get his old job back. He began by proving his fitness, running races for charity. This was followed by a series of battles with fire-service tribunals and appeal structures. The fire department said he was disqualified for no longer holding a heavy-vehicle license.

Finally, when he regained his license, Ian became the first-ever British fireman to be readmitted to the service following a heart attack. "I still eat the same things—although I've cut back on animal fats. And I exercise a lot. I've been back in the service for 8 years now, and the decision to readmit me has been proved correct because I've had no more problems. I hope it stays that way."

"I blacked out because a blood clot had stopped my heart, so I didn't remember a thing until I heard the cardiologist say to my wife, 'He may be brain-damaged because of the oxygen not getting to his brain.' But I was okay. I had short-term memory loss for a few days. People would say something, and I'd forget it, and they'd say it again, and again. But that soon righted itself."
Martin Beckwith

"My second attack in 1989 felt like a 10-ton truck parked on my chest."
Lowell Courtney; heart attack at 38, now 49

"I've never felt anything so painful before or since."
Pat Allan

"I was sitting down on the toilet when I felt an excruciating pain down my left arm and then through my legs. I started sweating profusely and then collapsed into a fetal position in the bathroom. If my wife hadn't come in then, I would have died."
Tony Brereton, former IBM manager; heart attack at 47, now 58

"I was telling the ambulance men it was just indigestion, when it hit me. It crept up my left arm to my shoulder, and I felt this clamping around my jaw and neck and a crushing chest pain. It was so intense—I would have been happy to die. I could hardly stay conscious."

Paul Allen, sales engineer; heart attack at 45, now 49

"I had a lot of trouble breathing and walking, but my doctors didn't put two and two together. I realized something was wrong when I was hit by this terrible pain and felt a huge weight on my chest—like an elephant was sitting on it. I'd never felt anything like it before."

John Bates, retired; heart attack at 51, now 54

"I woke with indigestion and heartburn, which spread across my chest and back. I became breathless and started sweating. It was so intense that I was doubled up. When the doctor at the coronary unit examined me he said, 'There's bad news and good news, John—you're having a heart attack, but you're in the best place to have one.'"

John Carter, mechanic; heart attack at 45, now 46

WHAT ARE THE CAUSES?

"I was a heart attack waiting to happen. I was smoking 15 a day, I'd gone 13 years with no exercise, I lived on fast food, I was very stressed because my marriage was breaking up, and I had a genetic predisposition because both my parents and all my grandparents had suffered coronaries. Also, my cholesterol level was far too high and I was working myself to the ground—16 hours a day running an extremely busy travel agency."

Lowell Courtney

"My job as an international business manager for IBM meant long hours and lots of travel. But the main cause may have been genetic. My father had the first of four heart attacks at 47 and died of a coronary thrombosis at 50. The difference was he went straight back to work and continued smoking."

Tony Brereton

"My father died at 57, his father had died at the same age, and three of my uncles went early—all from heart attacks. My mother also had heart problems. Following my attack, my brother was examined and had to have a quadruple heart bypass, which saved his life."

Paul Allen

PERCENTAGE OF HEART-DISEASE PATIENTS WHO COULD BENEFIT FROM ASPIRIN WHO ACTUALLY TAKE IT: 25

NUMBER OF HEART PATIENTS WHO MISTAKENLY USE A DAILY NONASPIRIN ANALGESIC: 1 IN 4

"My father died of a heart attack in 1979, but I didn't do anything for myself. I'm a toolmaker and sitting on the bench with a lit cigarette was just part of the job. I was smoking three packs a day. On the day of my attack, I'd just come home from buying a carton of 200."

Peter Batchelor; heart attack at 45, now 52

"I was eating what everyone eats—pies, fish and chips, burgers. If I knew then what I know now, I would have had a different diet."

John Bates

"It runs in my family—my father dropped dead at 52, and his brother had a heart attack at 48. But I was still drinking a lot, smoking 40 cigarettes a day, devouring fish and chips. Plus, I was working a lot of overtime—12-hour shifts with lots of stress and plenty of coffee."

John Carter

"I was an accountant working up to 18 hours a day, which meant I was under enormous stress. Over the years, I had various stress symptoms, in addition to a genetic predisposition to heart attacks."

Pat Allan

"I WAS AS HEALTHY AS A MAN CAN BE AT 52"

Mohammed Ashraf
Age 52
Building superintendent

Ashraf was proud of his reputation as the fittest man in his family. "I'd been going to the gym every morning for 12 years: treadmill, bikes, rowing. My weight was the same as when I was 20—161 pounds. My cholesterol level and blood pressure were both low, I've never smoked or drunk alcohol, and I didn't have a highly stressed job. So as far as I was concerned, I was as healthy as a man could be at 52."

One morning in 1998, as he was preparing to head off to the gym, Mohammed felt a sharp pain in his chest—a pain that rapidly became worse. "I couldn't breathe properly, and I was sweating profusely. I realized something was seriously wrong and asked my wife to call an ambulance."

Mohammed was admitted to intensive care. "The doctor immediately told me I was having a heart attack. I actually hadn't thought it could be that and was surprised—pretty shocked really—because no one in my family had heart attacks, and I was the healthiest of the lot. When he finished examining me, he shook his head and said, 'If you can get a heart attack, anybody can.' He seemed quite shocked himself."

Three days later, Mohammed spoke to another doctor. "I told her, 'I'm really disappointed that it could happen to me,' and she said that my gym work had saved me. I felt better about it after that."

He's since had no pain and has returned to his fitness routine. "I've made a few adjustments, though. I always study the labels on food before I buy them, and I will eat nothing containing saturated fat. I also take two aspirins every morning, to help thin my blood. And I've changed my attitude to life. The heart attack has made me realize how important my family is—I don't want to let them go."

HOW DO YOU COPE?

"The damage to my self-confidence was infinitely greater than the physical damage. I remember crying my eyes out because I'd thought I was gone at 39."

Lowell Courtney

"The way I look at it now is that heart-attack sufferers who survive, survive. It's not like living with cancer. Those people have far more courage."

Peter Batchelor

"For 18 months afterward, the slightest twinge would get me thinking 'Oh, now what's that?' I've suffered depression and a loss of confidence. I also struggled at work after being told on my first day back that I was a health problem and they didn't want to employ me any more. They made my life hell, but it took me 2 years to resign. My wife and daughters helped a lot. We've always been close, and now we're even closer."

Paul Allen

"The effect of the bypass operation really knocked me psychologically. It was traumatic because I came out having to be so careful. My wife, who was working, arranged for my mother to stay with me at home while I was recovering—I was really glad to have someone to talk to during the day, because I wasn't my old self. But within a month or two, as I improved physically, I was more or less back to normal."

Martin Beckwith

"The reason it knocks your confidence is that you don't know what you can and can't do. I needed a lot of reassurance; this came from joining a cardiac support group, where I met people a lot worse off than me."

Ian Atkinson, 56, administrative manager
for a laboratory-equipment manufacturer

"After the triple bypass, I came out with tremendous relief because I could breathe properly again."

John Bates

WHAT DOES IT TEACH YOU?

"I feel like I've been given a second chance, which means I'm no longer interested in chasing money. I still sell cars, but if it's freezing cold or raining I just don't go to work. It isn't that important anymore. I also appreciate my wife more."

Graham Beeson

"You develop a different view of life after a heart attack. Your emotions move closer to the surface, and unless you're prepared for it, it can be a strange thing. Family becomes more important, while things like money and career become less so."

Pat Allan

"It's a horrendous experience, but what comes out of it can be very positive. I see the funny side of life now. I laugh and joke more."
John Bates

"It made me realize I wasn't immortal. I've changed my approach to life. I'm still in the same job, but I won't work more than 48 hours a week. Basically, money isn't as important as it was before."
John Carter

"I was back at work after 2 weeks, and now I'm playing sports and living exactly as before. I never thought I would die, so it wasn't a life-changing experience. My view of myself and the world hasn't shifted. I'm the same person as before."
Brenton Joseph

"I IGNORED ALL THE SIGNS"

**Eaton Fallows
Age 43
Telecommunications operations
manager**

Fallows had always thought of himself as a man in good health. He had played for his local amateur soccer team up to the age of 40 and was forever being reassured about his health. "I weighed more than 210 pounds, but people would still say, 'You're not really fat, you're just big.'" He absorbed the compliments and ignored the doubts, despite the fact that his father died young from a heart attack.

"If I think about it now, my health situation was terrible and I was making it worse," he says. "I stopped exercising when I gave up soccer, I ate no fruit and lots of fatty foods, I was working late into the night in a high-stress job, and I was always out of breath."

One wintry morning in 1998, while he was scraping the ice off his car, his 41-year-old body finally rebelled. "First my arms felt weak, but I thought this was because of the cold. Then, when I was driving, I began feeling sick—really sick—so I stopped for a cup of tea." He then gave a lift to a colleague, Peter. "By that time, I was feeling violently ill: struggling to breathe, my arms feeling like lead. I guessed what was happening and said to Peter, 'I think I might be having a heart attack. You'd better call an ambulance.'"

He was soon being fed aspirin and injected with clot-busting drugs at the hospital. A cardiologist told him he'd been lucky and there was no lasting damage.

All the same, he was shaken by the experience. "You stop taking things for granted and feel more vulnerable. Each twinge frightens you." His attitude about his body has shifted substantially. "I've lost 49 pounds—I'm now down to 161 pounds, the same as when I was 27.

"I eat no red meat, lots of vegetables, and lots of fruit—five pieces a day. I walk 3 miles every morning and 5 on weekends, and sometimes I swim or use the treadmill. I've become known as the 'health policeman' and the 'cholesterol constable' at work because I can see heart attacks in the making."

HOW DO YOU PREVENT THE NEXT ONE?

"The doctor came to my bed and said, in this posh voice, 'Listen, old boy, unless you stop smoking, you'll die.' I was irritated, and it was absolute hell for 3 months, but it did the trick. The only way is cold turkey. I was lucky to get away with it, but I wouldn't like to challenge God in this way again."

Peter Bachelor

"I might share a bottle of wine on a Saturday night but no longer the six beers on Friday—and I haven't had Indian food for months. I can't do weight training anymore—I can't even change a tire—and I've only had one game of soccer since. But I walk for miles."

John Carter

"I joined a gym, I walk 25 to 30 minutes a day, and I cut my fat content drastically, so my weight fell by more than 70 pounds. Not smoking also helped."

Graham Beeson

"I run 15 miles a week and the odd half-marathon. It keeps the arteries open and fights angina."

Lowell Courtney

"When I got home from the hospital, we emptied the freezer because it was full of junk. Now it's five portions of fruits and vegetables a day, grilling not frying, no sausages or burgers, and lots of walking and swimming. I feel much healthier."

John Bates

"I remembered what happened to my dad, so I took a voluntary-retirement package from IBM at 50, stopped smoking, and gave up red meat. I now put in 30 hours a week as a volunteer at the local hospital."

Tony Brereton

Commit to Yourself

Duke University basketball coach Mike Krzyzewski shares his secret for a longer, stronger, better life

From *Leading with the Heart* by Mike Krzyzewski and Donald T. Phillips (Warner Books, 2000)

In January 1995, after barely one-third of the regular season, we had just been beaten by Clemson, 75-70, at Cameron Indoor Stadium in a loss that lowered our record to 9-3. After the game, our assistant coaches gathered at my house, as usual, to review and analyze the loss and figure out how we could get better.

"I want all you guys to sit down," I said to Mike Brey, Pete Gaudet, and Tommy Amaker. My wife, Mickie, was also in the room. Then I moved to a place where I could look directly into all their faces.

"I'm going to resign tomorrow," I said, after drawing a deep breath. "I've always believed that the group is more important than any single person. Duke deserves the best. Well, I can no longer do my best. I can't even be mediocre right now."

Over the previous several weeks, I had lost a lot of weight and had no energy or passion. I was a physical wreck, and I knew for me to continue would be a disservice to my team. It wasn't about quitting; it was the realization that somebody else could do the job better. I had to look after Duke, my program, my guys. It's what I learned in the military. If your people are engaged in competition and you cannot lead them, then you step back and let someone else lead. That was my thought.

Amaker, Gaudet, and Brey all expressed support but also encouraged me not to act rashly. "Take some time to think it over, Mike," they advised.

"I'm not sure if I want to coach anymore," I said.

"Well, Coach," said Tommy, "you know how you feel better than anybody. But as someone who played for you and worked for you—and with all due respect—I find it hard to believe that you don't want to coach anymore."

And then Mickie came up to me and gave me a hug. "I'm not going to let you do this," she said. "After all that you've accomplished, all that you've done—you're not going to go out like this."

ADVERSITY

This all had been building for quite some time—ever since the previous summer, when I started to experience pains in my left leg. I told my doctor that it was probably a pulled hamstring. So for 3 months, that's what I was treated for.

By September, the pain had not gone away, and Mickie reminded me that pulled hamstrings do not last that long. "You need to go to the doctor and get it checked out," she said.

My doctors informed me that I had a disk problem in my back and that the exercises I had been doing for that "pulled hamstring" were only making it worse. They recommended some new exercise therapy. But a few weeks later, on a recruiting trip to Kansas City, the disk ruptured, and I could barely walk by the time I got off the airplane. My doctors called in a prescription to kill the pain, and when I returned to Durham, they started giving me a series of shots to reduce the swelling.

But things didn't get any better. As a matter of fact, the numbness in my leg seemed to get worse. So I went to a neurosurgeon to have it checked out again. When he told me to stand on my toes with all my weight on my right leg, I did okay. But when he told me to do the same thing with my left leg, I collapsed to the floor. I was stunned.

"What does this mean?" I asked him.

"Well, you've lost your left calf muscle. If you don't want to walk around like Quasimodo for the rest of your life, you'll get surgery."

That scared me. And 2 days later, on October 23, 1994—8 days after basketball practices began—I had surgery to repair what turned out to be a severely herniated disk. After a few days, I began to feel better. I still didn't feel great, but any improvement was a sign to me that I should get back to my team.

The doctors advised me to go slow, to take up to 10 weeks of recovery time, and to severely limit my physical activity except, of course, for basic rehabilitation. But I said, "Hey, I'm feeling pretty good. I think I can come back in a week."

"Well," they responded, "then you have to do it on a limited basis. Maybe if you have a special chair there, it'll be okay."

So I got my way—and I was back on the court within 10 days.

Unfortunately, over the next 2 months, I really began to go downhill. I started losing weight. I was getting weaker. The pain in my back was getting worse. And I was exhausted all the time.

By this time, Mickie was furious at both me and the doctors. She didn't like the fact that I was ignoring all their medical advice—and she said the doctors were intimidated by "Coach K" and would not put their foot down to say no. "Any other patient who goes through that type of operation wouldn't be allowed to do what you're doing," she told me. And she was right.

But I kept right on forging ahead.

Our team went on a trip to Hawaii to participate in the Rainbow Classic, and we were fortunate enough to win two out of three games. But on the plane for that long 8-hour trip back, I had a terrible time. I couldn't get into any kind of comfortable position. My back was absolutely killing me. And I got no sleep during the entire tournament.

After the plane flight home, I felt completely worn down—both mentally and physically. I had all but stopped eating. I even had a conversation with a friend about my beautiful 9-year-old daughter, Jamie. "I thought Jamie was 14," he said. He was right. I wasn't thinking clearly enough to know how old my youngest daughter was.

Then we played the Clemson game, got beat—75-70—and I told the guys I was going to resign.

COUNTRY IN WHICH THE AVERAGE MAN IS MOST LIKELY TO DIE FROM DRINKING: **LITHUANIA**

LEAST LIKELY: **ENGLAND**

Two days later, when I woke up in the morning, I could barely move. I struggled to get up and shower, but then staggered back into bed. A little while later, I got up and shaved—and staggered back to bed. Then I tried to get up again, pulled on my coaching sweat suit, and fell back into bed.

Mickie saw me as a broken-down guy with sunken eyes and a stooped back. And she had had enough.

"I'm setting up an appointment with the doctor, and you need to be there," she said.

"I can't. I have to go to practice. I have appointments with the players. And then we're leaving for the Georgia Tech game. I don't have time."

"You don't have the strength," she said before leaving the room to call the doctor.

When she came back, Mickie informed me that the appointment was all set up for 2:30 that afternoon.

"But I told you that I have practice at 2:30!"

"Michael," she said, "I've never said this to you in our whole married life before, but it's me or basketball right now. If you don't show up at 2:30, I'll know what your choice was."

My first reaction to Mickie's ultimatum was anger. "Don't lay that on me," I thought. "Why is she doing this to me today? I don't need this on top of everything else."

But then, when I was driving to my office, I realized that to make a statement like that, she must have seen something that I didn't see—or didn't want to see. I not only trust Mickie, I love her. "I guess I better go to that appointment," I finally decided.

So I asked the assistant coaches to run practice, and I went to the 2:30 doctor's appointment. In my 15 years at Duke, it was the first practice I had ever missed. In fact, I had never before missed a practice in my entire coaching career.

That doctor's appointment was a turning point in my life.

A SEASON OUT

When I walked into Dr. John Feagin's office, he took one look at me and said, "You're going to the hospital. We're going to do a lot of tests, and we're going to see just where you're at right now."

He did not even examine me—I looked that bad.

"Okay," I said, "but will you at least let me go back to my office so I can tell the staff that I won't be able to go to Georgia Tech with them?"

Dr. Feagin agreed. "Make it quick," he said.

When I told the staff that I had to check into the hospital and miss the game, I broke down. "I feel like I'm deserting you guys," I said. "I'm sorry, I'm sorry."

It was one of the hardest things I've ever done. All my previous training taught me not to wave to the troops going away but to be with them. Now I had to let go—and it killed me to have to do it.

But the staff couldn't have been more supportive. "It's okay, Mike. It's okay. Go to the hospital. Let the doctors help you. We'll be okay. Don't worry about a thing. We love you."

So I was hospitalized and, as I underwent nearly every medical test known to man (everything from CAT scans to psychological analyses), I got worried. After all, [North Carolina State University's late basketball coach] Jimmy Valvano's cancer started with back pain. Was it possible I had cancer? I didn't have an answer. All I knew is that I had never felt so poorly in my life. Never.

Finally, though, the doctors told me that all the tests indicated my problem stemmed from trying to get back to work too fast after back surgery. I was trying to do too much too soon, they told me. I was driving myself into the ground.

To me, that meant that all I had to do was rest up a little bit. I was so relieved to hear that it was not cancer—or another slipped disk, or something equally as bad—that I immediately began to feel a little better.

"Okay, how long do I have to stay here?" I asked. "We've got a game on Tuesday. I should be able to make it, right?"

This time, the doctors were ready for me.

They decided to form a team so they would be stronger in telling me no. There were five of them. Five—the same number of players on a basketball team. The team consisted of Dr. John Feagin, the lead physician; Dr. Jean Spaulding, a psychiatrist; Dr. Ralph Snyderman, chancellor for medical affairs at Duke; Dr. Keith Brodie, former president of Duke and a close personal friend; and Dr. Jim Clapp, professor of medicine and director of the Duke Center for Living. They met several times as a group, conferred, and then called a meeting with me where they lowered the boom.

"First of all, we're in charge, not you," they said firmly. "You cannot coach for 2 weeks. Do you understand? You have to take the time to do postoperative rehab properly. At the end of that time, we'll reevaluate the situation."

For those next 2 weeks, I alternately rested and performed physical therapy twice a day. I was not allowed to go to any basketball games or practices. Heck, I wasn't even allowed to speak to any of the players or my staff.

Those 2 weeks were the most horrible time for me because the team began to fall apart. All I could do was sit at home and watch them lose ball game after ball game. I remember one game they played against Virginia at Cameron, in which they were ahead by as many as 25 points. Good, I thought, they're going to start winning again. I don't have to worry. But they ended up losing that game in double overtime—and I was devastated.

My guys were out there having a tough time and I was at home. There was a lot of anxiety on my part. "I need to get back," I kept saying to myself. "I need to get back."

When the 2 weeks were up, my physical therapist reported that I just was not getting any better. If anything, I was worse. Finally, the doctors called a meeting. "You're not trying to get better, Krzyzewski," they said. "You're trying to get back, and you're just making things worse. We need to reverse this process right now. You're out for the whole year. We don't want you to so much as think about coming back until next year. Do you understand? Is that clear?"

I was shocked. I could not fathom sitting out for the entire year. It had never even entered my mind.

But the medical team made the decision that this was what needed to happen. They looked me in the eye and told me so. I had no choice. Mickie was on their side and so were all my friends and associates.

The truth is that I felt relieved. I guess I needed somebody to tell me what to do, because I was blinded by my emotions and my commitment not to miss work. I guess it reminded me that even a head coach, like any other leader, has to remember that there are always other people around who can lead and that he should listen to them.

I went to my athletic director, Tom Butters, and told him the situation. "Tom, the doctors want me out for the rest of the season. They say I can't get better and coach at the same time. If you want me to resign, I'll understand completely. I'd feel guilty if I didn't tell you that."

After listening intently, Tom put his hand on my shoulder. "Mike, this is your job whenever you're ready to come back. It doesn't matter if it's to-morrow, 6 weeks from now, 6 months from now, or 6 years from now. This is your job. I don't want anyone else as Duke's basketball coach."

It was at that point that I started to get better. I finally realized that, for once in my life, I had to be committed to me—and me only. I had to do it in order to get my health back.

I had not taken care of myself. Now it was time to do so.

REMEMBER YOUR CORE

While I sat out the season, the Duke team fell apart and finished with a 13-18 record. Upon my return, I had to build the program back up—hopefully, to where it had once been. To do that, I had to accept the fact that the team had deteriorated because I had allowed us to get away from our core. Heck, I had actually deteriorated physically because I got away from my own core.

Sometimes, in our haste to accomplish, we forget why we're doing it. The truth is that I had violated the basic premises that originally allowed us to achieve all our success. Now I had to get back to them.

**PERCENTAGE OF DOCTORS
WHO HAVE NOT EXERCISED IN THE PAST YEAR:** 68

I pulled out the videotape of former point guard Quin Snyder's senior speech, and I wrote down the words he mentioned: *commitment, integrity, toughness, honesty, collective responsibility, pride, love,* and *friendship*. I placed the list in my notebook and carried it around with me. I vowed to myself that we, as a team, would get back to the core principles on that list—because that's what made us go. It certainly is what made me go. Getting back to those things would then lead to winning the Atlantic Coast Conference regular season, winning the tournament, going to the Big Dance, going to the Final Four.

I also thought back to the earlier days of my coaching career—even all the way back to when I was a kid in Chicago. I remembered that we didn't have organized leagues, that we didn't get trophies for winning. We just played the game.

We played because we enjoyed it. We played because we were friends. We played for innocence.

Then I realized, once again, that those basketball games were the vehicle for my relationships with my friends. And now, as an adult, coaching basketball is still my vehicle for relationships and friendships. In fact, coaching basketball is my vehicle for life itself—for the larger journey.

If the only reason I coached was to win college basketball games, my life would be pretty shallow. I coach not only because I love it but because I have the chance to teach and interact with young people.

At the end of every season, I don't think so much about the number of games we won or how far we got on the road to the national championship. Rather, I think about all the kids on the team and what we lived through together that year. I think about Chris Collins, Tony Lang, Jeff Capel, Cherokee Parks, Jay Bilas, and the scores of other guys who've played on our teams over the years. When I see one of them, whether it's in person or on television, I smile. I know I've impacted their lives. And they have certainly impacted mine—for the better.

Because of that view of life, because of those relationships, I have no baggage. I don't lie awake at night thinking about the national-championship games we did not win. I don't define my life by how many games we've won or by the dictum "I scored more than you."

Since I came back from my season out, I've constantly asked myself the question "What's your job, knucklehead?"

Answer: "I'm the Duke basketball coach. My job is to be the leader of my basketball program. My job is to be the husband and father of my family. Do your job, Mike. Do your job."

A person has to take care of his core. And my core revolves around my family and coaching basketball. It always has. In fact, I'm probably the only guy from the old neighborhood in Chicago who's doing right now what he wanted to do when he was 9 years old. I'm a lucky guy. I'm living my dream. And in my case, reality is better than the dream itself.

Today, I try to keep in balance all the people and things I love in my life. There are many games to be played and, hopefully, they're not just basketball games. There are dances to be danced, pianos to be played, and cheers to be cheered. I want to play those games, too. I don't want to be one-dimensional and have my whole life revolve around a series of screens and picks to produce a basket.

It's funny, but out of the dark days of that season came light and renewal. It was good to know that I was mortal. When life goes wrong for us, as it sometimes does, we just have to figure out what we can do better the next time around.

For me, it was not a season lost—it was a season found.

Long Live Your Liver

If it goes, you go. So here's how to keep your liver alive and well

By Zachary Veilleux

Your liver is like a small chicken. Well, at least in terms of size and weight. Otherwise it's completely different. It receives 25 percent of the blood your heart pumps—more than 2 quarts a minute. It can crank out 2 cups of fat-dissolving bile per day. Without it, you'd be unable to digest a meal or process fat. Your blood would run thick with sewage, and your cholesterol reading would break laboratory measurement devices. And yet your liver grabs none of the recognition that big-name organs just inches away enjoy—until something goes wrong.

Yours may already be in trouble. Like most men, you probably damage your liver almost daily and don't even realize it. Knock back a few too many on the weekends? Pop acetaminophen for every ache and pain? Chemical warfare against your liver. Keep it up and you could find yourself in a new battle—with liver disease, a condition that affects twice as many men as women and is more likely to kill you than atherosclerosis or high blood pressure. Need a new liver? Get in line. You may have to wait as long as 28 months. Or you can do something now to take care of the one you already have.

LOVE YOUR LIVER

Stop at six drinks. You're trying to avoid "fatty liver," a condition that occurs when you flood your liver with more alcohol than it can process. First, your body's beer filter swells with fat globules—hence the name—and then it turns a sickly yellow. "It can literally develop overnight," says hepatologist (liver specialist) Raymond Koff, M.D., of the University of Massachusetts Medical School in Worcester. Let your liver rehab for a few days and it'll usually recover, but keep bingeing and scar tissue will develop. And then you die—of cirrhosis.

Want to cheat death? Cut out the benders. "A man's liver has an alcohol threshold of 70 to 80 grams, or about a six-pack of beer," says Dr. Koff. "Drink less than that at one sitting and it's very unlikely that you'll get fatty liver." As for the damage caused by your pickled past, consider taking the herb milk thistle and drinking protein shakes (see page 178) to help patch things up.

Lose 10 pounds. That cummerbund of fat you're wearing may be squeezing your intestines in such a way that you aren't able to digest everything you eat. When this happens, bacteria will cause the leftovers to ferment, creating a homemade still in your colon. The result: fatty liver without the pleasure of getting loaded. The solution: Lose weight and eat fat-free yogurt. "Eating a daily cup of yogurt has been shown to have an antibacterial effect in animals, and it could minimize humans' chances of developing fatty-liver disease," says Mae Diehl, M.D., a professor of medicine at Johns Hopkins University in Baltimore.

Watch the acetaminophen. Every time you pop acetaminophen—the active ingredient in Tylenol—a harmful by-product is released. Your body can handle small amounts of the stuff, but large quantities all at once start destroying liver cells. "The problem with acetaminophen is that the toxic dose level is very close to the therapeutic dose level," says hepatologist William M. Lee, M.D., of the University of Texas Southwestern in Dallas. Dr. Lee recommends that men take no more than 2 grams per day. If you go over that limit and experience nausea, head to a hospital.

Never use acetaminophen within 48 hours of drinking. If you need something, take ibuprofen instead.

Check your medicines. If Tylenol can eat away at your liver, just imagine what a prescription drug can do. Depending on the drug, the by-products can be relatively harmless—or violently toxic, says Adrian Di Bisceglie, M.D., medical director of the American Liver Foundation. A few to watch out for: the antibiotic erythromycin, the antifungal ketoconazole (sometimes used to treat prostate cancer), and the high-blood-pressure drug Aldomet (methyldopa). If you're taking any of these or have been on any other prescription drug for an extended time, ask your doctor about scheduling a liver-function test.

Wash before eating. Unless you're an IV-drug user, there's pretty much only one way for hepatitis A to infect your liver: You have to eat crap—literally.

IT'S WORTH A SHOT

Hepatitis B can be transmitted by blood, saliva, or semen; and about 6 percent of men who pick up the infection go on to develop chronic liver disease. But what's really frightening about hep B is that most men don't know there's a vaccination that's 75 to 90 percent effective. "Everybody should have the vaccination," says Robert W. Haley, M.D., chief of epidemiology at the University of Texas Southwestern medical center in Dallas. The cost: about $150 for the three-shot series.

And you don't have to dine on contaminated food for that to happen; performing oral sex also puts you at risk. "Sex is a very intimate activity, and it's not unusual for fecal-oral exposure to occur," says Miriam Alter, M.D., of the viral-hepatitis division at the Centers for Disease Control and Prevention. Minimize your risk by showering together first. In the morning, hop out of bed and go get tested for hepatitis A. Not infected? Ask for the vaccine.

Think before you ink. If you're sober and you still want a tattoo, consider this: University of Texas Southwestern researchers found that patronizing a tattoo parlor makes you nine times more likely to contract the liver disease hepatitis C. "Hepatitis C is going to cause more American deaths in this century than AIDS," says study author Robert W. Haley, M.D. Even if the tattoo parlor sterilizes its equipment, there's still a chance that the needle will become reinfected by the time the artiste is ready to mutilate your body.

THE THREE-STEP OVERHAUL

Your liver may be the picture of health. Or it may look like Keith Richards's. Either way, giving it this makeover won't hurt, and it may heal.

1. Drop alpha-lipoic acid. It's not a hallucinogen; it's an antioxidant that turns up the production of glutathione, your liver's head janitor. Glutathione latches on to toxic gunk and makes it water-soluble enough to be flushed out through your kidneys. "We give patients who overdose on Tylenol a drug that stimulates glutathione production. It's the quickest way to rid the liver of toxins," says Savant Mehta, M.D., director of the liver-transplant program at the University of Massachusetts Medical School. For maximum liver scrubbing, take a 50-milligram alpha-lipoic acid tablet (sold in drugstores) twice a day.

2. Swallow some milk thistle. Popular in Germany—a country that's tough on livers—this herb is loaded with the compound silymarin. One research review concluded that silymarin may help heal liver damage caused by excessive alcohol consumption, infection with viral hepatitis, or exposure to certain toxic chemicals. "About half the patients in my clinic are taking it, but its efficacy remains to be proved," says Dr. Mehta. If you want to give it a try, check your local health food store for Thisylin by Nature's Way ($23 for 60 capsules); it's the brand used in most clinical studies.

3. Down a protein shake. Muscleheads know that guzzling protein drinks may help build bigger biceps. But how about building a really buff liver? According to a study review published in *Nutrition*, when rats were given a protein supplement, their damaged livers started regenerating faster than those of rats not given the supplement. "The thinking is that this would also apply to humans," says toxicology professor Harihara Mehendale, Ph.D., of the University of Louisiana at Monroe. Look for powders that get their protein from whey (not soy) and that list the essential amino acid glutamine as one of the ingredients.

KNOW THIS

Your Dentist Could Save Your Life

Researchers at the State University of New York at Buffalo believe that panoramic dental x-rays can warn of an impending heart attack or stroke. These x-rays often show the carotid arteries in the neck, the vessels that carry blood to the brain. Patchy, white spots in the carotids could indicate dangerous plaque buildup. "Only 2 percent of stroke victims have any warning signs," says Laurie Carter, D.D.S., Ph.D., one of the study authors. So ask your dentist to take a look at your carotids. If he sees anything on the x-rays that looks like calcified plaque, make an appointment to see your doctor right away.

Are You a Prostate-Cancer Kid?

Just how old was your old man when he had you? According to a Boston University study, men born to older fathers may have a greater risk of prostate cancer. Researchers studied 2,200 men over a period of 20 years and found that those born when their fathers were age 38 or older were 70 percent more likely to have prostate cancer than those born to younger dads. Study coauthor R. Curtis Ellison, M.D., speculates that older men's sperm may contain DNA abnormalities that cause prostate cancer. Dr. Ellison recommends that sons of older dads get screened for prostate cancer starting at age 40.

You versus Virus

You'll win if you're pissed. A recent Pennsylvania State University/ University of Nebraska study of 4,415 men showed that those with moderate levels of aggression (anything from fighting to run-ins with cops) had stronger immune systems than those who reported no aggressive acts. But don't go overboard. In a University of Maryland study, dominant, irritable men proved to have a much higher risk of heart disease. That's a shame, at least for Mike Tyson.

More Than a Snore

If she complains about your snoring, check your blood pressure. A recent study links breathing problems such as snoring and sleep apnea to hypertension. Scientists at Pennsylvania State University found that snorers are 50 percent more likely to have high blood pressure—and be at greater risk of heart disease and stroke—than silent sleepers. You may reduce snoring and lower your blood pressure by sleeping on your side, using a large pillow, avoiding alcohol, or losing weight.

Supplement SPF

Our official position is that working on your tan is a bad idea. But we know you're going to do it anyway, so here's a little protection edge. A German study published in the *American Journal of Clinical Nutrition* found that taking supplements of beta-carotene and vitamin E for at least 6 weeks prior to sunlight exposure helps protect the skin against sunburn. "The protective effects are comparable to the use of a sunscreen with a sun-protection factor of 2 or 3," says study author Wilhelm Stahl, Ph.D., of the University of Düsseldorf. The supplement sun-shield is nowhere near strong enough on its own but offers some preliminary protection. Researchers theorize that the antioxidants minimize the cell damage that plays a role in sunburn. Be sure to talk to your doctor before starting any supplement regimen.

Football Widows—Literally

The Dutch have taken the football-widow phenomenon to a new extreme. Researchers in the Netherlands found that men there died from heart attacks and strokes at a 50 percent higher rate during a 1996 championship soccer match than in the 5 days before and after the match.

Before you start fretting that the next sudden-death overtime you watch may trigger your own sudden death, remember this: The match that got those Dutch boys so agitated was a scintillating scoreless tie that France eventually won on penalty kicks. We never understood the appeal of soccer anyway.

DOWN THE PIKE

Software That Protects Your Hardware

If you're at high risk of heart attack, take note: A team of doctors and software engineers at the University of Pittsburgh is developing a computer program they believe will predict cardiac arrhythmia or sudden death up to 8 hours before symptoms appear. "We studied heartbeats prior to the onset of arrhythmia," says Kelley Anderson, M.D. The hope is that the program, which is based on the dynamics of cardiac cycles, will instruct a device to generate a warning signal and save lives.

A Painless Blood-Sugar Test

Diabetics may soon be able to monitor their health just by looking at their wrists. University of Pittsburgh researchers are testing an implantable wrist sensor that actually monitors blood-sugar levels. The implant contains fluorescent particles that glow when blood-sugar levels increase. "The glow isn't visible to the naked eye, but it can be measured through the skin," says Jerome S. Schultz, Ph.D., the sensor's developer. The implant, along with a watch that would provide continuous blood-sugar measurements, should be available within 2 years.

Camera in a Capsule

Scottish researchers are working on a tiny camera that will fit in a capsule and, once swallowed, film your insides. The pill will give doctors a director's-eye view and provide early warning about precancerous polyps or other problems. "Most of the technology exists but just needs to be integrated," says David Cumming, Ph.D., of the University of Glasgow.

**NUMBER OF YEARS
IT TAKES THE AVERAGE SMOKER TO QUIT:** 18.5

DOES IT WORK?

Booze Monitor

What man wouldn't want Precision Navigation's Digital Alcohol Detector ($50)? You blow into the monitor's sensor for 10 seconds, and it shows you how much alcohol is in your bloodstream. When we calibrated the detector against the machine police officers use, the handheld device gave us perfect readings. But even if the detector is accurate, other variables may throw off a reading, says Morris Chafetz, M.D., founder of the National Institute on Alcohol Abuse and Alcoholism. Our own tests prove why we wouldn't rely on it. It gave us different readings based on how far we held the monitor from our mouths. But if you're sober and use it correctly, testing a friend with the machine could help convince him to give you the keys. Click on www.precisionnav.com to order one.

Waterpik Flosser

Should you abandon your regular floss for this electric version? It claims to be easier than manual flossing. Stick the disposable plastic tip between your teeth and push a button, and with 10,000 strokes per minute, it'll remove plaque from between your teeth.

It's especially effective between teeth in the back of the mouth, where periodontal disease is most likely to develop, says Sig Socransky, D.D.S., chief of periodontology at the Forsyth Institute in Boston. So it may be a good idea to pick one up (for $25; 30 replacement tips are $5) if you have trouble reaching your back teeth. But if you don't, it's not as easy or as comfortable as regular floss, especially because it's a tough fit for people with tight teeth.

COOL STUFF

Cholesterol-Size Test

NMR LipoProfile

The level of your cholesterol is important. But a study found that the size of your cholesterol molecules is also an important indicator of cardiac risk. If your high-density lipoproteins (HDL)—the good molecules that carry cholesterol out of the coronary arteries—are small, they're less effective sweepers. And if your low-density lipoproteins (LDL) are small, they're more likely to get stuck in your arterial walls. Study author David Freedman, Ph.D., from the Centers for Disease Control and Prevention, recommends that people with risk factors test the size of their lipoproteins. The test costs $136, and your doctor can order it through North Carolina–based LipoMed (www.lipoprofile.com).

HDL Home Test

BioScanner 2000

If you're trying to raise your HDL levels, it pays to check your progress. Which would you rather do: Lance your finger or get a bypass? The BioScanner 2000 ($150) from Polymer Technologies Systems is the only FDA-approved home test for HDL. It's sold as a blood-glucose monitor, but buy the HDL testing strips at any drugstore ($18 for six) and it does double duty. Pick up a Softclix finger lance, too. To order, click into www.diabetes-testing.com or call (877) 870-5610.

Blood-Sugar Monitor

GlucoWatch Biographer

The GlucoWatch Biographer allows diabetics to monitor their glucose levels noninvasively. Instead of pricking their fingers a half-dozen times each day, they can let the AutoSensor on the back of this wrist device automatically take three readings per hour. It does this by drawing glucose from the fluid between skin cells, which in most cases is just as accurate as measuring it from blood. For more information on the $300 device (AutoSensor replacements are $4), click on www.glucowatch.com.

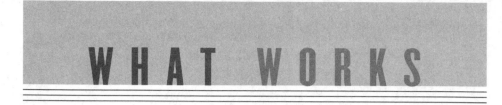

WHAT WORKS

With today's advances in medicine, most men are likely to live into their 80s, 90s, and beyond. As long as we can still hit the links and have great sex, we say bring on old age. The more years we have to do our favorite things, the better.

That's where this section of the book comes in. It gives you the tools to stop diseases before they stop you. It helps you take your health into your own hands to prevent everything from minor aches and pains to the top man-killers—all with one goal in mind: that someday your golf score will be lower than your age. Of course, golf lessons may help, too.

1. Find a doctor in your age group. A physician who's roughly your age—say, give or take 5 years—is facing the same health quirks you're facing. He'll be able to anticipate what tests and treatment you really need, says Jerome Grossman, M.D., coauthor of a report on medical errors for the National Institute of Medicine. For example, if you're in your late 40s, a 52-year-old physician will probably know exactly what you mean when you say, "My butt hurts after I have sex," while a 31-year-old M.D., staring at you with a mixture of revulsion and pity, might not.

2. Produce a reliable blood-pressure reading. No health test is more important or more frequently botched than this simple test, says Norm Campbell, M.D., president of the Canadian Hypertension Society. Here are the steps to keep your reading honest.

Use the right cuff. They come in five sizes. If your biceps measure about 13 inches, you need a regular adult cuff; if you're a *Men's Health* editor—meaning your biceps are bigger than 16 inches—you need a large cuff. In his study of 116 doctors, Dr. Campbell found that 40 didn't use a large cuff when necessary.

Check their form. Dr. Campbell found that 42 percent of the patients he studied were misdiagnosed as hypertensive due to the testers' casual technique. A few signs that they're doing a sloppy job: They don't let you rest for 5 minutes before testing, they don't take a reading from both arms, and they don't ask you to uncross your legs.

Have 'em do it again. If your blood-pressure reading is abnormal or hypertension runs in your family, ask the nurse to take three separate readings (1 minute apart) and then figure the average of the last two readings, says Dr. Campbell. This cuts the margin of error. If the reading is high, have your doctor schedule follow-up tests.

3. One more reason to get a flu shot. Researchers at the University of Texas have found that heart-attack survivors are one-third less likely to have a second heart attack if they get a flu vaccination before the flu season. The flu may contribute to inflammation that leads to rupturing of arterial plaques. It may also weaken your body in general, making you more susceptible to heart damage. "Those at risk of heart attack need to be especially careful about the flu," says Morteza Naghavi, M.D., lead investigator of the study.

4. Sideline yourself. Don't return to the game with a sore knee—playing sports when you have a joint injury increases your chances of developing osteoarthritis later in life. In a study of former soccer players, researchers at England's Coventry University found that 49 percent of them had moderate or severe osteoarthritis in at least one joint, compared with just 10 percent of men in the general population. "Stretching ligaments in your knee when they're already injured creates scarring and tissue damage that your body can never repair," says study author Andy Turner, Ph.D.

5. Spend more time in the weight room. Weights can make your biceps look good, but they're also good for your heart. Why? In addition to lowering cholesterol and blood-pressure levels, stronger muscles make physical exertion, especially lifting or carrying things, less taxing. "Stronger muscles result in a significant reduction in heart rate and blood pressure while you're carrying a heavy object," says Barry Franklin, Ph.D., director of cardiac rehabilitation at the William Beaumont Hospital in Royal Oak, Michigan. This may help you avoid straining your heart during exertion and possibly causing a heart attack.

6. Pay attention to chest pain. Here's a common last thought of a dead man: "Gee, this gas is bad. Next time, I won't eat the anchovies." The symptom that should make you call an ambulance, pronto: chest pain that lasts for more than 2 minutes. "It's the single most definitive sign of a heart attack," says James M. Atkins, M.D., professor of internal medicine at the University of Texas Southwestern Medical School in Dallas. And don't wait around, even if the chest pain is mild. "Doctors can reduce your risk of death if you reach an emergency room within 1 hour of the attack," says Dr. Atkins.

7. Snooze, don't lose. Next time your boss finds you curled up in the supply closet, point to the wisdom of the old country. The famous afternoon snooze in Spain (and most countries in Western Europe) is probably one of the reasons Spanish men enjoy a much lower rate of heart disease than we do; studies prove that taking an afternoon siesta causes a significant drop in blood pressure. That stands to reason; nobody can yell at you when they can't find you.

PERCENTAGE OF AMERICANS
WHO SAY THEY EXPERIENCE PAIN EACH MONTH: 89

8. Take a break. In a recent survey, researchers found that men who didn't take regular vacations were 30 percent more likely to die of a heart attack than those who did. Can't get away? For now, hang a light-blue picture on your wall; light colors have more of a calming effect than white.

9. Select painkillers carefully. Your chronically sore back may be responsible for your poor hearing. There's evidence that taking too many anti-inflammatory drugs can cause hearing loss, especially for those with existing problems. "Some of the drugs that can cause hearing loss or tinnitus are the most common headache medications, such as ibuprofen and aspirin," says otolaryngology professor Thomas J. Balkany, M.D., director of the University of Miami Ear Institute . Take acetaminophen instead, but eat something with it so it won't bother your stomach.

10. Develop a drinking habit. A high-fiber diet won't help keep you "regular" unless you wash down that roughage with water, says Michael D. Crowell, Ph.D., a professor of gastrointestinal physiology at the Johns Hopkins University School of Medicine in Baltimore. It gives the fiber something to soak up, which softens your stool. Cola doesn't count, by the way. The sodium in it draws water out of your bowels. And lay off alcohol when the train won't leave the station. Booze slows down gastric emptying—which is why drinking wine with dinner makes you feel full, says Dr. Crowell.

11. Save yourself from blood clots. Blood tends to pool below your waist, where clot-busting enzymes don't circulate efficiently. The result: Your legs are prone to blood clots, which can then travel to your heart or brain—with disastrous results. Here are two ways to avoid them: (1) Take two aspirin before a long flight. It'll thin your blood and reduce the risk of clots. (2) Get up for frequent strolls on planes. Walk around as much as possible when you're on a flight that's more than 4 hours long—and not just to avoid your talkative seatmate. Strolling keeps the blood moving in your legs, preventing it from pooling. If walking isn't possible, repeatedly flex your leg muscles every half-hour, starting with the feet and squeezing up into the thighs, suggests Stanley R. Mohler, M.D., director of aerospace medicine at Wright State University in Dayton, Ohio. Massaging your legs with your hands (in the same sequence) will help, too. Finally, wear loose clothing; the last thing your leg veins need is a tight waistband.

12. Eat, drink, then fly merry. An American Heart Association study found that eating a light meal and drinking an hour before a flight can increase circulation within the body by 20 percent, doubling the amount of blood flowing to the brain. Those changes may be enough to eliminate most flight-time headaches and illnesses.

NUMBER OF YEARLY EYE INJURIES CAUSED BY TOILETS: 327

13. Keep kidney stones in check. Here's how.

Measure your pee. If you're at risk for developing stones and you're not peeing at least a half-gallon of urine a day, you're not drinking enough fluids, says urologist Stephen W. Leslie, M.D. So keep a water bottle handy, and make regular deposits at the urinal. It'll pay off better than your 401(k).

And have it analyzed. Your doctor can test your urine's calcium and acid content to see if you're prone to developing stones, says Dr. Leslie. If you are, diet changes and medication can reduce your risk. And always save any stones you pass; they're great keepsakes, and they provide prevention clues, too.

14. Switch toothpaste to prevent canker sores. Canker sores are like party crashers in your mouth—you don't know where they came from, and you just want them to go away before they ruin everything. These mouth ulcers are typically caused by trauma, an allergy, or stress, but a detergent called sodium lauryl sulfate (SLS) in most over-the-counter toothpastes may also be to blame, says Kenneth Burrell, D.D.S., of the American Dental Association. One theory is that SLS dries out the protective mucus in your mouth, making you more vulnerable to canker sores. If you have frequent sores, switch to an SLS-free paste such as Rembrandt Natural.

15. Size up your shoes. Dutchmen's wooden shoes help them maintain strong feet, but that doesn't mean you should start whittling, says New York City podiatrist Stuart Bernstein, D.P.M. The benefits accrue because those shoes are designed with wide arch and toe compartments that don't constrict the feet. "Genetic foot disorders aside, men in many cultures suffer foot problems because they wear tight-fitting shoes," explains Dr. Bernstein.

16. Pick honey over sugar. The Irish have a lower incidence of diabetes than Americans, and some researchers think it's because they use honey instead of refined sugar in cooking and flavoring their food. "Honey takes longer to digest than sugar, so it requires your pancreas to produce less insulin," says Glenn Geelhoed, M.D., author of *Natural Health Secrets from around the World.*

17. Learn to take a punch. For times when a drunk argues his point with his fists, boxing trainer Andy Dumas—whose father sparred with Jake LaMotta—showed us the best way to take one on the chin.

Shrink into a small target. Turn sideways (left foot forward for righties) and bend your knees slightly. Keep your elbows in, your hands up, and your head toward your chest.

Deflect it. Catch an incoming punch with an open hand, almost as if you were snagging a line drive. Your free hand will be available for delivering a counterpunch.

Absorb the shock. Turn your head away; that'll lessen the impact and keep your nose, teeth, and soul patch intact. If you're still standing, laugh derisively. Resume stance.

ANY QUESTIONS?

Cough Medicine

Why does my doctor want me to cough during a hernia check?

—J. B., Palos Heights, Ill.

Well, someone has to break the uncomfortable silence.

A cough also helps your doctor feel for torn muscles, says New York City internist Stuart Fischer, M.D. Your doctor has to place his hand on your scrotum to feel the base of the inguinal canal, which runs from the outer part of the scrotum up into the abdomen. Normally, the upper and lower parts of the canal are separated by a layer of muscle. But if you have a hernia, this muscular barrier is torn, allowing the intestine to sink into the lower part of the canal. Coughing puts pressure on the abdomen, causing the intestine to press southward through the canal. If the doctor is able to feel the intestine with the tip of his finger, you have a hernia. Doing this test yourself in public places, however, will only get you arrested.

A Stone's Chance

My father has passed several kidney stones, and he describes the pain as being worse than a gunshot wound. Are stones hereditary?

—J. O., Dothan, Ala.

Not only was your dad's stone really painful, but he had to walk himself to the hospital—uphill, both ways.

As for you: "Some kinds of kidney stones are hereditary; some aren't," says kidney specialist Neil Kurtzman, M.D., of Texas Tech University Health Sciences Center in Lubbock. "You'd have to find out which type your father had." Two common types, calcium stones and uric-acid stones, aren't hereditary. Another common type, calcium oxalate stones, may run in families.

But even if genetics isn't on your side, you're not doomed. For instance, drinking lots of water—$1\frac{1}{2}$ to 2 quarts a day—can significantly reduce your chance of developing stones. Talk to your doctor about other preventive strategies. It's important to consult a professional on this: The very things that can prevent one type of stone can increase your risk of others.

"Son, about Your Inheritance"

My dad had cancer. How can I find out if I'm at greater risk of developing it?

—S. S., Lake Charles, La.

Researchers have identified the genes for colon, thyroid, and kidney cancers and are close to finding those for leukemia as well as prostate, lung, and bladder cancers. But the only test currently available to detect a cancer-causing gene is for colon cancer. Since this disease is the third-leading cause of cancer deaths in the United States, the American Cancer Society recommends that everyone start regular screenings at age 50.

But if you have a family history, you should see your doctor. Beginning stages of colon cancer can develop as early as age 30. Seeing a genetic counselor and being tested for the gene (it's a simple blood test) could help determine whether these early screenings are necessary.

Having a gene for colon cancer doesn't mean you'll develop it; it just puts you at higher-than-average risk. The National Cancer Institute (www.nci.nih.gov) can help you find a local counselor who can conduct the test.

Sick of Yourself?

I work out at lunch, so every day my sweaty clothes are trapped in my gym bag for hours before I get home. Could my clothes and my bag make me sick?

—J. W., Binghamton, N.Y.

Your dark, moist gym bag may be an ideal breeding ground for bacteria, but those are your own bugs. That's different from the way people typically get sick: by rubbing their nose or eyes after touching other people's stuff, says microbiologist Joan Slonczewski, Ph.D., of Kenyon College in Ohio. When bacteria feed on the perspiration residue left on your clothes, they produce waste—a waste that stinks more than the john at Taco Bell. Try chucking a fabric-softener sheet in your bag to cover up the aroma until you can find a washing machine. Or just leave your bag outside. Nobody's going to steal it, and the air will mask the smell of the bacteria residue.

PART SIX
STAY TOUGH

MUST READS

Anger: Your Secret Weapon

The right kind of rage can improve your life

By Tom Zoellner

Last March, Peter Bradley, a 39-year-old construction contractor from Missouri, forced his way into the cockpit of an Alaska Airlines MD-80 and went berserk. Luckily, crew and passengers subdued him before he could send the plane into the Pacific. The press was quick to tag it as a particularly nasty case of "air rage"—the nouveau syndrome that makes hassled coach passengers abuse innocent flight attendants. It's a high-altitude version of road rage, the late-'90s syndrome that turns a normal man into a finger-flipping, pistol-waving killer when he's stuck on route 88 in his K car. News accounts hardly mentioned that Bradley was likely suffering from encephalitis and hallucinations when he stormed the cockpit. It didn't matter. He fit a neat profile: the hostile, pissed-off modern man who becomes violent if served a plastic cup of warm club soda.

WHY IS EVERYONE SO SHORT-TEMPERED? a recent front-page headline in *USA Today* wondered. The story solemnly warned of rampant tailgating on U.S. highways, livid fathers assaulting high-school baseball umpires, men no longer opening doors for ladies. "Leading social scientists say the nation is in the middle of an anger epidemic that, in its mildest forms, is unsettling, and, at its worst, turns deadly," the story reported. We're witnessing a "general breakdown of social conventions, of manners, of social controls," which is turning us into "a culture of vulgarity," adds one quoted source from Cornell University in New York City.

Somewhere in Montana, Elvis is having a good laugh.

The notion that we're all homicidal powder kegs and that our parents' world was friendlier than Mayberry is, pretty obviously, nostalgic fiction. There is a lack of hard data to support the rage theory, but there are plenty of schlock surveys and anecdotes about increased crankiness. For example, the *USA Today* article cited a recent USA Today/CNN/Gallup poll that found 79 percent of people believe that, basically, society is becoming less polite and nobody has manners anymore. A good follow-up might have been to ask the respondents if they think teenagers act like jackasses.

Likewise, most of the data cited to support the upswing of road rage come from a 1997 report from the American Automobile Association, which stated that the number of "aggressive driving" incidents had increased by 60 percent between 1990 and 1996. The problem is, the numbers used in the report were drawn from a very narrow sample of newspaper stories, police reports, and insurance-company claims.

"A lot of events defined as road rage in the report have nothing to do with rage," says attorney Michael Fumento, of the Hudson Institute in Washington, D.C., an organization that studies public trends. He notes that the invention of the term *road rage* has simply made police more likely to describe as "rage" the petty B.S. we've always done—like weaving through lanes or flashing the headlights at the slow codger up ahead.

"If you look over the course of history, there was chariot rage, there was horse rage, there was stagecoach rage," says David Murray, Ph.D., director of the Statistical Assessment Service in Washington, D.C. "People have always engaged in furious roadside disputes. The difference is, we didn't draw boundaries around it and call it a trend."

In fact, statistics from the National Highway Traffic Safety Administration actually show that U.S. highways are becoming kinder and gentler. Fatal

GREAT BURSTS OF ANGER IN HISTORY

Circa A.D. 30: Jesus throws over some card tables.

1776: We mail a note to King George III telling him to kiff our aff.

1864: General Sherman orders his troops to retreat at Chattanooga, where they are trapped by Confederate fire. Realizing that retreat would mean suicide by artillery, the men mutiny and charge. Sherman takes credit for the victory.

1936: Jesse Owens forgets to be inferior in Berlin.

1944: "Nuts."—General Anthony McAuliffe's reply to the Nazis when they ask him to surrender his surrounded 101st Airborne Division in Bastogne, Belgium.

1946: Trials at Nuremberg.

1962: President Kennedy tells Khrushchev to get those missiles out of Cuba—now.

1963: Federal officers clear Alabama governor George Wallace from a doorway so two kids can go to school.

1965: "Get up and fight, sucker!"—Cassius Clay to supine Sonny Liston.

1969: The outfielder Curt Flood is traded from St. Louis to Philadelphia. He doesn't like this, so he goes to the Supreme Court. Now there's a free-agent system.

1969: Apollo II touches down on the moon. The word *cosmonaut* is now about as frightening as *Boris Badenov*.

1978: Arthur Blank and Bernie Marcus are fired from a Handy Dandy hardware store in California. They start a new store called Home Depot.

1981: Reagan warns Iran that the hostages had better be back on U.S. soil before he takes office. They are, on his inauguration day.

car accidents declined by almost 14 percent between 1990 and 1997, even though licensed drivers increased by 15.7 million during that period. What's more, you're four times less likely to die in a car accident today than your dad was in 1966. There may be enraged maniacs on the highway, but they're driving a little more carefully—and a lot less drunk.

The similar drop in violent crime also contradicts the rage theories. If everyone is so damned angry, they've become much better at refraining from beating the hell out of each other. Aggravated assaults dropped by 38 percent between 1993 and 1998.

But the worst consequence of the rage hype isn't just a lot of baseless paranoia. It's that it's tarnished the good name of anger.

"Anger is a virtue, not a vice," says Florida psychologist and stress researcher Nick Hall, Ph.D. "It's a tremendously useful tool." Like any sharp-edged instrument properly used, anger has served mankind brilliantly through the centuries. Without anger, we might still be wandering around Europe hoping nobody would see us sneak into church. Or, according to a lot of old men with buzz cuts, we might be buying tea and crumpets with Deutschmarks.

"Anger makes a statement to the world that you won't be a victim," says Virginia psychologist Doyle Gentry, Ph.D.

And it's an effective statement. A billion years of biology has instilled one lesson in you: Without a temper, you won't survive in a hostile environment. Stronger pond slime will eat you. Your neighbor will steal your wife. Your boss will continually step on your face. If you can't get mad, you have no chance.

"Anger protects you and the people close to you," agrees sociology professor Michael Obsatz, Ph.D., of McAlester College in St. Paul, Minnesota. Being passive is tantamount to being a victim, as any friendly New Yorker

THE MACHINERY OF ANGER

1. You walk out of a bakery and see that your windshield has been smashed.

2. Your amygdala, a small structure near your brain stem, activates to release a surge of aggressive hormones into your blood.

3. The amygdala then delivers neuroactive peptides to the rest of your brain, which quickly produces the white-hot fight-or-flight response: Run or kill? The higher your baseline testosterone levels are when you're calm, the easier it is for your amygdala to trip this response.

4. The neuroactive peptides trigger your adrenal gland to dump a massive amount of adrenaline into your bloodstream, causing your heart rate and blood pressure to shoot up. You're raring to kill. Your sweat glands are activated. All muscles brace. You're shaking. Your pain sensitivity is almost nil. You fill out a police report.

SOURCE: Emil Coccaro, Ph.D., University of Chicago

will tell you. And ultimately, it's also just as unhealthy as being a fist-pounding lunatic.

"Repressing healthy feelings of outrage can play hell with your heart and even lead to long-term depression," says psychologist Warner Burke, Ph.D., of Columbia University in New York City. A recent medical study reported in the journal *Health Psychology* found that men who persistently suppressed their anger had higher blood pressures than those who vented it constructively.

The key to maintaining your health amidst life's infuriations, says Burke, is to learn to react with "controlled anger." That's the benevolent brother of the red-faced rage that Gentry calls "toxic anger."

The tangible difference? With controlled anger, you become like a leopard on the Serengeti; adrenaline sharpens your senses and summons your instincts, giving you sufficient clarity to focus on producing the result you want—be it a dead gazelle, a humiliated opponent, or an upgraded hotel room. In contrast, toxic anger just makes you a hostile moron who spews like a fire hose, acting without any specific goal.

"Toxic anger clouds your judgment so all that's left is a primitive urge to hurt someone," explains Gentry. Uncontrollable anger is also deadly; a study in the journal *Circulation* found that men with high levels of anger were twice as likely to suffer heart attacks as other men. That's largely because it produces frustration, which is just impotent anger, instead of results.

How do you mold destructive anger into a useful weapon? It's not easy. You know good anger when you feel it, and you get better at producing it with practice. Follow these steps to improve your odds.

Give your anger a specific mission other than revenge. You need to produce positive results, not just ground-down teeth. If you've been fired wrongly, or if the neighbor kid drove his bike into your Mustang, take a few seconds to figure out what you really want other than revenge. A fat settlement? A reinstated reputation? A new car and a restraining order on the hellion? Devise a plan to get it, then use your anger to spur your efforts. Dumb anger only wants immediate revenge—namely, a lot of pain and suffering to besiege the offending party. If that's your primary goal, you're wasting your anger on a frivolous cause that won't really benefit you, says psychiatrist Redford B. Williams, M.D., of Duke University in Durham, North Carolina. "The gift of anger is that it focuses your powers on getting what you truly deserve," he explains.

Attach a moral cause to it. "Empathy-aroused anger" is the healthiest and most powerful form of controlled anger; it occurs when you're out to right a wrong that was inflicted on somebody other than you. This situation helps free you of the personal need for revenge but leaves you capable of immense focus and effort. It makes you dangerous to enemies but benign to yourself—

and this is anger's most blessed state. So don't be miffed because the manager at Tub City won't honor an extended warranty on your washer-dryer; get hot because he's probably screwed a dozen single mothers this same way.

Be aware of your physical changes in stature. You have a healthy dose of controlled anger when you're outwardly calm but feel 3 inches taller and 25 pounds heavier, says Gentry. To the most primitive parts of your brain, this means you have no fear of being drawn into a fight or of losing one.

Bomb somebody. When University of Minnesota researchers analyzed the personality traits of the first 41 U.S. presidents, they found that the greatest ones (probably all but Jimmy Carter) manifested the distinct signs of being, well, disagreeable bastards. This makes a lot of sense. Nobody is going to march off and die for a nice guy.

How to Win a Fight

A man's life is filled with conflicts. Here's how to come out on top in all of them

By Ted Spiker

In any monumental battle, there are no ties. You slay Goliath or die, you pay the sticker price or you don't, you win custody of the DVD player or she does. Whatever your fight—whether it's physical, verbal, or both—you need only a few swift moves at the right moment in order to win. Here's expert advice for learning how to successfully fight . . .

A SPEEDING TICKET

Remember this: Asking for forgiveness helps when you're loitering in purgatory, but not when you're pulled over. Telling the officer that you're very, very, very sorry only gives him what he wants: a confession, says attorney David Brown, author of *Beat Your Ticket: Go to Court and Win*. If the officer asks you if you know how fast you were going, respond by asking him to tell you the speed. If you say you don't know, that means your actions are indefensible. But some states don't have absolute speed limits, so you might be able to prove in court that for that time of day, and on that road, 68 was a safe speed.

YOUR BOSS

Win arguments with him by making him think he's the genius. "Nobody likes to lose. The key is to make the other side think they've won while you get what you wanted," says defense lawyer Alan Dershowitz. Do it by planting the answer you want. Instead of spurting out your opinion, form a question that lets your boss feel as if he came up with the solution himself. "Do you think hiring a bunch of interns might give us lots of cheap labor and access to our key customer group?"

A DRUNK

He pushes you, so you cock your right fist back and prepare to punch. But that windup gives him time to duck or to block the punch. Instead, surprise him with a quick left jab. "When you get jolted with a jab in the face, it's like running into a door. You don't expect it, and the punch goes all the way down the spine," says Angelo Dundee, former trainer to Muhammad Ali. Another benefit: Most of the power actually comes from your legs and hips, which are stronger than your arms and shoulders. To throw a strong jab, turn 90 degrees so your left side is facing the thug, then snap your left fist into his jaw. Proclaim, "I'll beat you so bad you'll need a shoehorn to put a hat on." Then run.

CITY HALL

Extreme methods of protest—like streaking down Main Street—attract the TV cameras. But they do little to change the city's plans for the new outhouse factory. "These tactics can make life miserable for public officials, but they may also make people mad and create a backlash," says political-science professor Jack Nagel, Ph.D., of the University of Pennsylvania in Philadelphia.

Instead, find personal ties to influential public officials. Eventually, a gym buddy or co-worker will know a golf partner whose mother is the cousin of the mayor's secretary. Or something like that. Politicians are more likely to act when they know a person who has to smell the outhouses every day.

THE PAIN

Your legs hurt, you're exhausted, and your nipples are bleeding. Either you've had one hell of a date, or you're approaching mile 18 of a marathon. Here's how to beat leg cramps, at least: Get off to the side of the road and lie on your back. Hoist your legs into the air and "spin" them bicycle-style for 1 minute. That'll help flush out the lactic acid that may have accumulated in your oxygen-starved muscles.

NINE GUYS AT ONCE

In basketball, rebounding wins games, and the other nine guys on the court will push you, elbow you, or Three Stooges you so they can grab the ball. For a defensive rebound, keep your eye on the ball until it's released,

PERCENTAGE OF PEOPLE WHO SEEK REVENGE: 20

says 6-foot-10 Darrall Imhoff of the United States Basketball Academy. Then do this.

- Move your nondominant hand behind you as you turn to face the basket.
- Jam that hand into the gut of the guy you're guarding.
- Lean slightly backward so your butt anchors him in that position while you grab the rebound. Don't lean too hard. A good offensive rebounder will step back, and you'll fall.

YOUR WIFE

If you're arguing with emotional or stubborn foes, your priority is reducing their stress, says Lt. Bill O'Leary, commander of the hostage-negotiation unit for the Vermont State Police. Lt. O'Leary's crew has succeeded with these hostage-negotiation tactics during domestic arguments.

Ask open-ended questions. "Why are you upset? I'm 10 minutes late." That lets her vent, which eventually calms her down. If you have a comeback for everything ("Bug off; I'm only 10 minutes late"), that'll enrage her more.

Give her subtle encouragement. Say "Okay" and "Uh-huh" as she's talking. It tells her you're listening (even if you aren't). That makes her more agreeable to your position. Once her anger is spent, you can address the real problem, calmly.

A MAN WHO'S TALL

Your best strategy: Get him on the ground, where his height isn't an advantage, says John Perretti, who competed as a kickboxer at 139 pounds and is now the producer of Extreme Fighting. Use a fake punch to the head to get him off-balance, then reach for his legs, like this:

- Step toward him with your dominant leg between his feet.
- Wrap both arms around his knees.
- Keep your back foot to the side and drive him to the ground with your shoulder.
- Stabilize him by shoving your knee into his armpit.
- Punch him with your elbow to catch him off-guard, then get the hell out of there.

AN UMPIRE

When an ump calls you out, don't make Ray Charles jokes. Raising your voice means you'll be ignored, says Merle Butler, national director of umpires for the Amateur Softball Association. "Go to the fellow who made the call, and ask if he would ask his partner if he saw it," Butler says. Umps are more willing to change their minds if you don't pit them against each other or try to show them up in front of the crowd.

AN OFFICE RIVAL

If you're in the midst of a knockdown in front of the boss, you can convince your foe to concede with subtle, nonverbal cues. Nod your head or say things like "Surely, you agree that the terra-cotta-urinal idea isn't a success." That strategy forces your opponent to say yes, Dershowitz says. The more he says yes, the more he subconsciously believes he agrees with you, and the better your odds of winning in the end.

CUJO

When a dog threatens you, stop moving and take your sunglasses off; dogs think shades make you look threatening. And smiling won't work because it looks as if you're baring your teeth. If backing away doesn't do it and the dog attacks, offer a piece of clothing. Past that point? Submit, cover your head, and play dead. All dogs except trained attack dogs view submission as the end of a fight.

A THUG

He doesn't like the way you look or the way you looked at his tattoo-flaunting honey. When he asks if you have a problem, turn sideways so your shoulder is pointing to him. Put your hand up as if you're signaling someone to stop. Then, look him in the eye and in a confident, low-pitched voice, say, "It's cool, man." That should back him off. The body language is strong enough to assert your power without appearing like a threat or a challenge, says John Hall, founder of Smart Escape, in Cincinnati. If your confrontation escalates to the point at which the thug grabs you by the collar and starts to strike you, grab his collar and pull him toward you so he has no room to punch, Hall says. Then tackle him so you'll be able to hit him and break free.

AN UPHILL BATTLE

A good strategy for winning a tough argument: Concede your weakness first, says *How to Argue and Win Every Time* author Gerry Spence. If you try to hide your weakness, your opponent will be able to uncover it and use it against you to make his point—and make you look stupid.

YOUR MOM

There are only two weapons that work in a fight with Mom. One is guilt. The other is helplessness. But if you're willing to stoop that low, consider tackling lesser opponents. Like your mother-in-law.

The New Depression

They're young, educated, affluent, and successful. They're men who should be happy . . . and don't understand why they're not

By Joe Kita

David Ramsey just built a new house—3,100 square feet of custom living space set on an acre of land in the North Carolina woods. He has a pretty, young wife with long, brown hair, and the money she makes as an attorney pushes their annual income well into six figures. They travel a lot together, vacationing in Puerto Vallarta, Maui, and the Cayman Islands.

David Ramsey also has two blond sons, ages 7 and 2, who consider Dad their hero. There's a full-time nanny to take care of them when he and his wife aren't around. And although he often works long hours, it's for no one but himself. As the owner of a distributing business, he's his own boss.

Yes, David Ramsey has it all. Yet in his bedroom, locked in a nightstand, is a black Glock 9 millimeter that he can't seem to chase from his thoughts. Although he's never slipped in the magazine and put the barrel to his head, he's thought about it—more than once.

And David Ramsey has just one question: Why?

From his car phone, Ramsey, 39, calls to ask a question that tens of thousands of men like him are asking: "Why aren't I happy?"

"From the outside looking in, my life is unbelievably great," he says. "Right now, for instance, I'm driving through Fayetteville, North Carolina, and it's an absolutely beautiful afternoon. Not one soul has said an unkind word to me all day, and I'm heading home to spend the evening with my family. Yet I'm not happy. I never am. And I can't understand why."

Ramsey is not alone. After we heard similar complaints from dozens of friends, co-workers, and relatives—and finally were unable to dismiss their grumblings as so many midlife crises—we posted a small ad on the *Men's Health* Web site that read, "We're looking for unhappy guys with perfect lives. If you have a great job, a great family, a great house full of great stuff, but you're still feeling unfulfilled and, at times, even miserable, we'd like to hear from you."

It was a tiny baited hook, but the attention it drew was remarkable.

"I'm definitely in a rut," wrote Dennis, 30, a regional vice president, new homeowner, and proud father. "I have every reason to be happy with my life, yet I feel lost."

"I'm an anesthesiologist," wrote Andrew, 39. "Been married for 9 years, couple of houses, dog, snowboard, kayak, just spent 3 weeks vacationing in

Australia. But I'd chuck it all to be as happy as I was in medical school. It seems when I had less, I felt better."

The e-mails go on and on, stacks of them. Evidently, there are a lot of dissatisfied men out there, guys who you'd never guess were unhappy, men who would otherwise evoke feelings of admiration and even jealousy. They come forward tentatively, ashamed about complaining. Not all of these men are suicidal, of course, but they can't see themselves continuing like this indefinitely. Happiness is a reward they've earned, and they're tired of waiting to claim it.

THE PROBLEM NO ONE'S TREATING

Most of us understand the symptoms of depression: the lack of energy, of appetite, of sheer will; the manic moments of confusion; the retreat into drugs, alcohol, or isolation. But that's overt depression, says psychotherapist Terrence Real, author of *I Don't Want to Talk about It*. There's a second type, one that even many psychologists don't recognize. It's called covert depression or, as it's known clinically, dysthymia.

Overt depression is what we expect from a mood disorder. It's "a state of profound impairment, utter despair, thorough debilitation," Real explains. "A truly depressed man would lie in bed in the morning, staring at the ceiling, too apathetic to drag himself off to another meaningless day."

First identified in 1974, yet seldom reported on afterward, dysthymia is far less obvious—both to the sufferers and to the people around them. "It's the life of quiet desperation that Thoreau wrote about," says Real. "Most men don't view it as a disease but as a weakness. It is a disorder of self-esteem." Its textbook symptoms include at least 2 years of depressed mood, plus at least two of the following: poor appetite or overeating, insomnia or oversleeping, fatigue, low self-esteem, poor concentration or difficulty making decisions, and hopelessness.

"I've had a certain level of dissatisfaction for the past 6 years," says Dale, 42, a wealthy insurance agent. "But it has only started getting to me recently. It's a slow burn of increasing intensity."

"Any person with a chronic sense of unhappiness or dissatisfaction in spite of the success and happiness in his life almost always has a mood disorder and often has dysthymia," says pharmacology and psychiatry professor Richard C. Shelton, M.D., of Vanderbilt University in Nashville. "The condition is grossly underrecognized and undertreated, especially among men."

The reason it has received so little popular attention is because of the shame men feel about it. Not only are we far less likely than women to seek professional help for depression but, for reasons of pride or simple embarrassment, we won't even discuss it.

"It's hard to talk to friends about this, because they don't understand how

I could have anything to complain about," admits Tony, 34, a debt-free, college-educated newlywed with a prestigious job in San Francisco. "In fact, I've gone to therapists, and even they just sort of look at me as if to say, 'What's your problem?'"

Although men like these may tell themselves they're just a little down, that nobody can be happy all of the time, such rationalization is inaccurate.

"Humans are, by nature, a happy breed," says *Happiness* author David Lykken, Ph.D., a professor emeritus of psychology at the University of Minnesota in Minneapolis. "That's because happiness is protective. Happy people get sick less often and get well sooner than unhappy people. It's an adaptive trait. The typical person has above-neutral feelings of well-being most of the time."

After extensive research, Lykken has concluded that each of us has a "happiness set point" that is genetically predetermined. Our moods may occasionally rise above or fall below this point, but eventually we all return to it. And in most cases, it's well above neutral. When someone feels chronically unhappy, there's something wrong.

What's perplexing is why so many young, successful men are suddenly noticing their unhappiness.

"Let me give you an analogy," says dysthymia sufferer Stephen Braun, author of *The Science of Happiness*. "Before the invention of eyeglasses, what was considered normal eyesight was probably on the blurry side. But as soon as glasses were invented, normal vision became 20/20. I think we're at the same stage with happiness. With so many new and effective antidepressants available, any mood that's the least fuzzy is being viewed as abnormal."

Add to this such social factors as the recent booming economy and low unemployment, and the result is less for men to worry about and strive for. When the living is so easy, happiness should be an affordable commodity. Its continued slipperiness is disconcerting.

"I took a psychology class in college in which the professor had us write a letter to ourselves listing all our goals," says Jon, a teacher with two advanced degrees. "He told us to call him in 10 years, and he'd mail the list to us. Well, I did, and I'd nailed every one—the degree, the job, the marriage, the kids, the house, the car. I'm 36. So, now what?"

And there's another factor: pop culture. "The degree of upbeatness on television, for instance, is incredible," says pharmacology professor Steven Treistman, Ph.D., of the University of Massachusetts Medical Center in

CHANCE THAT THE AVERAGE MAN WILL SUFFER FROM DEPRESSION: 1 IN 22

12 WAYS TO GET HAPPY FAST

1. Drive to a hardware store and buy a couple of gallons of light-blue latex paint, a roller, and a stepladder. Head home and—quickly, vigorously, and without much care for cleanliness—paint the porch ceiling. Not only will the exercise lift your mood but research also shows that staring at the color blue will relax you. (Bonus: According to Pennsylvania Dutch legend, a blue ceiling will keep flies away from your porch.)

2. Look in the Yellow Pages for the nearest Chinese restaurant that delivers. Call and order the ginger chicken with broccoli. According to *The Green Pharmacy* author James Duke, Ph.D., ginger and broccoli may temporarily help relieve depression.

3. Call up an old friend and suggest a spur-of-the-moment road trip—to some weekend college basketball game, to the nearest warm-weather golf course, to Toledo, wherever. The point is to spend a lot of time in the car driving somewhere, throwing garbage into the backseat, and just being men.

4. Rent one of those giant metal Dumpsters. Tell 'em to park it in the backyard, within chucking distance of an upstairs window. Then methodically work your way through the house, throwing out all the accumulated crap in your life. In the end, you'll feel lighter, like you're starting over.

5. For the next few minutes, act happy. Grin, laugh, waggle your eyebrows, walk with a bounce in your step, whistle. According to *The Pursuit of Happiness* author David G. Myers, Ph.D., people who are manipulated into smiling feel better instantly. "Going through the motions can trigger the emotions," he explains.

6. Walk around the block, do 20 pushups. . . . Aerobic exercise is just as effec-tive as antidepressants in lifting depression, according to a new study conducted at Duke University. Researchers had 156 volunteers exercise, take Zoloft, or do both for 4 months. Everyone experienced significant reductions in depression. The exercise group also had lower relapse rates than the other two.

7. Call your local community college and request a copy of its spring catalog. Pick a non-credit course you've always been interested in but never had time to pursue, then register for it. New challenges + new expertise = new enthusiasm.

8. Go to the supermarket and buy the thickest, juiciest filet mignon you can find. Then take it home, dig out the charcoal grill, and fire it up. (Never mind that it's the middle of January.) Let the aroma waft through the neighborhood. Sit on a lawn chair and drink a beer. You are now in touch with your primal self. Soon, you will find it easier to smile.

9. Make a list of five things you're going to accomplish before the end of today. Write them down; put them in your pocket. Get in the habit of doing this every day. One thing all happy people have in common is that they feel in control of their lives.

10. Go to bed before 10:00 P.M. tonight and sleep until at least 6:00 A.M. tomorrow. Repeat for the next 7 days. Being happy is often as simple as being well-rested.

11. Imagine that the plane crash took Barbra Streisand and Celine Dion instead of Buddy Holly and the Big Bopper.

12. Picture all of your co-workers naked. Okay, not all of them. Maybe just two.

Worcester. "Every other commercial has people singing and dancing, as though that's the way everyone lives." Against such a yardstick, even mild happiness can seem negative.

A BLURRY GRAY ZONE

Dysthymia isn't something you typically can conquer on your own. Although it's relatively easy to treat with the right kind of professional help, it's very difficult to recognize and manage by yourself. Unlike classic, overt depression, which barges into life and usually lasts between 1 and 2 years, dysthymia sneaks in and lingers for 10 to 20 years, says Dr. Shelton. In some instances, it never goes away. Although it does not always lead to more serious depression, he says that under stressful circumstances it makes depressive episodes more likely to occur. In fact, it's usually when a person seeks help for one of these episodes that the underlying dysthymia is detected.

Unfortunately, when men do muster the courage to seek help, their trouble isn't always pinpointed. One study found that 67 percent of overtly and covertly depressed men were misdiagnosed by their doctors. William Pollack, Ph.D., director of the Center for Men and Young Men at McLean Hospital/Harvard Medical School, blames this on biased assessment criteria that miss common male symptoms ("Women get weepy, men get busy") and on stubborn macho stereotypes that incline physicians to prescribe fortitude rather than psychiatric care.

Real's theory, drawn from more than 20 years of practicing family therapy, is that men cope with covert depression by masking its symptoms. Typically, they use work, exercise, spending, and drinking. Because it's considered unmanly to admit sadness, Real says, men try to distract themselves from it with behaviors that bolster self-esteem.

"The less time I have to think about how I feel, the better," says Dennis, the regional vice president. "So I keep busy and immerse myself in my work. The more down I feel, the harder I drive myself."

"I go to the gym," says Andrew. "Exercise makes me feel dramatically better and gives me a sense that I can control my mood."

Coping strategies such as these are effective in the short term, but they eventually backfire, says Real. Either the behavior itself becomes addictive and destructive (alcoholism, bankruptcy) or one of the crutches unexpectedly snaps (athletic injury, loss of job). With no support left for the ego, overt depression can result.

The danger of masking persistent feelings of unhappiness is that it can become life-threatening. According to Dr. Shelton, suicide rates for long-term covert depression and short-term overt depression are similar (about 10 percent of untreated cases).

The thought of suicide is what finally prompted Braun, the 43-year-old author, to recognize and treat his dysthymia. "I was driving along one evening, and I had this sudden feeling of pointlessness," he recalls. "I had no reason to be sad. And yet, I had this powerful sense of meaninglessness. And as I eased onto the exit ramp, a black thought bubbled up: I could just kill myself. That's when I knew something was wrong."

Braun sought psychiatric help, experimented with various antidepressants, and eventually came to an important realization. "Mood disorders are like an eclipse. The center is totally black, then there is a much bigger area, a penumbra, around that black center. If the center is depression, then that surrounding area is dysthymia. The tricky thing is, there's no sharp boundary between normal and dysthymic. It's a blurry, gray zone."

THIS WAY OUT

If you've read this far, you're probably either nodding your head in self-recognition or thinking of someone you know who has all these symptoms. The problem is, the way out of dysthymia can be just as labyrinthine as the way in. Here's where to begin.

Take a quick emotional inventory. As we've seen, men often cover up their depression by working longer, training harder, or drinking lots of beer. If you find yourself constantly doing one of these and not deriving any pleasure from it, there could be an underlying problem, says Pollack.

Find someone to spill your guts to. If your wife or girlfriend is the supportive type—meaning she's not the kind who'll either (a) tell you to grow up or (b) blame herself—she can probably help. But you should also seek out men whose integrity you trust. You just might find someone who's feeling exactly the same way.

Define what has real meaning for you. Write down three goals you'd like to realize by this time next year. But here's the catch: Don't make them materialistic. Not a higher salary, not a nicer car, not a boob job for the missus. Instead, stay away from fickle, performance-based self-esteem and pick three goals with inherent meaning, such as spending more time with your kids, getting to know your parents better before they die, or developing a closer relationship with your wife.

Get help if you need it. Eighty percent of people who are treated for depression, regardless of type, report substantial relief. "I've had men say to me, 'I can't believe I lived my whole life that way,'" says Real. "They never knew what being happy felt like." The best treatment, studies show, is a mix of psychotherapy and antidepressants.

PERCENTAGE OF AMERICANS WHO ADMIT THAT THEY TALK TO THEIR CARS: 68

Real says men require a different kind of therapy than women—not the sappy, stereotypical, "tell me everything you're feeling" brand but a more dynamic, opinionated style of coaching. To find a therapist like this, he recommends interviewing candidates. Call around and ask two questions: Do you have experience helping men reconnect, and do you have an active or passive style? And demand progress. "If you're in therapy for 6 months and you feel 5 percent better, that's not good enough," he says.

Speak to your doctor about St. John's wort. Some claim that this herb is useful for treating depression. Studies are not conclusive, but side effects are

IT COULD BE WORSE . . .
You Could Be This Guy

Bob Lozier of New Canada, Maine, awoke early one morning to find that an 800- to 900-pound rutting bull moose had demolished his 1998 Oldsmobile Aurora. Twisted metal, broken glass, blood, hair, and "moose fluid" were everywhere. The horny bull also tried copulating with the decorative pillars in front of his house, resulting in sizable damage and more telltale "moose fluid." Lozier slept through the entire incident.

Aaron Caudill, 28, of Morehead, Ohio, talked his girlfriend into performing oral sex on him in a photo booth at Paramount's Kings Island family amusement park. What he didn't know was that a monitor outside the booth publicly displayed the images being taken, which quickly attracted a curious crowd of kids and their parents. When he realized what was happening, Caudill jumped out of the booth and tried covering the monitor with his hands. The couple was arrested and charged with public indecency. Caudill, who had been hoping to land a teaching job after recently graduating from college, suddenly found work a little hard to come by. He and his friend were later sentenced to 80 hours of community service.

Nathaniel Bradley, 82, of Tabor City, North Carolina, was robbed of $3,000 by a 27-year-old woman who asked to use his phone, stripped naked, then demanded sex. "I said, 'Listen, girl, I'm 82 years old. I'm not having no sex,'" Bradley told police. Disappointment evidently turned to anger as she grabbed the money and fled.

Or one of these lucky guys who stepped into infamy by becoming recipients of the Darwin Awards (www.darwinawards.com):

Khay Rahnajet, a dimwitted Iraqi terrorist, didn't pay enough postage on a letter bomb. It came back with "return to sender" stamped on it. Forgetting it was a bomb, he opened it and was killed in the resulting explosion.

Antonio Mendoza, an attorney from La Grange, Georgia, had to have a cell phone surgically removed from his rectum. "My dog drags the thing all over the house," he explained. "He must have dragged it into the shower. I slipped on the tile, tripped against the dog, and sat down right on the thing." The operation, which took more than 3 hours, was complicated by the phone cover's having opened slightly after insertion. It also rang three times during surgery.

Martyn Eskins of Elyria, Ohio, thought he'd quickly eradicate the cobwebs in his basement by using a propane torch instead of a broom. The resulting fire burned the first and second floors of his home.

minor, so it may be a good first step for those hesitant to take antidepressants. Clinical psychologist Frank Dattilio, Ph.D., of the University of Pennsylvania School of Medicine in Philadelphia, points out that you need to take it for 2 to 4 weeks (300 milligram doses three times daily) before you see any improvement.

Don't be afraid of antidepressants. Most of the men we spoke to were hesitant about resorting to drugs, but Real says they're worth a shot. "This isn't heroin," he says. "If you try it and either it doesn't do much for you or the side effects are awful, then stop. But at least you'll have given it a try."

Stay challenged. Men are not maintainers, we are builders. (That's why vacuuming holds no allure for us.) We are happiest when we're creating something—a career, a home, a family. Make sure there's always a project on your workbench, something new you're trying to accomplish.

"Here's my best advice, as someone who's been through it," says Braun. "First, do everything you can to eliminate stress and conflict in your life. If you have a bad relationship, try to make it better. Second, if you're still not feeling very good, then get yourself to a doctor. But don't just accept the first drug he gives you. Try different ones. Be open to the idea that happiness can have something to do with chemistry."

"Men like these often see themselves as inadequate or as losers," concludes Real. "But I consider them pioneers. Their unhappiness is not a personal failing but a thirst. By their very dissatisfaction, they're saying the old male roles no longer work. They're eventually going to help us move beyond those old ideas to healthier values. In that respect, I think they're heroes."

Find a Good Challenge

It's time to bust out of a rut

**From *The* Men's Health *Longevity Program* (Rodale)
by the editors of *Men's Health* Books**

Get out a pad of paper, and make two lists. In the first list, itemize all the things you have always been curious about or interested in knowing more of but have never gotten around to studying. Perhaps you're fascinated with dinosaurs or the Civil War or the writings of Ernest Hemingway or how to cook a good Chinese meal or how to play the saxophone.

In the second list, include all the physical feats you have always fantasized about but have never gotten around to doing. Maybe you dream about running a 10-K race or biking 100 miles or taking up skiing or bench-pressing your weight or climbing a 12,000-foot mountain.

Pick the one item from each list that appeals the most to you. Grab a calendar. Figure out what the date will be 6 months from today. Mark your calendar: That's the date by which you'll complete the easier of the two tasks. Go 3 months farther, and mark the date by which you will complete the second item.

Figure out exactly what it will take to fulfill these goals. Convince yourself that you are going to do it. You *will* do it. Tell your wife, your kids, whomever that you are going to do it. By telling someone, you make the goal even more real. Now, get started. And don't look back.

Riddle for the day: What do a herd of cows, a life without challenge, and poet Robert Frost have in common?

Answer: They choose a path each day.

Cattle follow the same route through the pasture, day in and day out, until they wear a groove in the grass. The familiar path is comforting, easy to follow, and not at all taxing on what little brains they have.

When our lives take predictable patterns—get up, work, exercise on the treadmill, eat supper, read the paper, sleep, get up, and so on—we can wear a groove right through the calendar. When we live that way, the rut we make in our lives isn't too different from that cow path.

As for Robert Frost, well, you knew this was coming: He wrote the poem "The Road Not Taken," in which the narrator looks at two roads leading into the woods and decides to head down the less-used route. "And that has made all the difference," he concludes.

Frost knew all about choosing a challenge. After dropping out of Dartmouth and Harvard, he wound up teaching and working on a poultry farm in New Hampshire. He tried to get publishers interested in his poetry, but found little success.

At the age of 38, he faced a momentous decision. He could head into middle age with his chickens. Or he could sell the farm, pack up his stack of unpublished poetry, and head to London with his wife and four kids to look for a more receptive audience. He followed the uncertain path, won four Pulitzer Prizes, became his country's unofficial poet laureate, and got to read his work at the inauguration of President John F. Kennedy.

We're certainly not telling you to chuck your job and write poetry (unless that's what you really want to do), but you should find a challenge each

PERCENTAGE OF AMERICANS WHO SAID THEY WERE IN A GOOD MOOD WHEN ASKED BY RESEARCHERS: 83

PERCENTAGE OF AMERICANS WITH ANNUAL INCOMES BELOW $20,000 WHO RESPONDED THIS WAY: 72

ROCK AROUND THE TIME CLOCK

As you seek new experiences from day to day, don't forget to challenge yourself in those 8-hour chunks of time that you call work. John Sena, Ph.D, coauthor of *Work Is Not a Four-Letter Word*, offers a few pointers on giving your job a jolt.

• Though it may sound like a bad idea to volunteer for more work, ask to cover some of a co-worker's tasks when he's out of the office. It can shake up your normal routine—and it may actually make you glad that you have *your* job and not the other guy's.

• Watch for unaddressed problems at the office and think of solutions. Ask for assignments that can teach you new skills.

• When you hit a lull during the day, read a professional magazine, journal, or other material relating to your work. You'll get a break from your normal tasks, and you may even learn the latest news before your boss does.

and every day that gives you a new reason to jump out of bed in the morning, whether you are starting a family and career or enjoying retirement. The daily gauntlets that you throw down for yourself will keep your mind and body honed to a razor's edge and can protect your health, happiness, and sanity.

DRIVE YOUR TRAIN OF THOUGHT OFF THE TRACKS

Imagine the blizzard of the century descending upon your town, covering the roads with 3 feet of snow and trapping you in your home. For days, you'd eat the same foods, breathe the same air, and stare lethargically at the same wallpaper. After enough time deprived of new stimulation, you'd likely fall prey to cabin fever.

That same process can happen to your life—no blizzard needed—when you slip into an easy yet mind-numbing routine. One year passes, then another. You get the hang of it; it feels good. No, not good, exactly. It feels *comfortable*. Decades pass. But your life remains at a sort of standstill. "The longer one is in a particular position or lifestyle, the more likely it is that the lifestyle or position will become habit," says psychologist David Abramis, Ph.D., of California State University, Long Beach. "And once something is habitual, it's harder to change."

But sometimes, a guy wakes up one morning and wonders what he's been doing all this time (it happens at a certain age). By golly, he'd better start living! But he ain't no Robert Frost. Instead of finding an outlet in poetry, he decides he needs a girlfriend, a red sports car, and an earring, in no particular order. When he gets it all out of his system, our guy can be left looking at a broken family, an empty savings account, and a sheepish face in the mirror.

Let's be clear: The idea is to shake up your routine before you hit the extremes of either falling into a slumber or feeling the need to turn your whole life on its ear. "You should be mixing time spent doing comforting, familiar things with time spent sprinkling in challenging new things," says Powell Lawton, Ph.D., senior research scientist at the Polisher Institute of the Philadelphia Geriatric Center. "It doesn't take a whole lot of zestful sprinklings to make life interesting."

Challenges do more than add a shot of jalapeño pepper to a bland burrito of a life. Research has shown that people who throw themselves into new activities often have better problem-solving skills.

Novel adventures can also keep your mind and body from deteriorating as you age. Challenges trigger the release of endorphins and other brain chemicals that lift your mood. And mastering new skills—from learning a musical instrument to solving crossword puzzles—strengthens your brain by encouraging cells to make new connections.

THE WAY TO CHANGE

Think about what you did the past 5 Saturday nights. If you can't remember or you did the same thing all 5 nights, you may be slipping into a rut, suggests Sidney B. Simon, Ed.D., author of *Getting Unstuck: Breaking Through the Barriers to Change*. You can attack your complacency with several different approaches: physical, over-the-top physical, and mental and creative.

Physical. A good place to start challenging your regular routine is at the gym. If you regularly do one exercise—running, for instance—a mix of sports can give you the cross-training you need to avoid injury and keep from burning out. Toss in activities that use different body parts, such as using a rowing machine for your arms, bicycling for your legs, or swimming for everything. If you normally do just aerobic workouts, throw in some weight training. If you're a dedicated lifter, mix in some lung-busting aerobic exercise.

Of course, you don't have to make exercise a solitary pursuit. Join a martial arts class to build your coordination, focus, and ability to kick someone in

NUMBER OF VACATION DAYS THE AVERAGE GUY GETS EACH YEAR: 13.5

NUMBER OF VACATION DAYS HE ACTUALLY TAKES: 5.5

PERCENTAGE OF AMERICANS WHO CHECK IN WITH THEIR OFFICES WHILE ON VACATION: 96

the head. Hook up with a running club and make plans to run in a 10-K. Join a sporting league at your workplace, or ask about adult team sports at your local YMCA, chamber of commerce, or university.

Over-the-top physical. The next time you flip through the channels and secretly admire the young, facially pierced lunatics who put their butts on the line by rock climbing, skateboarding, and leaping from planes on snowboards, remember that you're never too grizzled to get up and join them. Here are some cases in point.

- "Banana" George Blair still water-skis in his mid-80s—barefoot. Sometimes he does it with the tow rope clenched between his teeth. He learned to ski like this when he was 46. Oh, he skydives and snowboards, too.
- Sam Gadless's 92-year-old legs hauled him across the finish line of the New York City Marathon in a little less than $8\frac{1}{2}$ hours. He might have run it even faster if he hadn't lost several weeks of training time after being hit by a car. He plans to be the oldest man ever to finish the race when he runs it again at the age of ripe, old 94.
- Earl V. Shaffer hoofed the whole Appalachian Trail, which spans more than 2,000 miles between Georgia and Maine, at the age of 29. But that wasn't the really impressive part. He did it again 50 years later, when he was 79.

If you don't know where to go to find high adventure, you may want to consider Outward Bound, a nonprofit educational adventure group. This program offers courses like backpacking, rock climbing, sailing, and other outdoor activities. While they design the activities with an eye on safety, you're expected to join in the challenges. We know a veterinarian in his mid-50s who ended his trip with a mile-long swim through the choppy Atlantic. At the beginning, it was everything he disliked. At the end, he knew he was ready for more challenges. Check out www.outwardbound.com.

Mental and creative. When you think back on your education, which teachers captured your attention? The ones who shuffled you and your bored classmates through repetitive drills and fact-memorizing sessions? Or the ones who taught physics with wind-up toys and covered medieval literature by explaining the bawdier parts of *The Canterbury Tales*?

Now that you're an adult, you can choose to take only the classes that fire up your brain with cool and unusual challenges. Here are the kinds of evening courses that community colleges around the country are offering these days: "Acupressure Self-Care," "Secrets of the Wolf," "Basic Car Repair," "Starting an Investment Club," and "Be a Home Builder or Learn to Hire One." Pick up a course catalog from a university, community college, or extension campus in your area to see if they have anything that strikes your interest.

STARTING EASY

Sometimes, before you can face up to a big new challenge, you need to ramp up with some small ones. Here are simple, seemingly unimportant things you can do on any given day that can put you on the path to grander changes and goals.

• When you leave work, head in the opposite direction from your usual route. Find your way home while driving on as few of the roads that you normally use as possible.

• Go to the gym and do only unfamiliar exercises. Join a kickboxing or abdominal-workout class, or hop on that thigh-strengthening machine that you've never seen a guy use. Or ask a trainer for his favorite exercises and instructions on doing them right.

• Pick up an international magazine and read it from cover to cover, or find a foreign-language cable station and watch it for 15 minutes. Even if you have little idea what's going on, you can see what people in other cultures find interesting and entertaining. At worst, you might find a destination for your next big vacation.

• Go to an ethnic restaurant that you've never before tried. Ask the waiter to select an array of dishes that represents the best of the chef's work. If you want to keep it inexpensive, limit the choices to appetizers, soups, and salads.

• Go online to see if you can track down classmates from high school. When you succeed, send an e-mail telling them how great your life is.

You could also spend your spare time learning a creative skill that would impress your friends, like painting a life-size oil portrait of the Three Stooges, cooking a skillet of Thai chicken, or picking up a guitar at a party and wowing the crowd with a little Aerosmith.

Think these creative endeavors are beyond you? Maybe they are. But if you don't try, you'll never know. While we tend to think that only a gifted few have creative gifts like these, most of us have some degree of artistic abilities—we just need to develop them, says psychology professor Dean Keith Simonton, Ph.D., of the University of California, Davis.

Check out the art, music, cooking, and drama opportunities that your local educational centers and art councils offer. And don't forget that your odds of meeting a nude model jump much higher when you're in an art class.

KNOW THIS

Nod Off the Road

A late night at work can impair your senses as much as drinking a couple of shots. Researchers at the Environmental and Occupational Health Research Center in New Zealand examined a group of 39 people, forcing some to stay awake for 28 hours and others to get drunk. "After about 18 hours of being awake, the subjects' mental and physical skills were impaired as much as when they had drunk two or three glasses of wine," says Anne-Marie Feyer, Ph.D., one of the researchers.

The Downside of Anger

A study at Ohio State University suggests that there is a link between hostility and the chemical homocysteine—both thought to promote heart disease. Researchers found a compelling correlation between levels of hostility and homocysteine in 64 healthy people. High levels of the chemical may damage the inside of arterial walls, leading to plaque formation. Catherine Stoney, coauthor of the study, believes that hostility and stress temporarily elevate homocysteine.

We know, you just read about the benefits of anger on page 192. Here's how to be hostile *and* healthy: Add beans, spinach, and orange juice to your diet. They contain folic acid, which helps control homocysteine levels.

Feel Bad for Bullies

The meatbag who gave you daily wedgies in high school probably had bigger problems besides bad teeth and illegitimate siblings. Researchers in Finland studied 16,410 kids ages 14 to 16 and found that bullies have higher rates of depression and suicidal thoughts than other kids. So you can forget about ripping off his toupee at the reunion: He probably won't even show.

NUMBER OF TIMES
THE AVERAGE GUY CALLS IN SICK EACH YEAR: 4.7

Does Juicy Fruit Make You Smarter?

Forget to wear pants to work again? Chew gum, say some Japanese scientists who found that gum chewing may boost brainpower and in turn reduce memory loss. So why were those Bazooka Joe comics way over our heads?

Cool Anxiety Relief

According to recent news reports, some Germans are paying big bucks to spend a couple of minutes pretending they're Thanksgiving turkeys: sitting in a freezer—naked. Wearing only gloves, slippers, and bandages to cover frost-bite-prone spots (the wimps), they chill out for 1 to 3 minutes in a $-166°F$ freezer and claim that this reduces their stress. Turns out their idea isn't all that far-fetched, says Kathy Birkner, Ph.D., of the Pain and Stress Center in San Antonio. Cold temperatures increase the level of serotonin in the brain, making you feel calmer. A simpler way to cool down: Put an ice pack wrapped in a towel on the back of your neck for 15 minutes.

DOWN THE PIKE

What's Manly Also Keeps You Sharp

Researchers at Rockefeller University in New York City believe that testosterone supplements may eventually help prevent Alzheimer's disease. Their study, published in the *Proceedings of the National Academy of Sciences*, found that extra testosterone added to nerve cells inhibited the process of plaque formation in the brain. The testosterone appears to curtail the enzymes that form the beta-amyloid protein that creates the plaques, says study author Paul Greengard, Ph.D. Previous studies have shown that supplements of estrogen may help prevent the onset of Alzheimer's disease in women. Researchers have not yet begun testing their findings in animals, and Greengard cautions that it may be years before the testosterone supplementation is approved for Alzheimer's patients.

A Feel-Good Device?

Twenty U.S. medical centers are testing a brain implant called the Vargus Nerve Stimulator that may help patients manage previously untreatable cases of depression. The implant sends electrical pulses into the brain stem, stimulating activity and increasing bloodflow to areas known to regulate depressive symptoms.

Safer St. John's Wort on the Way

Nature's Prozac is about to become safer. The antidepressant herb has been thought to prevent antibiotics from working. Now researchers in the United States and the United Kingdom are hoping to engineer a new form that will be able to calm depression without interfering with other drugs.

PERCENTAGE OF ADULTS WHO SAY THEY'RE SO SLEEPY DURING THE DAY THAT IT INTERFERES WITH DAILY ACTIVITIES AT LEAST A FEW DAYS A MONTH: 43

DOES IT WORK?

Covert Ops Fantasy Spy Camp

Most fantasy camps are just an expensive excuse for overweight 50-year-old men to toss baseballs to even-more-overweight ex-ballplayers. Now there's a camp for men who wish they were spies instead of shortstops. At the Covert Ops fantasy spy camp in an Arizona desert, guys pay $7,000 for 6 days (or $3,800 for a weekend) to learn how to shoot, drive, and fight like a spy. They even stage a mock hostage rescue and are tagged with a code name! You could call (800) 644-7382 to book a trip. Or you could just rip up this page and eat it.

Sweat Solutions

Whether you're giving a speech or making off with the company copier, excessive sweating usually means that your nervous system is revved up. And your palms may be getting stuck with the wet part of the fight-or-flight response. We rate the solutions.

The pseudo-solution. Practitioners of Eastern medicine say that compresses of walnut and sage leaves may relieve symptoms. Downside: Like Judd Nelson, this remedy rarely works.

The quick solution. Try some antiperspirant on your palms before any big moment. The aluminum chloride in antiperspirant thickens the sweat pouring out of the sweat ducts and plugs them up with thousands of gooey corks. Downside: It's only a temporary fix.

The drug solution. Glycopyrrolate—a drug used during anesthesia to ensure a regular heartbeat—is often prescribed to control sweaty hands. Downside: One of the side effects is dry mouth, which is okay if you drool, too.

The drastic solution. A surgical procedure called endoscopic thoracic sympathectomy can fix your hands permanently. Downside: Besides the estimated $8,000 price tag that insurance usually won't cover, there's also the unpleasant side effect of compensatory sweating in your groin.

COOL STUFF

Valerian Value

Leave the sleeping pills for troubled former child stars; you're better off popping the herb valerian. "It improves the quality of sleep without the morning grogginess you get from sleeping pills," says pharmacologist Norman Farnsworth, Ph.D., of the University of Illinois in Chicago. Before you start, here's how to get the most out of it.

Take it for 2 weeks. You can't take valerian for 1 night and expect results. "It needs to be taken until it builds up to a certain level in the blood," says Eric Heiligenstein, M.D., clinical director of psychiatric services at the University of Wisconsin at Madison. The nightly dosage should be between 150 and 300 milligrams.

Buy the cheap kind. Avoid the more expensive valerian supplements that have additional ingredients or herbs. There's no research showing they'll improve your sleep, and some may actually prevent your body from absorbing the valerian.

Use "valerian root," not "valernic acid." Some manufacturers make each capsule or tablet with the same amount of valernic acid—the compound they believe is responsible for the herb's sleep-inducing powers. But researchers don't know yet if it has any sedative effect separate from the rest of the herb.

Surgical Preview

Tune in to The Learning Channel if you're scheduled for surgery. A recent Austrian study of 100 people showed that patients had less stress—and needed less postsurgery pain medication—if they watched a video of a similar surgery before their own. Seeing how procedures work helps patients better cope with the surgery, says lead study author Stephan Doering, M.D.

NUMBER OF TIMES THE AVERAGE GUY WILL GET FIRED: 2

NUMBER OF TIMES HE'LL QUIT: 9

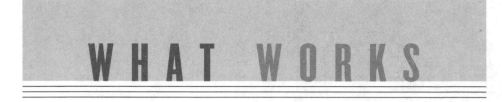

WHAT WORKS

America has a new favorite pastime: watching contestants match wits on such game shows as *Who Wants to Be a Millionaire?* and *The Weakest Link*. What does our latest fascination with these prime-time puzzlers say about us? The smart kid in the class is no longer the nerd. And what makes him smart? That's right: He knows when to use a lifeline.

Consider the following pages your lifeline to boosting brainpower. These tips will keep you mentally sharp, help you outwit your opponents in life, and reduce the stress and fatigue that cause brain fog. They'll position you ahead in today's man-outsmart-game-show world so that when you give Regis your final answer, you can be confident it's the right one.

I. For starters, quit watching those game shows. There's a good reason the TV is called the boob tube, and it has nothing to do with breasts. Researchers at Kansas State University, Manhattan, found that people who watched just 15 minutes of television had diminished brain-wave activity, an indication that their minds were turning off. How else could you sit through a rerun of *Eight Is Enough?*

"For the most part, the images on that screen just flow through you without enhancing your life," says *Smart for Life* author Michael Chafetz, Ph.D. He recommends making at least 1 night a week a no-television night. That might be a good time to take a night class.

2. Consider the waffle cone. Ask yourself, "What could the world really use right now?" Posing this question may just lead your innate sense of inventiveness to new creations, says Harvard University psychology professor Ellen J. Langer, Ph.D. Quickly write down a whole host of ideas. Don't prejudge them, just get them down on paper. From there, you can branch off into different directions.

Sometimes, a great idea is simply an old idea turned on its head. For example, ice cream was once served on top of a flat waffle. Some confectionery genius got the idea to fold that waffle into a funnel and, bingo, the waffle cone was born.

3. Pour your drink down the sink. Since alcohol can easily get between your mind and the information you want to remember, you should cut back on drinking if you're having trouble with your memory. While we still don't know the exact effects that just a few drinks a day have on your recall, drinking until you're tipsy definitely puts you at risk for memory loss, says Barry Gordon, M.D., Ph.D., author of *Memory: Remembering and Forgetting in Everyday Life*.

4. Learn to handle information overload. If you have trouble remembering information because torrents of it pour on you from all directions, try this exercise a few times a week. Read a book with the volume on a nearby television turned up. Put the book down and watch TV for several minutes. Then, read the book some more. After 10 minutes of switching your attention, turn off the TV, put down the book, and see how much you remember from each source, say Houston neuropsychologist Fran Pirozzolo, Ph.D. Gradually, your ability to tune out distractions should improve.

5. Practice your math skills. It wasn't that long ago that you did math problems either in your head or with a slide rule. Then came cheap calculators, and now you're lucky if you can count your toes. When you're at the cash register, make a game of figuring out the change you're due before the clerk punches the sale button. Balance your checkbook in your head. Check it with a calculator afterward until you're sure of yourself. "If you use a calculator every time you have to add three numbers together, your mental abilities are going to suffer," says Thomas Crook, Ph.D., director of Memory Assessment Clinics in Scottsdale, Arizona.

6. Give your memory a workout. You can keep your memory strong by memorizing lists whenever possible instead of writing them down, says psychology professor Alan S. Brown, Ph.D., of Southern Methodist University in Dallas. While helpful, a written list can be a crutch that reduces your ability to remember information. The next time you make a grocery list, leave several items off and try to keep track of them in your head.

7. And test it. How much of the stuff that you learn will you retain? Test yourself with this quick-and-easy peek into your memory capacity. Read over this list for 1 minute, then try to recall as many of the 10 words as you can.

Pickle
Mailbox
Artist
Lipstick
Button
Shovel
Table
Engine
Balloon
Nickel

AMOUNT OF TIME THE AVERAGE GUY SLEEPS ON A WORK NIGHT: 6.9 HOURS
AMOUNT OF TIME THE AVERAGE GUY NAPS ON THE JOB EACH WEEK: 1 HOUR, 7 MINUTES

The average number remembered for each age group is eight or nine for people up to age 30, seven or eight for those 30 to 39, six or seven for those 40 to 49, five or six for those 60 to 69, and four or five for those 70 or older.

If you did better than average for your age group, great. We'll look for you at the blackjack table in Vegas, next to Rainman. If you didn't do better than average, don't panic. There's great variability in how people perform on memory tests. If you totally bombed, see your doctor to rule out any organic problems.

8. Sleep solo, sleep better. When you really need to get a good night's sleep, head for the couch. A recent study shows that people sleep more restfully when they sleep alone. Researchers at Loughborough University in Leicestershire, United Kingdom, monitored sleep in 46 couples for 8 nights by fitting each participant with a wristwatchlike device that measures body movement. Half of all movements by one partner triggered a movement by the other within 30 seconds. The conclusion: Sleeping alone elicits a more peaceful sleep. Other findings:

- Men move around more than women during sleep.
- Older couples were less disturbed by their mates' activity than younger couples, suggesting that one gets used to his partner's movements during sleep.
- People whose partners were away for a night went to bed earlier and slept longer and more peacefully. Despite this evidence, most couples claimed they slept better with their partners than without them.

9. Schedule wake-up calls for 7:22 A.M. People who wake up earlier than that have higher levels of the stress hormone cortisol all day, according to researchers at Westminster University in London. The early risers complained of worse moods and more headaches than the later wakers.

10. Enforce Eastern Standard Time. If you're traveling within the United States for only a few days, maintain your normal sleeping schedule—you won't have to readjust your body's internal clock. Going overseas? Arrive in the morning—seeing the sun will help you reset your body clock to local time.

11. Declare Monday a decision-making holiday. Making tough judgments after a weekend of relaxation is not only bad policy—Monday is the least productive day of the workweek—but also risky since Monday is when you're statistically most likely to have a heart attack. Push off the big decisions until Tuesday—your brain will be sharper and your body better able to cope with the stress.

12. Personalize your workspace. Decorate your office space with a few personal items—books you love, family photos, souvenirs from vacations to the Antarctic.

"It will give you a sense of place and a feeling of security and ownership," says architect Peter Juanpere, who designs executive offices for Intec Group.

Also, create separate areas for working, holding meetings, and reading. And consider installing an aquarium—water is soothing.

13. Beat office enemies. They're a fact of business life. Here's what to do about 'em.

Your enemy: The back-slapping, loudmouthed, howyadoin' phony who drives you nuts because he plays himself up as he knocks you down.

Your tactic: Press him for specifics in front of the boss. These fellows talk a lot—but don't have the information to back it up. He'll fumble for answers when you ask nonconfrontational questions like "How much?" "How'd you do that?" or "What did the client say?"

Your enemy: The boss's secretary and gatekeeper who makes your life hell because she can.

Your tactic: Take her to lunch. It's old-fashioned, but hey, it works, because ultimately she just wants to be liked. One simple gesture can buy you a trouble-free 6 months.

Your enemy: The boss who continually steals your ideas and takes credit for your work.

Your tactic: When it's your turn to talk about the project, say subtle things like "I appreciate how much Bob helped me on the project." It gives the boss the credit he's craving but still tells the whole group who did all the work.

Your enemy: The two-faced woman who trashes your boss to you, then trashes you to the boss over drinks.

Your tactic: Confront her by asking, "I heard you had a problem. What exactly was it?" She'll deny the remarks, but don't brawl or you'll look like the bad guy. Consider your confrontation a warning so that she'll pick on someone else. And don't bitch to your boss to clear your name; you'll look defensive and paranoid.

Your enemy: The woman in accounting you had a fling with, who now hates you because you ended it.

Your tactic: Talk to her more than ever, says Paula Ann Hughes, dean of the graduate school of management at the University of Dallas. If you ignore her, you'll just upset her even more. You can cut down on office buzz—and risk of a harassment suit—by maintaining a decent relationship with her.

PERCENTAGE OF MEN WHO SAY THEY READ THE BIBLE EVERY DAY: 29

ANY QUESTIONS?

Early Riser

I often wake up in the middle of the night and have trouble falling asleep again. Is it better to toss and turn, or just get up and start the day?

—D. C., New York City

If it's more than a couple of hours before the alarm, try to get back to sleep, says William Kohler, M.D., medical director of the sleep center at St. Vincent Hospital in Billings, Montana. If you're still awake after 20 minutes, get out of bed and do something that bores you. (We suggest needlepoint or reading Gore Vidal.) Go back to bed when you feel tired. But if you wake up at 6:00 A.M. instead of 7:00, just hit the showers and get on with your day—there's not enough time to dip back into deep sleep. Note: If you're doing this all the time, talk to your doctor. This is a common symptom of depression.

Sleep Light

What can I do to train my body to need just 4 to 6 hours of sleep?

—B. D., San Francisco

Unless you're trying to inflict medieval torture on yourself, it's not a good idea to cut down on shut-eye. You may be able to shorten sleep for a few weeks, but you won't be able to live by it permanently.

Seven to 8 hours of sleep a night fuels peak mental performance. Anything less can lead to a weakened immune system, stress risks, and increased aging. When you have a late night, compensate with an extra hour or two of sleep the next night. For the follow-up night, it's best to allow yourself to wake up naturally, rather than set the alarm: Your body will judge how much catch-up rest you need.

PERCENTAGE OF PEOPLE WHO GRIND THEIR TEETH WHEN THEY SLEEP: 8

PART SEVEN
GET BETTER FAST

MUST READS

All Your Symptoms Explained

We know your symptoms. We've had most of them (this week). So follow along as we help you tell the doctor precisely what's wrong

By Rebecca Kleinwaks

When you go to the mechanic, you talk mechanic language. You say your engine has a ping, a sputter, a rattle, or a grrrrch. Then you beg the guy not to steal all your money. We say, do the same thing when you go to the doctor. We asked a bunch of M.D.'s how to describe symptoms so they'll know what the hell you're talking about.

CHEST
"Deep, Aching Pain, and Pressure Like I'm Wearing a Heavy X-Ray Vest. My Left Arm Feels as if It's Fallen Asleep."
Possible problem: A heart attack. A blocked artery has cut off blood to your heart. Chew an aspirin tablet and call 911. The aspirin will prevent a fatal clot; chewing it will make it work faster, says Richard A. Stein, M.D., a spokesman for the American Heart Association. Don't wait to see if it works before calling an ambulance.

"It Hurts to Breathe, as if I Were Stuck at the Bottom of a Dogpile."
Possible problem: Asthma. Smoke or some other trigger has caused your airways to swell and the muscles to contract around them, making it hard to breathe. Grab a cup of coffee on the way to the doctor. The caffeine will open your bronchial passages by relaxing the muscles that surround them.

"Burning Pain behind My Sternum, as though I'd Barfed and It Only Came Halfway Up."
Possible problem: Acid reflux. The muscle that lets food into your stomach and keeps acid from leaving has improperly opened, allowing gastric juice to shoot into your esophagus. Pick up a pack of Juicy Fruit—gum helps you produce saliva, your body's version of Pepto-Bismol. And stay away from peppermint, which aggravates the condition. See your doctor if you suffer frequently, since chronic reflux can be a sign of esophageal cancer.

STOMACH
"A Wicked Stitch in My Right Side That's Getting Worse. Some Jabs Take My Breath Away."

Possible problem: Appendicitis. A virus has infected your digestive tract, causing inflammation; or the tube connecting the large intestine and the appendix is blocked by trapped stool. See a doctor—the only treatment is surgical removal. But before you get there, avoid taking painkillers or laxatives. Aspirin or acetaminophen can mask your symptoms, and laxatives can create pressure in the digestive tract, bursting the appendix.

"A Burning in My Gut, as if I'd Swallowed a Lit Cigarette."

Possible problem: A peptic ulcer. H. pylori bacteria or overuse of anti-inflammatory drugs has created a hole in your stomach lining that's irritated by stomach acid. Don't drink milk to soothe the pain. It contains proteins that stimulate acid secretion. Eat a piece of bread instead, to sop up excess acid. And see your doctor. Antibiotics can permanently cure 80 to 90 percent of peptic ulcers.

"Sharp, Pinpoint Pain 6 Inches above My Belly Button."

Possible problem: Gallstones. Little rocks of bile are created by excess cholesterol in your gallbladder. See a doctor to decide on drug treatment or surgery.

HEAD
"My Head Feels like an Enormous Lemon That's Being Squeezed."

Possible problem: A tension headache. Stress or fatigue has caused blood vessels in your temples to constrict. Hit the gym. Exercise increases scrotonin, a neurotransmitter that research shows dampens pain.

"Intense Pain along My Eyebrows That Gets Worse When I Lean Forward."

Possible problem: Sinusitis. An infection has caused nasal membranes to swell, trapping mucus in the sinuses over your eyes. When you lean forward, the added pressure increases the pain. Place a hot, wet washcloth over your eyes and cheekbones, and take a decongestant. The moist heat will shrink the swelling and promote drainage. Keep a hankie nearby.

"Intense Pain on One Side of My Head. I'm Nauseated. Beams of Light Feel like Needles in My Eyes."

Possible problem: A migraine headache. Blood vessels outside your skull are dilating and swelling. Put one hand in a bucket of ice water, make a fist, and swirl it around. We're not kidding. This will cause the dilated vessels to constrict, easing the pain, says neurologist Egilius Spierings, M.D., of Wellesley Hills, Massachusetts. If you get migraines frequently, see a doctor for a prescription.

PENIS
"When I Pee, It Feels as if I Were Passing a Golf Ball."
Possible problem: Enlarged prostate. As the prostate grows (it happens to many men if they live long enough), it compresses the urethra, the tube through which urine passes. The result is the same as when you step on a garden hose. Talk to your doctor about taking a saw-palmetto supplement. A study in the *Journal of Urology* found that 106 milligrams a day reduces symptoms. If this doesn't work, ask your doctor about prescription medication or surgery.

"I'm Peeing Battery Acid."
Possible problem: Gonorrhea, a sexually transmitted bacterial infection. See a doctor for antibiotics. Take your partner with you to be tested.

"It Feels as if My Penis Were in a Noose."
Possible problem: A urinary-tract infection. Bacteria from the digestive tract spread to your bladder, and the inflammation makes it feel constricted. If the infection goes untreated, the kidneys may be next. Antibiotics will clear up the problem within a day or two, but in the meantime, put a heating pad on your abdomen. It will relieve pain by relaxing muscles and bringing fresh blood to cart away infection.

RECTUM
"As if Someone Used a Tire Pump to Inflate My Gut."
Possible problem: Constipation. Stress, dehydration, or lack of fiber has jammed your colon. Have coffee and an apple, and drink more water. If constipation is frequent or you also have cramps or abdominal swelling, see your doctor.

"Like I Have Poison Ivy In My Butt."
Possible problem: Hemorrhoids. Constipation, weight gain, or excessive straining during bowel movements has caused veins to bulge around your anus and within your lower rectum. This causes itching, burning, and pain in the area. Sit in warm water for 10 minutes twice a day, advises Lester Rosen, M.D., professor of clinical surgery at Pennsylvania State University. This relaxes the anal sphincter muscle, allowing protruding hemorrhoids to recede.

**MALE-ONLY STUDIES FUNDED
BY THE NATIONAL INSTITUTES OF HEALTH: 244**

FEMALE-ONLY STUDIES: 740

BACK
"A White-Hot Poker in My Lower Back."
Possible problem: Kidney stones. Hard masses can develop when your body absorbs too much calcium from food and empties the excess into your urine. It hurts because they block your pee tubes. Drink 2 to 3 quarts of water a day until the stone passes. The water dilutes stone-forming chemicals in your urine. If you've had kidney stones before, see your doctor.

"Like the Muscles Are All Twisted and My Spine Is Locked in One Position."
Possible problem: Degenerative disk disease. Excessive use or injury has damaged the disks between your vertebrae. The body tries to heal them by laying down calcium deposits in the spine, causing you pain and stiffness. Take a pain reliever. If you have spasms, lie on the floor on your back with your knees bent at a 90-degree angle. This position takes the pressure off your back, disks, and nerves, says Philip Greenman, D.O., professor of physical medicine at Michigan State University in East Lansing. Twenty minutes in this position provides hours of relief.

THROAT
"Wheezy, with a Burning in My Chest When I Cough. I Also Bring Up Big Green Hawkers."
Possible problem: Bronchitis. Tobacco smoke, a virus, an allergen, or bacteria have inflamed the airways in your lungs. Acute bronchitis will probably clear up on its own in a few days. But if it happens consistently over a 3-month period each year for 2 years or longer, it is chronic bronchitis, a lung-cancer risk factor that's usually caused by cigarette smoking. See your doctor and throw away the butts.

"My Throat and Lungs Have Been Disk-Sanded."
Possible problem: Pneumonia. An infection has caused your lungs to fill with pus and other liquid. This makes you short of breath and causes you to cough up thick mucus. It can result from one of more than 30 different bugs. Get to the doctor. The drugs used to fight pneumonia are determined by which germ you're fighting.

"A Scratchy Feeling in the Back of My Throat. And I Itch."
Possible problem: Allergies. Your body is trying to wash away allergens like dust or pollen by increasing production of mucus and tears. The itch is your body's reaction to the chemical it's using to fight the invaders. Eat jalapeño peppers. Spicy foods keep the mucus flowing freely while bolstering your immune system.

"Tired and Achy All Over, Like I Have the Flu."
Possible problem: The flu. Rest completely the first 2 days, when the virus is attacking full-force, then gradually increase activity as you get stronger. To avoid catching the bug, see your doctor this month for a flu shot.

MOOD

"Everything Is Unfocused, as if I Were Looking through Gauze."

Possible problem: Clinical depression. The neurotransmitters in your brain that your nerves use to communicate with one another have become unbalanced. See your doctor.

"Completely Gassed All the Time, and I Can't Remember Anything. I'm Always Cold."

Possible problem: Hypothyroidism. Your body mistakenly attacks the thyroid gland, screwing up your metabolism. Get a blood test. Treatment is in the form of a tiny pill, but you'll have to take it for the rest of your life.

How Doctors Treat Themselves

What happens when the medical experts suddenly become the patients? Here's what you can learn from them

By Duane Swierczynski

Most of the time, it's cool to be an expert. People respect you. Children cheer when you walk by. Dogs stop to lick your hand. So do journalists.

But sometimes, it's not so cool to be an expert. Sometimes a certain higher deity grows tired of your know-it-all bravado. And sometimes this certain higher deity decides to play a little prank on Mr. Expert.

That's what happened to the five medical specialists you're about to meet, each of whom woke up one day and discovered he had the very condition he had spent his adult life treating. Ironic? You bet. But it's also a chance to learn something, since these men weren't about to settle for second-rate care. Here, in their own words, is what the pros did when they became the patients—and what you should do if the deity ever decides to play a prank on you.

DIAGNOSIS: HEART MURMUR

Douglas Zipes, M.D., Distinguished Professor of Medicine and Chief of the
Division of Cardiology at the Krannert Institute of Cardiology at Indiana University;
President of the American College of Cardiology in Bethesda, Maryland

I was having a routine physical for a life-insurance policy when the G.P. told me, "You have a heart murmur."

Now, at the time, I was a 59-year-old cardiology professor who just so happened to be a heart-rhythm expert. So I told him, "You're full of expletive deleted. Give me that stethoscope."

But the G.P. was right. I could hear it myself, through three layers of clothing. I had a mitral-valve prolapse, which means that a faulty valve in my heart was steering blood in the wrong direction. Left untreated, it would spell serious trouble for me in years to come. I'm very knowledgeable about the problem—I write about it, teach about it, lecture, and so on. Still, I touched bases with my colleagues at major institutions, and their opinions were unanimous: I should have surgery.

Before the surgery, I found a cardiologist here at the university and asked for a heart catheterization. This was to both pinpoint the mitral-valve problem and peek at the coronary arteries. I reasoned that since I was going to undergo major heart surgery, we might as well look at the coronaries because they can be bypassed at the same time. You know—a little lube job, change the oil. Fortunately, my pipes were clean.

I chose a surgeon at another university hospital. We spent an hour talking the day before the operation. This was important to me, not to mention to my wife, who is not a cardiologist. You'd think I'd already know this stuff. But I did and I didn't. Many of my patients go through this, but I'm not hands-on for the surgery; I'm not a surgeon.

Was I nervous? Sure. As a cardiologist, I know very well that while the cardiovascular surgeon can be absolutely superb, I'm in the care of a system. By that, I mean the anesthesiologist, the person who runs the bypass machine, the nurses in the OR—everyone is part of a system. And if that system breaks down at any level, I'm the one who has the repercussions. And indeed there was a problem.

After surgery—which went well, by the way—I had a temporary pacemaker pacing my heart. The first evening after the surgery, a nurse came in to hang an IV.

"I'm giving you some magnesium," she said.

Now, I know that a low magnesium level can cause major heart-rhythm problems. I have to think that somebody somewhere said, "If there's one

WHAT TO ASK YOUR SURGEON

What is the exact procedure? "In my heart operation, they had my arms way above my head for adequate exposure," says Douglas Zipes, M.D., president of the American College of Cardiology in Bethesda, Maryland. "Consequently, my shoulder was very sore when I woke up. Had they not warned me about that, I'd have wondered what had happened."

What can I expect right afterward? Heart surgery also changed Dr. Zipes's ability to sign checks—but not in the way you think. "The fine finger movement of my right hand was significantly reduced for 2 weeks," he says, "probably from the shoulder stretch. I couldn't even sign my name legibly." These kinds of aftereffects are good to know ahead of time.

What kinds of physical activities will I be allowed to do after surgery? "I couldn't lift anything heavier than 10 pounds, and I wasn't allowed to drive my car for a month," says Dr. Zipes. These little details are important in planning your postoperative life.

person we don't want to give heart-rhythm problems, it's Zipes. So let's give him IV magnesium."

I asked the nurse, "Why not milk of magnesia? Hell, it'll help my bowels, and you won't have to do the IV."

"No, the doctor said IV," insisted the nurse.

"All right."

The nurse hung the IV, and almost immediately, my heart was jumping all over the place. I looked over at the heart monitor and realized that the pacemaker was malfunctioning. The magnesium had altered the function of the pacemaker, which was now pacing my heart in a dangerous way. In the extreme, it could have killed me. So I fiddled with the controls on the pacemaker.

The nurse walked in and said, "You can't do that!"

"Well, where's the doctor to correct this?

"We paged him. No one's here yet."

"I'm changing this myself." I immediately corrected it and took care of the problem.

And had I not done that—who knows what might have happened?

DIAGNOSIS: CHRONIC BACK AND NECK PAIN
Richard Guyer, M.D., Spine Surgeon and Cofounder
of the Texas Back Institute in Ft. Worth

My first attack was in my late 20s. I was stretching to hang up a plant, and suddenly I had severe, severe back pain like I'd never experienced before. It was ironic because I had just begun my orthopedic residency. I'd see these patients in clinic, and I'd think, "Oh God, what are these people complaining about?"

Hanging that plant, I knew.

Looking back on it, I know what I did wrong. I stretched and twisted at the same time—which is how many people end up hurting their backs. I didn't know much about the treatment of backs back then; I just took some aspirin and hoped it would go away. Only later, when I became a spine surgeon, did I understand what I really needed to do—and what I continue to do whenever my back and neck pain flares up.

First, I back off. If I'm doing yard work and I feel some twinges in my neck or back, I'll stop. Next, I'll take anti-inflammatories. (Of course, I have access to prescription drugs, but over-the-counter stuff, such as ibuprofen or Aleve, will work just as well.) Finally, I'll do some basic stretching exercises—what we call the Mackenzie exercises—for the lower back.

Traditionally, back doctors would recommend the Williams exercise, in which you bend forward, or lie on your back and pull one knee up, then pull the other knee up. (This is also known as flexion.) But the Mackenzie is an extension exercise. You stand up and extend your back backward, or do a pushup with your hips still on the ground. That's what works for me, but keep in mind that everybody's different. One stretch isn't working? Try the other.

When my back bothers me while I'm doing spine surgery, I'll put on a lumbar corset and try to change positions frequently. If it's really bad, I'll ask the nurse to bring a stool for me to put one foot on so that my hip is flexed. This changes the rotation of the pelvis ever so slightly, and often that's enough to make me feel better.

When I'm examining a patient, I normally bend over. But if my back is bothering me, I'll squat down on my hips and knees so I can keep my back straight—basically, I'm using good body mechanics. (Yes, I should do that all the time, but I don't.) In my Suburban, I have one of those little inflatable lumbar supports. I'll fill it up, release the air after 20 minutes, then fill it again later.

The key is to let your back change position, because there's nothing worse than having to stay in one position too long. The body likes motion. It will complain if you keep it in one position for long periods.

My patients feel better once they realize I endure the same kinds of pain they endure. I certainly don't wonder "What are they complaining about?" anymore.

DIAGNOSIS: INFLUENZA
Jack Gwaltney, M.D., Head of the Epidemiology and Virology Department at the University of Virginia in Charlottesville

When I have the classic symptoms during a known flu epidemic—in other words, when I feel like I've been hit by a truck, and I have a fever, a sore throat, and general malaise—I get anti-influenza medicine into my body as soon as possible. I keep some in my medicine cabinet so I don't have to wait around to get a scrip filled.

There are four prescription drugs: The older ones are amantadine and ri-mantadine, and the newer drugs are Relenza and Tamiflu. They're all effective at reversing the illness and making it much milder, but you really need to take them within 24 hours of when the symptoms start. After 48 hours, they won't do you much good.

You can predict these things, by the way. Flu occurs only at certain times of the year: typically after Christmas, and most often between January and the end of March. If you're in good general health, see if your doctor will pre-scribe some antiflu medicine for you before the season. It makes sense: These drugs are safe, and they're most effective when taken immediately. Your doctor should know this and won't want to have you waiting around for an appointment or a diagnostic test.

ODDS THE AVERAGE GUY WILL CATCH THE FLU THIS YEAR: 1 IN 3.5

AVERAGE NUMBER OF DAYS HE'LL SPEND IN BED BECAUSE OF FLU: 5

If your doctor refuses and you feel the symptoms start, call him immediately. At this point, he should call in a prescription to your drugstore right away so you can take the medicine as quickly as possible. Besides, in a flu outbreak, if everybody goes in to see the doctor, he's going to be swamped anyway.

HOW TO TRACK A WILD FLU

Really want to avoid the flu? Track its whereabouts by region at the Web site of the Centers for Disease Control and Prevention (www.cdc.gov/ncidod/diseases/flu/regions/senusmap.htm). For instance, you'll find that Alabama, Kentucky, Mississippi, and Tennessee were hit the hardest by the flu in 2001. Make it your new office pool!

You can even take this antiflu medication if you're going on a ski trip next week and you don't want to get sick. Say you didn't get the vaccine, but now the flu is in town and your kids are sick. You should get the vaccine and then go on the flu medicine until the vaccine takes effect—roughly 12 days. It won't hurt you a bit. These are safe medicines.

If you have chronic lung disease, you should get a vaccination every year. What if you aren't vaccinated and the epidemic starts? You can go in and get a vaccination right away, but remember: It's not going to kick in for about 12 days. So have your doctor give you a 2-week supply of one of these drugs, and take it until the vaccine begins to work.

And what if you miss that magic window of opportunity? Take ibuprofen and cough medicine, stay in bed, and drink plenty of fluids. Those things will help you, but they're not as effective as nipping it in the bud.

DIAGNOSIS: BLOWN-OUT KNEE
Chuck Bush-Joseph, M.D., Associate Professor of Orthopedic Surgery
at Rush-Presbyterian–St. Luke's Medical Center in Chicago
and a Spokesman for the American Academy of Orthopaedic Surgeons

I was playing basketball, full-court. I tried a crossover dribble on a fast break, and heard a pop. I knew immediately I had ruptured my ACL—the anterior cruciate ligament. The sound and feel were just how my patients have described it so many times.

You see, ACLs are a specialty of mine. I did a sports-medicine fellowship, and all I really do is knee and shoulder reconstruction here at Rush-Presbyterian. I teach medical students, fellows, and national courses all the time. I mean, this is my game.

And there went my other game.

I didn't even see a doctor for a day or two. I was in denial, I guess. After a couple of days, I cooled off and had my associate Bernie look at it. I had an MRI to see if I had cartilage damage or not—which I did not. Because it was in the middle of summer, I really wanted to hold off on having surgery.

With isolated ACL tears, there's no acute rush for surgery. If you tear your ACL, say, while skiing in Colorado, many mountain doctors like to operate on you before you go home. But you're honestly better off delaying surgery until the swelling goes down, you regain motion in the knee, and the pain is gone. Usually, that's within 1 to 3 weeks.

I waited until summer was over. Let's face it, you're pretty uncomfortable for 5 to 6 weeks after surgery. In the middle of summer, you suddenly can't go to parties or picnics—you can't do anything, really.

Soon enough, it was time. Bernie was actually a little more nervous than I was. But I had ultimate confidence in him, and things went as expected.

I followed the same recovery program that I'd been giving my patients for years: Sign up for a full rehabilitation program of exercise with weights, stationary bicycles, and elliptical trainers. But I did learn two things from my experience that will help my patients even more.

First, in that first 24 to 48 hours after surgery, you are completely immobile and utterly dependent. Make sure your girlfriend will be with you for a couple of nights. Believe me, you'll need her.

Second, it's going to hurt like hell for a couple of days. I give my patients much more pain medicine than I used to. Certainly for the first week or two after surgery, it's important to do everything you can to make patients feel more comfortable, to allow them to get more sleep and be able to do their rehab exercises without too much pain. This flies against that old doctor's mentality of "Get off pain pills right away."

DIAGNOSIS: PROSTATE CANCER
Archie Hewett, M.D., a Prostate-Cancer Expert Who Has Practiced Urology for More Than 40 Years and Still Performs Prostate Surgery in Ft. Smith, Arkansas

About 3 years ago, I had a routine prostate-specific antigen (PSA) exam. That's when I noticed that my PSA level had risen from 3.5 to 5.0. My son is also a urologist, so he biopsied me. The pathologists in town were a little hesitant to make a confirmatory diagnosis, so we sent the biopsy to a leading pathologist in Florida—one whose specialty is prostate biopsies, particularly those that are somewhat tenuous. He said yes, this is cancer.

Now, at that point I was 67, in excellent health, still actively practicing medicine. My son and I had performed numerous radical prostatectomies, and I was well-apprised of the risks. This was my business. And now, suddenly, my life.

NUMBER OF MEN WHO JOIN THE RANKS OF NEW HIV CASES EACH YEAR: 28,000

PERCENTAGE OF THOSE MEN WHO WERE INFECTED THROUGH HOMOSEXUAL SEX: 60

I decided to have the surgery.

I should explain my options. Today, there are basically four treatments: radiation therapy, hormone therapy, radical prostatectomy, or opting to do nothing. Brachytherapy—a form of radiation therapy—is the latest. That's where we implant 60 to 120 radioactive seeds into the prostate. However, in 1997, there wasn't too much brachytherapy being done. It's really only become popular within the past 2 years. And there still isn't any long-term data on its effectiveness.

It's my belief that for a fairly young man in good health, a radical prostatectomy, in which the gland itself is removed, is the way to go. It offers the best possible survival rate—somewhere in the 90-percent range. Incontinence and impotence can be a problem, but rehabilitation is possible. And I can tell you from personal experience, mild incontinence is a small price to pay for being alive.

My next step was finding a doctor. This is very important since a great deal depends upon the surgeon's ability to preserve the nerves in the penis so it can maintain erections as well as preserve your continence. I looked around for a good physician. My urologist friends mentioned Dr. William Catalona, an extremely well-respected urologist at Washington University in St. Louis. I had read several of Dr. Catalona's articles on prostatectomies. I called him, and he agreed to perform my surgery, which took place in June of 1997.

Fortunately, the operation was a complete success. When I returned from surgery, they immediately had me on my feet. There's a long hallway in the ward, and Dr. Catalona walked me around every hour or two. Apparently, one of his patients had had trouble with a blood clot, so to prevent this—and to get the blood circulating in your legs—they have you up walking very early.

One problem with radical surgery is wearing that catheter for 2 weeks. That gets old pretty fast, but you need to allow the bladder to heal. And of course, there was the incontinence. At first, you wear Depends. As your control improves,

HOW TO FIND A PROSTATE-CANCER DOC

According to Archie Hewett, M.D., a prostate-cancer expert who has practiced urology for more than 40 years and still performs prostate surgery in Ft. Smith, Arkansas, the key is to find patients who've had a radical prostatectomy and grill them. Here are the questions to ask.

What kind of results did you have? Fortunately, Dr. Hewett had one of the most skilled prostate docs in the country on the case. As a result, he didn't have much pain and was able to recover with nothing stronger than acetaminophen (Tylenol).

Did your doctor take care of you and stand by you during any problems? You want a doctor who will be responsive if you have incontinence and erectile problems later—not to mention keep an eye on follow-up prostate-specific antigen tests.

What's his track record? The more radical prostatectomies he's done, the better. Fewer than 100? Skip Doogie Howser and try someone else.

you wear smaller and smaller pads until finally they're no longer necessary.

However, my experience helps me to better advise my patients. I especially encourage them to get their PSAs checked every 3 months. If your PSA stays at 0.0 for 2 years, there's a 95 percent chance you're cured. Dr. Catalona keeps up with me. I send him my PSAs regularly.

I'm glad I made the choices I did. So far, my PSA has been 0.0. I think I'm cured of my disease, my quality of life is good, and I still practice actively.

In fact, I'm doing a radical prostatectomy tomorrow.

Bulletproof Your Health Plan

Health-insurance pitfalls that could bankrupt you, if you let them

By Ron Geraci

Don't get blindsided by land mines lurking in the fine print of your health-insurance plan. Two choices: (1) spend an hour scouring that little policy booklet you got from human resources (yeah, they'll send you another one), or (2) for about $50, hire an agent from the nonprofit Alliance of Claims Assistance Professionals (877-275-8765; www.claims.org) to peruse your policy for these common pitfalls.

THE PLAN DOESN'T COVER THE TREATMENT THAT MIGHT SAVE YOUR LIFE

Every policy has a list of exclusions—procedures and treatments that aren't covered. For example, many policies refuse to pay for chiropractors or psychological counseling. Some won't cover an MRI (magnetic-resonance imaging), a common diagnostic scan. "Some very restrictive policies don't even cover x-rays," says Susan Dressler, president of the Alliance of Claims Assistance Professionals.

Most important, many plans won't pay for any "experimental" drugs, surgical procedures, or treatments. And who gets to decide what's experimental? That's right, the insurer. "The insurance company can refuse to pay for any test or treatment that it claims isn't in widespread use yet—even if the approach obviously works," warns Jay Wolfson, Dr. P.H., J.D., director of the Florida Health Information Center in Tampa.

What to do: If you have an individual insurance policy (that is, you're self-employed), you can get rid of troublesome exclusions by simply paying a higher premium to cover a particular potential cost. In job-sponsored plans, however, the exclusions are pretty rigid. You have three choices, says Wolfson. Switch insurance plans, or ask your human-resources director to pressure the insurer or plan administrator to change the policy, at least in your case (if not for every employee). Failing that, you could buy a separate insurance plan that'll cover whatever the primary plan does not.

IF YOU FORGET TO MAKE A CALL, YOU GET SCREWED

Health-insurance policies have dozens of traps that can reduce your coverage. They're usually listed under "provisions" in your insurance booklet. For example, many policies require you to get a second opinion before undergoing any type of surgery. So, if you're rushed to an ER with stomach pain that turns out to be a hot appendix, be sure to have somebody call your primary-care doctor within 48 hours—or even better, as soon as possible. "One client of mine will be forced to pay $29,000 for an operation because he forgot to make a 5-minute phone call," says Dressler.

What to do: Most people break rules because they never knew they existed. Take a magnifying glass to your policy booklet. "If you break a regulation, you'll most likely need to prove that it was an emergency situation," says Wolfson. Letters from specialists and witnesses help. Hire an attorney if the stakes are high.

YOU HAVE $500,000 WORTH OF COVERAGE AND GET $1,000,000 WORTH OF SICK

Many policies have a measly lifetime cap of $500,000—meaning that's all you can be reimbursed for, ever, no matter what. A family man needs more than that paltry sum. "One problem pregnancy or an accident could wipe you out. Even a lifetime max of a million bucks is uncomfortably thin," says Dressler. "If you have an accident, you can spend that very quickly." A $5 million cap will let you snooze soundly. If you're single, a $2 million cap is adequate.

What to do: If the insurance company won't allow you to upgrade the lifetime cap on your company-sponsored plan, consider buying supplemental umbrella insurance. An additional $1 million may cost about $300 to $500 a year, says Dressler.

YOUR NEW POLICY WON'T COVER THERAPY FOR YOUR TRICK KNEE

Sometimes, new plans consider long-standing ailments—like high blood pressure, high cholesterol, or your daughter's asthma—to be "preexisting con-

KNOWLEDGE IS POWER

Can't understand your health coverage? Here's where to find help.

Health Insurance Association of America: www.hiaa.org, (202) 824-1849
American Association of Health Plans: www.aahp.org, (202) 778-3200
American Association of Preferred Provider Organizations: www.aappo.org, (202) 220-3111
National Committee for Quality Assurance: www.ncqa.org, (888) 275-7585
Links to state health-insurance departments: www.insure.com/links/doi.html

KEEP WHAT YOU EARN
God bless the USA, not the IRS

We at *Men's Health* believe in our republic—and our families. Result: The IRS gets every nickel the law requires, and not a penny more. When calculating your medical expenses, don't overlook these deductions.

Programs to help you quit. If you pay for an accredited stop-smoking program, write it off. Don't try, "That video library calmed my nicotine cravings."

Travel to a medical summit. If you have a condition that requires you to stay on top of the latest medical research, you can deduct the cost of attending a conference and the cost of getting there. Hotel and meals aren't deductible.

Pills you pop. If you're a self-medicating supplement man, the IRS will hammer you if you try to deduct your vitamin E, folic acid, and garlic tablets. But if your doctor says (or rather, writes down) that these are treatment for a high-cholesterol condition, you might get away with deducting a few bottles.

ditions" and refuse to cover them for up to a year (or possibly forever). You get whacked with big doctor and medication bills.

What to do: Be certain the new policy specifically states that you'll have "continuity of care and continuous coverage" for any problems you already have, says Wolfson. If it doesn't, ask your human-resources director to compel the insurer to give you a written waiver stating that it will cover your family's preexisting health issues. If the insurer won't play ball, ask your new boss for a hiring bonus, which you'll spend to extend your former employer's insurance (through a program called the Consolidated Omnibus Budget Reconciliation Act, or COBRA) until the new policy starts covering the conditions in question. Know the exact cost before you ask for the bonus; those stinging COBRA premiums can be $6,000 or more a year.

THE KIDS' COVERAGE QUITS
BEFORE THEY HAVE COVERAGE OF THEIR OWN

Some policies cover children until they're 23, others 21, and others 19. Some policies will underwrite your kids as long as they're full-time students (which means in high school, or taking 12 to 15 college credits a semester). Frighteningly, some plans cancel child coverage the minute Junior moves out of your house—even if he's as young as 16.

What to do: If your company coverage drops your kids—and they can't get cheap health insurance through a college or employer—call your insurance agent and ask about getting a short-term indemnity health plan. Since teenagers rarely get things like emphysema, coverage should run only about $40 a month. Or, if they're generally healthy, consider a catastrophic policy that will pay for care in the event they have a serious accident or illness, but not a sinus infection or a Sunday-morning hangover.

YOUR PAYCHECKS STOP COMING IF YOU BREAK YOUR HEAD IN A SOFTBALL GAME

If your health plan doesn't have a long-term-disability provision that'll pay you at least 70 percent of your salary for 5 years, think about buying coverage separately—unless your savings account is fat enough to shake the Dow. This safety net is vital if you can't work.

What to do: "If you're 45 and fit, it pays to buy long-term-disability coverage now," says Dressler. You'll pay relative peanuts for it ($200 a year), and you'll avoid being forced to cough up $4,000 or so for brand-new coverage when you're 60, a mistake most men make. Suggest that your parents look into this additional coverage, too, advises Dressler. If it pays at least $100 a day for nursing-home care, it could prevent them from having to sell their house to finance a long stay in an assisted-living facility.

Interpreting DocSpeak (Hint: "Good" Means "Bad")

Read this, and you'll never be stumped by your doctor again

From *The Hypochondriac's Guide to Life. And Death* **(Simon & Schuster) by Gene Weingarten**

Every profession has its conventional euphemisms. Butchers sell "chopped sirloin," not "ground cow." Even journalism, which is supposed to be about truth telling, occasionally resorts to bull hockey. Newspapers will write about a "developing nation" even when the nation about which they are writing is not developing at all, inasmuch as it has a rooster-based economy. Euphemism is the driving force behind the classified ad.

> **What it says:** "Cozy starter home"
> **What it means:** House is size of men's room in Exxon station
> **What it says:** "Attractive benefits package"
> **What it means:** Janitorial salary
> **What it says:** "Runs good"
> **What it means:** Owner is idiot

The language of medicine is similarly deceptive. When doctors say a test result was "positive," that means it is bad. "Negative" test results are good. A "thrill" sounds cool, but if a doctor hears one when listening to your heart, you might keel over at any minute. An "ecchymosis" sounds revolting, but it is only a black-and-blue mark.

Among themselves, however, doctors tend to speak plainly. Surgeons will refer to a "peek-and-shriek," which is, literally, an open-and-shut case: Look in, blanch, close him up, let him die. Doctors will say a patient belongs to the Hi-Five club, meaning he has HIV. Doctors can be real cards.

But when they are speaking in front of patients, doctors have learned the opposite skill—creative euphemism. They learn it as interns, when they are making "rounds." Rounds occur when a learned doctor in a teaching hospital goes from room to room trailed by a pack of lickspittles in lab coats who leave behind them an oily trail of sycophancy. Everyone must discuss each case in the presence of the patient. The lickspittles want to show off by exhibiting intuitive diagnostic skills, but they must do so in a manner that does not alarm the patient. They cannot say, for example, that Mr. Achenbach is "decomposing faster than a pile of fish heads in the Kalahari." They would say Mr. Achenbach is "an excellent candidate for palliative treatment" (see page 241).

Doctors never lose this tendency to obfuscate in front of their patients. Most people will ignore this, figuring that if there is something the doctor needs to tell you, he will get around to it in due course. Some people might even be grateful for the doctor's delicacy and diplomacy. This is not true of the hypochondriac, who is constantly looking for validation of his fears. He will assume everything the doctor says is a subterfuge to hide the ghastly truth about his condition.

DOCTOR: Good morning, Mr. Achenbach.
PATIENT: I am dying, right?
DOCTOR: I haven't examined you yet.
PATIENT: But it looks bad, doesn't it, Doc?
DOCTOR: We are talking on the telephone.

This sort of suspicion causes needless worry for the hypochondriac. There are only a handful of terms doctors routinely use to disguise bad things, a few dozen terms that are really, really scary but that you might not recognize. Here they are.

What They Say	What It Sounds Like	What It Means
A "mass"	A solemn religious event	Cancer
A "lesion"	A scrape	Cancer
A "mitotic process"	Some damn technical thing	Cancer
A "neoplastic involvement"	A trinket from the dollar store	Cancer
An "opacification"	Giving in to Hitler	Cancer

NUMBER OF MEN WHO DIE FROM HEART DISEASE EACH YEAR: 354,000

NUMBER OF MEN WHO DIE OF STROKE EACH YEAR: 158,000

Yes, cancer is the leading cause of medical euphemisms; but it is not the only terrible thing that medical language is designed to hide.

What They Say	What It Sounds Like	What It Means
"AMI"	College where you can major in pig husbandry	A heart attack, or acute myocardial infarction
A "CK leak"	Calvin Klein takes a whiz	A heart attack. Refers to release of an enzyme that accompanies the death of heart muscle. Cardiologists love this term
A "calculus"	Something hard that you want to pass	Something hard that you don't want to pass. This is a calcified stone in the gallbladder or kidney
A "demyelinating process"	Getting salt from seawater, saving the peasants of India	Multiple sclerosis
"Secondary lues"	Reserve infielder from Dominican Republic	Syphilis, featuring crusty, weeping sores

Other medical terms are designed to hide the significance of bad symptoms.

What They Say	What It Sounds Like	What It Means
"Exquisite"	Wonderful	Horrible. Describes pain that is incapacitating. A patient in "exquisite" pain is often whimpering and drooling
A "bruit"	Fat guy. Beats up Popeye	An unexpected sound when doctors listen to an organ. It is usually bad. Heart bruits, for example, can indicate CK leaks
An "adventitious" sound	To your benefit	To your detriment. Adventitious sounds are bad lung sounds
"Ronchi" and "stridor"	*Star Wars* characters	Specific adventitious lung sounds; they can signal anything from a cold to a tumor
A "deficit"	A little red ink	A big red flag. A deficit means an insufficiency of something, often signaling serious illness. An "oxygen deficit" in the body is sometimes followed by coma, brain injury, a vegetative state
A "vegetative state"	Kansas	Brain death
An "accident"	Oops. Ha ha.	Oops. Bye-bye. A grave event in your body. A cerebrovascular accident is bleeding in the brain
"Decompensated"	Docked	Decked. It means the failure of a system—whatever ails you has reached the point that the organ in question is no longer able to maintain basic body function. If you have compensated liver disease, your liver is functioning well enough to sustain life. If you have decompensated liver disease, it is not

What They Say	What It Sounds Like	What It Means
"Discomfort"	Discomfort, as from an itch	Pain, as from insertion of a penis catheter
An "embarrassment"	A faux pas	A sudden, dramatic problem caused by an interruption to circulation or a drop in blood pressure, occasionally produced by bad diagnostic technique. Feeling for a pulse on the carotid artery at both sides of the neck at the same time, for example, can sometimes cause unconsciousness, as if the patient were being hanged (See "syncope" on page 242)
A "dissection"	Something bad that happens to a frog	Something bad that happens to you. It's a spontaneous ripping and rending of tissue, as though it is being unzipped by God. When it happens to your aorta, you often die
An "event"	A party	No party. A bad thing. A thrombotic event, for example, is a stroke
"Iatrogenic"	A play by Aristophanes	Describes an illness or injury caused by medical treatment or diagnostic procedures. For example, sometimes a spark caused by a colonoscope will accidentally ignite intestinal gas, causing an explosion in the body. It can be fatal. And disgusting
"Idiopathic"	Duh	Duh. When doctors diagnose an illness as idiopathic, it means they have no idea what is causing it
An "insult"	Injured feelings	Injured flesh, often grave damage. In the autopsy report, for example, JFK's head wound was described as an "insult"
"Palliative treatment"	Some sort of treatment	No treatment. Doctors have given up on a cure. At best, they will do something final and dramatic, like amputating a gangrenous limb or creating a permanent colostomy. Usually, though, palliative treatment means doping you up until you die
"Precocious"	Mozart	Mozart did not have huge, hairy genitals at the age of 4, so far as we know. Medically, a precocious development occurs unnaturally early and is usually a very bad sign. Precocious puberty, for example, occurs in pineal hyperplasia syndrome, or tumors of the hypothalamus. Kids get adult-looking genitals at age 4. No, it is not cool
"Progressive"	Modern, forward-thinking, socially conscious	Deadly. A "progressive" disease is one that is progressing, inexorably, despite treatment. Multiple sclerosis is often described as "progressive"

What They Say	What It Sounds Like	What It Means
"Resection"	Restore, put back, fix	Cut away, amputate
"Tamponade"	Women's personal-hygiene procedure	Restrictive pressure on the heart, causing reduced bloodflow to the body, breathlessness, and sometimes syncope (See below)
"Syncope"	Thelonious Monk	Thelonious Monk OD's. Syncope is fainting, unconsciousness
"Prodrome"	A dirt-floored stadium in some toilet of a town, outfitted for tractor pulls and demolition derbies	The early stage of a disease. It is often deceptively mild. Prodromal symptoms are sometimes described as "premonitory"
"Premonitory"	You may already be a winner!	You lose. If a symptom is premonitory, it seems trivial, but isn't. You know: hiccups, cancer
A "bad result"	A bad result	A very bad result. This is universal DocSpeak for "death"

Fire in the Hole

How to extinguish heartburn

From *Staying at the Top of Your Game: A Man's Guide to Peak Performance* (Avon Books) by Timothy Gower

You start the day with a large cup of coffee and a smoke. Then for lunch, you inhale a giant Italian sub with onions and hot peppers. Dinner? A mega-order of Buffalo chicken wings—washed down, naturally, with several pitchers of beer. As you lie down at night, you get heartburn so bad it brings tears to your eyes. You figure it's the spicy chicken-wing sauce, on top of those onions and peppers. Perhaps. More likely, "it's the fat and the smoke and the alcohol," says Jorge Herrera, M.D., assistant director of the University of South Alabama Digestive Health Center in Mobile. And if you're overweight, that just about seals your fate.

Some 60 million Americans get it once a month: the intense and fiery sensation in the chest, sometimes accompanied by a battery-acid backwash in the mouth. It can cause hoarseness or a sore throat and has even been linked to asthma and—in rare but scary cases—cancer. Heartburn is one of the most

PERCENTAGE OF FREQUENT HEARTBURN SUFFERERS WHO SAY THE PAIN "GETS IN THE WAY OF SEX": 34

common physical complaints, but it's also one of the most easily treated. Ignore it at your own peril; this simple nuisance can degenerate into a troubling, even grave, condition.

Each day, the average person's stomach churns out about 8 ounces of hydrochloric acid, a corrosive compound that's also found in industrial solvents (albeit in higher concentrations). Sounds awful, but since the stomach is lined with a layer of protective mucus, the acid doesn't cause pain or discomfort, so long as it stays where it belongs.

Stomach acid is a vestige from early man, who probably needed it to protect his stomach from bacteria in the mammoth tartare he had for lunch. You don't need stomach acid to digest food; most digestion goes on in the small intestine. But your stomach is awash in the caustic juice anyway, which wouldn't be a problem if not for a quirk in the human digestive tract: the relaxed sphincter. Specifically, the lower esophageal sphincter, which acts as a valve at the juncture of the esophagus and stomach. When you swallow food, it relaxes, or opens, long enough for chewed-up particles to pass through the slender chute connecting the mouth and stomach. Then it quickly closes, to guard the tender lining of the esophagus from the swirling acid bath below.

Occasionally, the valve opens when there's no food to swallow. That's not entirely a bad thing; you couldn't belch if it didn't. However, a valve that doesn't seal tightly can allow the acid bath in your belly to wash up and burn your esophagus, a phenomenon known as *gastroesophageal reflux*.

MANY CAUSES, MANY CURES

Everyone refluxes at least a few times a day. But not everyone gets heartburn. How come? It's hard to say. "There is no single cause of heartburn," says gastroenterologist Joel Richter of the Cleveland Clinic Foundation. In some people, Richter says, a leaky valve leaves the gullet exposed to acid for prolonged periods. Others have unusually acidic stomach contents; even a splash on the esophagus leaves them swearing off spicy foods for life. Finally, for some people the problem seems to be an exceptionally sensitive esophagus.

Fittingly, there is more than one way to fight heartburn. Your choice of weapons ranges from simple lifestyle changes to powerful medicine. But don't use a howitzer to kill a mosquito. Try a few simple strategies for dousing heartburn before moving on to the heavier artillery.

Hose down the flames. For some people, a glass of water is all it takes to rinse acid off the esophagus.

Mind your menu. Food is the instigator when your chest ignites, of course, but the culprits aren't always so obvious. Again, heartburn triggers vary from one person to the next, as does the manner in which they inflict misery. Citrus fruits, coffee, and anything tomatoey can burn the esophagus on the way to the stomach.

But a weird stew of seemingly unrelated foods can cause heartburn in a different way. Such foods seem to stimulate the release of hormonelike substances that can make the esophageal valve wobbly and ineffectual, says gastroenterologist Donald Castell of the Graduate Hospital in Philadelphia. The list includes chocolate, garlic, onions, peppermint, and milk. For some people, any high-fat dish will do the dirty deed; booze, too. Make note of what you ate before you developed heartburn, and avoid it, if you can.

Mind your portions. When you wolf down an entire pizza, your stomach expands, which may widen the opening to the esophagus. A little restraint will help.

No more late-night suppers. Lie down after eating and you lose gravity, one of the forces that keeps food from traveling back up the esophagus. Post-meal acid levels take at least 2 hours to subside. If nocturnal heartburn wakes you frequently, try to elevate your upper body while you snooze; acid is less likely to creep upward. An extra pillow won't do the trick, though. Buy an under-the-mattress foam wedge, or try this strategy recommended by the American College of Gastroenterolgy: Slip a four-by-four under the legs at the upper end of your bed. You may want to nail a pair of jar lids, top down, onto the wood, to keep the legs from slipping.

Loosen up. A too-tight belt can raise abdominal pressure, forcing contents upward and into the esophagus.

Butt out. Smoking dries up saliva, which would normally protect the esophagus from acid.

OVER-THE-COUNTER MEDICATIONS

When watching your diet and tinkering with your headboard don't work, there are literally dozens of OTC heartburn aids to choose from. We've come a long way since the days of "plop, plop, fizz, fizz."

Antacids. The brand names—Alka-Seltzer, Maalox, Rolaids—are almost as well-known as Coca-Cola and McDonald's. These candylike pills and milky cocktails contain salts—aluminum, calcium, magnesium, or sodium—that rapidly bind with stomach acid to form a neutral compound. Bottom line, you still reflux, but the fluid doesn't burn. Antacids work fast, but the relief lasts

CURRENT PERCENTAGE OF CANCER PATIENTS
WHO LIVE AT LEAST 5 YEARS AFTER DIAGNOSIS: 60

PERCENTAGE IN 1980: 50

only an hour or so. As your stomach contents move along into your intestines, so do the neutralizing agents. If your stomach pumps out more acid, heartburn can return. Take an antacid right after you eat a meal that may give you heartburn. Taking an antacid before eating is useless since it will probably exit your stomach before the acid onslaught.

Rafting agents. They work by forming a layer of foam, or "raft," atop the stomach contents. The best known is Gaviscon. These agents keep acid from splashing upward and into the esophagus. They can ease symptoms for up to 4 hours, as long as you don't lie down; go horizontal and the foam shifts position, clearing the way for acid's entry to the esophagus.

H$_2$ blockers. These former ulcer drugs are now considered state-of-the-art heartburn beaters. Zantac 75, Tagamet HB, and the other so-called H$_2$ blockers all work the same way: by interfering with histamine, a chemical messenger that tells the stomach to make acid. They put out the fire for 3 hours or more—but take at least 30 minutes to start working. They're pricey, too.

Richter says there's no harm in taking an H$_2$ blocker before eating *and* an antacid right after to stop heartburn completely. But he quickly adds that OTC preparations are suitable only for *occasional* heartburn. More frequent heartburn may signal a more serious condition. If you . . .

- Gobble Tums like Pez and keep a bottle of Maalox in your desk
- Can't seem to pinpoint your heartburn to any one food
- And fight the postprandial flames twice a week or more

. . . you may have a variety of heavy-duty heartburn known as gastroesophageal reflux disease, or GERD. Dial up your doctor, soon—your after-meal malaise may be causing other health problems. GERD can damage the esophagus and lead to some ugly complications, including painful esophageal ulcers and esophagitis, an inflammation that can narrow the opening of the stomach, making food get stuck. Some epidemiologists say GERD is a leading risk factor for cancer of the esophagus.

Furthermore, about 80 percent of asthma sufferers also reflux, according to San Francisco gastroenterologist Kenneth McQuaid. In many cases, the breathing disorder can be caused by stomach contents backing up into the esophagus and spilling into the lungs.

PRESCRIPTION DRUGS AND BEYOND

Currently, there are four options for GERD patients. Prescription-strength H$_2$ blockers were once standard therapy, but increasingly, doctors are turning to newer, more potent drugs. And in very serious cases, they're even recommending surgery.

Promotility agents. Drugs like Propulsid increase the speed at which the stomach empties, giving acid less chance to cause trouble. They may also make the valve seal more tightly, which cuts down on the amount of reflux that can splash into the esophagus.

Proton-pump inhibitors (PPIs). Like H_2 blockers, these drugs reduce acid, but they are far more powerful. PPIs, such as Prilosec and Prevacid, interfere with histamine *and* several other chemical messengers that signal cells in the stomach to produce acid. Block all three messengers, and you virtually halt acid production. Some doctors worry that an acid-free stomach is not such a good thing, but there's no evidence to suggest that's true.

The last resort. In fundoplication surgery, doctors wrap a portion of the upper stomach around the esophagus to form a collar. When the patient's stomach fills up with food, it compresses the esophagus, cinching off reflux. According to surgeon Garth Ballantyne of St. Luke's–Roosevelt Hospital Center in New York City, surgery can cure GERD in 95 percent of cases. An older version of the procedure involved a 6- to 10-inch incision, a lot of pain and blood, and a long recovery. Today, fundoplication is far less invasive and requires just five tiny incisions.

KNOW THIS

Headache-Hypertension Connection

Researchers have long known that severe high blood pressure can cause headaches. But a recent report published in the *Archives of Internal Medicine* suggests that even slightly elevated blood pressure may cause headaches. When people with moderately high blood pressure were given a pressure-lowering drug, they reported fewer headaches than a placebo group. The differences suggest a blood pressure–headache link, according to Lennart Hansson, M.D., of Uppsala University in Sweden.

New Drugs to Fight Cancer

The first of a new class of drugs has been shown to slow tumor growth by selectively killing cancer cells—without damaging healthy cells. Researchers studied 96 patients who had prostate-cancer recurrences after prostatectomy and found that Exisulind, a selective apoptotic anti-neoplastic drug (SAAND), acted like a cancer-cell off switch. "Exisulind makes cancer cells undergo apoptosis—programmed cell death," says lead researcher Erik Goluboff, M.D., of the Columbia University College of Physicians and Surgeons in New York City. He believes that SAANDs, which should start to be available early next year, will increase the effectiveness of surgery, hormone therapy, and radiation therapy.

Hot-Tub Help for Diabetes

Researchers at the University of Colorado think hot tubs may be therapeutic for people with type-2 diabetes. Eight volunteers soaked in a hot tub for a half-hour 6 days a week, for 3 weeks. Result: Blood sugar dropped enough to produce a 35 percent reduction in diabetes-related complications. One subject decreased his necessary dose of insulin by 18 percent. "My theory is that the hot tub increases bloodflow to the skeletal muscles and simulates the effect of exercise," says Philip Hooper, M.D., one of the researchers. Talk to your doctor before trying hot-tub therapy. If you have foot-numbness problems, you may burn yourself. And diabetics are often at greater risk of infections.

Or You Could Ditch the Cat

If you have asthma, you have our sympathy. If you have a cat allergy, you're our hero. If you have both, ask your doctor about Accolate, an asthma medication that may also alleviate cat-allergy symptoms. Researchers at Johns Hopkins University in Baltimore put people in a room with a lot of cat hair. Those who had taken the active ingredient in Accolate had far less dramatic responses to the cat stuff.

Faster Hemorrhoid Healing

Researchers from Leicester Royal Infirmary in England have made a great discovery: a less painful technique for hemorrhoid removal. In a procedure called stapled hemorrhoidectomy, a surgeon removes anal-lining tissue from higher up in the bowel than a conventional hemorrhoidectomy, so "it doesn't excise any pain-sensitive skin," says David Hemingway, M.D. The surgeon closes the incision with tiny staples. A study published by Dr. Hemingway and his colleagues in *Lancet* found that patients who had stapled hemorrhoidectomies left the hospital faster than patients who had conventional surgery. They also returned to their normal activities in about half the time. If you're scheduled for a hemorrhoidectomy, ask your doctor about the staple option.

St. John's Thwart

The popular herbal remedy St. John's wort may decrease the effectiveness of drugs. Researchers from the National Institutes of Health gave eight healthy volunteers the anti-HIV drug indinavir—first by itself and then in combination with St. John's wort. The addition of the herb led to significantly lower blood levels of the drug—decreases from 49 percent to as high as 99 percent. "St. John's wort revs up the rate at which the drugs are metabolized," says Stephen Piscitelli, Pharm.D., "and so may decrease their effectiveness." Talk to your doctor about how this herb might interact with or undermine your medicine. And see page 215 to read about a more drug-friendly St. John's wort in the pipeline.

Is That Bandage Moving?

Instead of making your skin crawl, maggots could save it. Bandages embedded with live maggots have healed 5,000 skin patients at the Princess of Wales Hospital in Bridgend, United Kingdom. The larvae attack infection caused by MRSA—a virus resistant to antibiotics.

DOWN THE PIKE

Four out of Five Dentists Recommend It

American Dental Association scientists are currently developing gum, toothpaste, and even candy that will reverse tooth decay, causing cavities to heal on their own. Look for them in 5 years.

Colon-Cancer Double Whammy

Growths in the colon often become cancerous. But low-dosage combinations of two drugs—one old and one new—could one day be a treatment for polyprelated colon cancer. Scientists at Wyeth-Ayerst Research Laboratories in New York made the breakthrough discovery after combining sulindac, an older drug, with a newly developed drug, EKI-569. "Mixing 25 percent of each drug's standard dosage prevented polyp growth 95 percent more effectively than using either drug alone," says researcher Philip Frost, Ph.D. Lower doses of sulindac have fewer side effects, too, making it easier for patients to tolerate over the long haul. A clinical trial on the safety of the drug combination is planned.

Fresh Breath, Clean Lungs

Researchers at the State University of New York at Buffalo have developed a mouthwash that alters the taste of cigarette smoke. The new mouthwash reacts with nicotine, altering its flavor and making it taste unbearably bad. "The taste is so awful that in a test of 20 hard-core, long-term smokers, most couldn't get past the first puff," says Sebastian Cianco, D.D.S., who developed the product. The mouthwash lasts 3 to 4 hours and has no effect on the tastes of foods. Look for it this year.

Cocaine Combat

Researchers at Yale University have cleared two hurdles in testing a cocaine vaccine. Animals given the vaccine showed a decrease in self-administration of cocaine, and recent human trials found that the vaccine produces antibodies that bind to cocaine. According to Thomas Kosten, M.D., the principal investigator, upcoming human trials will show whether those antibodies can actually help people overcome addiction by inhibiting the high the drug produces.

Anti-Cancer Magnets

Researchers at UCLA Medical Center think magnets may help make chemotherapy more effective. They added particles of iron to a chemotherapy drug before injecting it into an artery feeding a tumor. Then they put a magnet right over the tumor and drew the iron-laced chemicals to it. "This type of technology may mean the therapy can be concentrated right on the tumor site," says Scott Goodwin, M.D., one of the study authors. It may not only make the medicine more effective but also reduce side effects. The study was the first in a series needed to get FDA approval for the procedure.

NUMBER OF MEN WHO DIE FROM CHRONIC LUNG CONDITIONS EACH YEAR: 57,018

INCREASE IN CHANCE OF DYING FROM A CHRONIC LUNG CONDITION IF YOU SMOKE: 10 TIMES

PERCENTAGE OF LUNG-CANCER DEATHS IN MEN THAT ARE LINKED TO CIGARETTE SMOKING: 90

DOES IT WORK?

Scalp Surgery

For years, we've told all bald men the same thing: Accept your fate, avoid the comb-over, and keep the rest of your hair short. Then comes disturbing news like this. An Italian plastic surgeon is smoothing out bald guys' heads. The doc, Paolo G. Morselli, M.D., claims the ridges that some men have on the sides of their heads can make them look aggressive or violent—he calls it the Minotaur syndrome. So he sucks out fat tissue and superficial layers of the temporalis muscle. Only a 5-millimeter scar remains.

It sounds simple enough, but we're skeptical. There can be significant swelling because of the muscle removal, and numbness can last up to a month. Plus, there's the danger of hitting a facial nerve and paralyzing part of the forehead, warns Bernard Markowitz, M.D., associate professor of plastic surgery at the University of California, Los Angeles, who reviewed Dr. Morselli's paper. Our bottom line: You need this surgery like you need a hole in the head.

Johnson & Johnson Advanced Healing Strip

These bandages use Compeed Moisture Seal technology, which turns fluid from the cut into a protective layer of gel. This shortens healing time, allowing you to continue running from the cops.

It works because skin cells work better to repair an injury when the area is moist. Plus, the gel keeps the bandage from pressing on the wound. "This causes less skin damage," says Billy Trolan, M.D., a California emergency-room doctor.

The extra healing power is great for cuts or scrapes with uneven edges. If you have a straight cut, like one from your ex's pocketknife, the wound heals pretty fast on its own. The new strips cost a lot (about $4 for 10 bandages; regular Band-Aids cost $2.50 for 30), but we found them more flexible and water-resistant. Which is great if you're cut on your . . . well, never mind.

COOL STUFF

Bacteria at Work

Microscopic Medicinal Robots

Researchers at Utah State University are developing microscopic robots that can clean blocked arteries and zap individual cancer cells with drugs. Even more impressive, the robots will be powered by live bacteria attached to the blades of a tiny motor. As they swim, the bacteria will push the motor's blades, turning the propeller and moving it forward. "Right now, we plan on using E. coli or salmonella, since they have fairly long life spans and tend to be the best swimmers," says Alicja Copik, one of the robots' designers.

New Tonsil Technology

Microwave Tonsillectomy

If a doctor says your tonsils should come out, you can have them surgically removed. But that process can lead to severe pain and bleeding. A new procedure called microwave tonsillectomy can eliminate recurrent tonsil infections without surgery. "We stick a small computer-controlled probe inside your tonsils and zap them with high-powered radio waves," says Mansoor Madani, D.M.D., director of the Center for Corrective Surgery in Bryn Mawr, Pennsylvania. "As the tissue heats up, it can shrink by up to 60 percent." For more information on the procedure, visit www.snorenet.com.

A Pump for Prostate Cancer

Viadur

Until now, patients with advanced prostate cancer often had to get a testosterone-suppressing injection every few months. But the FDA has just approved a new product that will make life easier for them. Viadur is a matchstick-size pump that is implanted in the upper arm and continuously releases the testosterone-depressing drug leuprolide into the bloodstream for a full year. Prostate-cancer patients won't have to see their doctors solely for injections anymore.

WHAT WORKS

No matter your occupation, marital status, or bank account size, living your life is like playing in the major leagues. You need to be in the best of shape to stay in the game and keep winning. So when you're sidelined by injury or illness, you want to get your health back fast before some upstart takes over your position. Whether you're benched by a headache or something as serious as prostate cancer, these tips will keep you at your best so you don't get thrown out at the plate.

I. Use caution with painkillers. If your headache doesn't go away after you down a few aspirin, don't attack it the way you attack buffet lines. "Taking more ibuprofen, acetaminophen, or aspirin to compensate can actually make symptoms worse by causing a rebound headache," says Merle Diamond, M.D., associate director of the Diamond Headache Clinic in Chicago. Dr. Diamond suspects that extra doses may create a false tolerance for pain. When the pills wear off, normal pain may feel exaggerated. Or with pills that contain caffeine—such as Excedrin—you could feel pain because caffeine causes the blood vessels in your head to constrict and then swell. Stick to two nonprescription pills every 4 hours; don't take them every day.

2. Heal your wounds. Road rash hurts bad enough. It'll sting even worse if you try to disinfect it with hydrogen peroxide. Try rinsing the abrasion with the same stuff you use on contact lenses—saline solution. It'll wash away bacteria and keep the wound feeling cool, says Tom Newberg, assistant trainer for the Seattle Mariners. To help the area heal quickly, apply a mixture of Neosporin antibiotic ointment and zinc oxide two or three times a day. Keep it covered with nonstick gauze.

3. Hijack a hangover. Before you embark on your alcohol adventure, leave two aspirin tablets on the bathroom floor, right where you'll find them later

NUMBER OF MEN WHO DIE OF PROSTATE CANCER EACH YEAR: 32,000

OF I,000 MEN SURVEYED OVER THE PHONE ABOUT PROSTATE CANCER, PERCENTAGE THAT THOUGHT WOMEN HAVE PROSTATES: 21+

(don't do this if you have a history of stomach problems, or small children or pets that could find them). To blunt the headache that comes with your hangover, down them with a large glass of warm milk, which will help you sleep. Do not, under any circumstances, take acetaminophen or ibuprofen when you're drunk. You may damage liver cells. Finally, sleep naked—it may help you avoid getting the sweats.

4. Rub yourself the right way. Spend too much time in front of your computer? For headaches and eyestrain, apply small circular pressure to your temples with the two middle fingers of each hand. To fight frowning, use your first and second fingers like scissors: Press them against your forehead, squeezing the skin in a cutting movement and working toward your temples. To create soothing darkness, cup your hands over your eyes for a few minutes.

For palm strain and headaches, apply circular pressure with your thumb over the opposite palm and around the base of the opposite thumb. Knead the muscle on the back of your hand between your thumb and index finger. Then, stretch your fingers by holding each one at the base and pulling it firmly, sliding and twisting your grip upward. Stroke across one palm with the heel of the other hand. Glide back, repeat, then work in the opposite direction.

5. Lower-back pain? First assess, then attack. Back pain is more than a convenient excuse to skip boccie-ball practice; it actually sends 14 million people to the doctor every year. Start your diagnosis here.

Is the pain shooting from the center of your back out to one side?

This is probably a muscle spasm. Any movement—bending wrong or sleeping in an awkward position—can cause it. If untreated, it can lead to a muscle strain. Apply ice at 20-minute intervals for several hours.

Are you suffering from tightness in the middle of your lower back?

It's most likely a muscle strain, says Kevin R. Stone, M.D., U.S. ski-team doctor. Strains are generally caused by poor posture, weak abdominal muscles, or rushing into exercise without warming up. Stretch and ice it two or three times a day. If you don't feel better in 3 weeks, see a doctor.

Do you feel extreme pains off to one side of your central lower back?

Could be kidney stones. Men with a little extra weight will feel this right next to their love handles. Start drinking extra water (to flush the stone) on your way to the doctor.

Do you have a sharp, shooting pain starting in your back and extending below the knee?

It may be a herniated disk, which is a swelling of the cartilage separating two vertebrae. The onset can be sudden or gradual, affects only one leg, and intensifies to a shooting sensation when you sneeze or cough. Golfers are especially susceptible because swinging causes the spine to bend and twist. You may need surgery. See a doctor.

6. Avoid these combinations of foods and drugs. If man were always afraid of mixing weird things together, there'd be no such thing as chili or Angelina Jolie marriages. But when it comes to combining foods and drugs, take care not to mix the following.

Drug You're Taking	Foods You Should Avoid
The antibiotics doxycycline, tetracycline, or ciprofloxacin	Dairy products. Calcium may make it harder for your body to absorb the drug. Wait 2 hours after taking the medicine before downing any dairy
High doses of an antacid made with aluminum hydroxide, such as some types of Maalox and Mylanta	Milk with vitamin D. It could lead to milk-alkali syndrome, which causes calcium deposits in the kidneys, says Michael Hogue, Pharm.D., of the American Pharmaceutical Association. Worst-case scenario: kidney failure
Either of the asthma/pulmonary drugs Slo-Bid or Theo-Dur (theophylline)	Cola, coffee, and other beverages containing caffeine. Doctors suspect that the caffeine can worsen the drugs' side effects, including nausea and dizziness
The antidepressant Parnate (tranylcypromine)	Aged and fermented products, such as cheeses, smoked fish, and Chianti. These have high levels of tyramine, which when combined with the drug, can increase blood pressure
The anticoagulant Coumadin (warfarin sodium)	Green leafy vegetables. They contain large amounts of vitamin K, which can put you at risk of blood clots when combined with this medication
The high-blood-pressure medication Plendil (felodipine)	Grapefruit juice. It inhibits the medication from breaking down in your liver before it's absorbed, so you might end up with a double or triple dose

7. And understand the side effects of the drugs you take. When you use medicine, you know you might experience side effects. But drowsiness and nausea are one thing; growing breasts is quite another. To tell if the weird stuff that's happening to you is a symptom of your sickness or a side effect of your drug, check www.nursespdr.com for complete descriptions of nearly 1,000 drugs. Then talk to your doctor; he can prescribe a different medication if you're having unwanted reactions to a certain drug, like maybe one of these . . .

CHANCE THAT AN AMERICAN'S *STREPTOCCOCUS PNEUMONIAE* INFECTION IS RESISTANT TO PENICILLIN: **1 IN 4**

Drug	The Fine Print Says You May Have . . .
Digoxin, spironolactone (congestive heart failure)	Breast enlargement. These drugs alter a man's hormone levels—digoxin increases estrogen, and spironolactone decreases testosterone. It's a fairly common side effect in older men
Prednisone (allergies, asthma)	Hallucinations, at high doses. Rare. "I had a patient who said he saw Jesus on TV—literally, that Jesus was sitting on top of his TV," says pharmacy professor Bruce Canaday, Pharm.D., of the University of North Carolina in Wilmington
Trazodone (insomnia)	Priapism. Prolonged erections happen occasionally if the drug reacts negatively with the neurotransmitters and the vascular system of the penis. Sounds like it'd be fun—for about 20 minutes. After that, it's hell
Versed, propofol (short-term sedation for medical procedures)	Mistaking dreams for reality. Rare. These drugs can alter your normal sleep cycles, which is what makes it seem that the nurse is holding a riding crop

8. Before deciding on a prostate-cancer treatment, ask your doctor the following questions.

How advanced is the prostate tumor?

If cancer hasn't spread outside the prostate, a radical prostatectomy (surgical removal of the prostate) will probably work—but only 58 percent of men are diagnosed this early. If there's evidence that it has spread, or if the scores on two standard prostate tests are elevated—a prostate-specific antigen (PSA) count greater than 10 or a Gleason score higher than 7—there's more reason to try radiation therapy, says radiation oncologist Alan Pollack, M.D., of the M.D. Anderson Cancer Center in Houston.

How quickly will the tumor grow?

A physician can predict this with several diagnostic tests, such as determining how swiftly the PSA count has risen. Faster-growing tumors need more aggressive treatment.

What has been the success rate in other men the same age with similar tumors and treatments?

Ask the doctor to contact urologist Ashutosh Tewari, M.D., of the Josephine Ford Cancer Center in Detroit. He's one of the creators of the Neural Network, a database of 5,000 prostate-cancer patients treated from 1980 to 2000. It allows doctors to compare a man's profile (using such factors as age, race, PSA score, symptoms, and family history) with thousands of case histories. "It's useful in determining the grade of your tumor and how successful a certain treatment will probably be," says Dr. Tewari, who fields about 50 requests a month. About 2,000 of the database patients are African-Americans, who are far more vulnerable to prostate cancer. Doctors can reach Dr. Tewari at (313) 874-6722 or atiwari1@hfhs.org.

What have clinical studies shown about my specific treatment?

Search for the latest published research at www.ncbi.nlm.nih.gov/ (click on the PubMed button). Look for recent studies that tell the relative effectiveness of the therapy and its side effects.

This step is especially important if a doctor suggests a new procedure; if there's no clinical proof that it's the best option, ask him to justify his hunch.

Is it worth enrolling in a clinical trial?

If you have advanced prostate cancer, consider joining a clinical study. "The first men to be successfully treated by a new drug or procedure will be in a study, and you might as well be among them," says oncologist Joel Picus, M.D., of Washington University in St. Louis. Hundreds of trials are testing refinements to FDA-approved drugs and well-studied procedures, which eases the guinea-pig factor. For a listing of clinical trials, call the National Cancer Institute at (800) 422-6237, or click on the oncology link at www.centerwatch.com.

ANY QUESTIONS?

Standard Deviation

My doctor says I have a deviated septum. How did this happen, and do I need to do anything about it?

—G. M., Sweetwater, Tex.

A deviated septum means that the cartilage and bone dividing your nostrils are deflected to one side. You probably know how this happened better than we do; it's usually caused by a childhood fall or a frat-house sucker punch. It's a pretty common thing—about 80 percent of us have it—and it is not at all dangerous, says otolaryngologist John Coniglio, M.D., of the University of Rochester in New York. But it is annoying: It can cause snoring, sinusitis, chronic congestion, frequent nosebleeds, or headaches. If that sums up your typical day, you may need your septum straightened. (Getting hit from the other side won't do it.) The simple outpatient procedure takes about an hour, and it's covered by most insurance plans.

Night Sweats

I always wake up in the middle of the night drenched in sweat. What causes this, and how do I stop it?

—D. F., Dalton, Ga.

Maybe the kids are playing a cute little "Let's mess with Dad's heart medication" prank. A common—yet potentially serious—cause is sleep apnea, a condition in which the upper airway becomes obstructed at night, according to Jonathan Schwartz, M.D., director of the Integris Sleep Disorders Center in Oklahoma City. "We're not sure why, but nearly half of our sleep-apnea patients also experience night sweats," says Dr. Schwartz.

PERCENTAGE OF MEN AGES 51 TO 60 WHO HAVE ENLARGED PROSTATES (BPH): 50

PERCENTAGE OF MEN PAST AGE 80 WHO HAVE BPH: 90

Your first step should be a visit to your doctor, who may refer you to a sleep-disorder clinic. Treatments for sleep apnea include weight loss, decongestant drugs, and a nasal mask that keeps the airway open by blowing air to the back of the throat.

Does the Medicine Stay Down?

The other night, I took a dose of an antibiotic and then vomited a little while later. Should I have taken another dose right away?

—N. K., Denver

Sometimes a sick body just doesn't seem to appreciate the one thing that could make it better. The truth is, your body will have absorbed some of the medication even after a few minutes, so don't pop another. "Not unless you see a pill come back up entirely intact is it safe to take another dose," says Mike Cohen, president of the Institute for Safe Medication Practices.

Smart Wart Removal

I have two plantar warts on my foot. Do doctors still burn them off, or is there a less barbaric method of removing them?

—J. T., Dearborn, Mich.

Plantar warts can be cut out, frozen, treated with a topical acid solution, or removed with a laser, says Houston podiatrist Ronald Lepow, D.P.M. (The hot-poker method didn't make his list.) The technique your doctor uses depends on what kind of warts you have. A single wart can be treated with any of these methods, while a cluster of warts is best treated with a laser or acid. "It's not as scary as it sounds," says Dr. Lepow. "We use a local anesthetic to numb the area, and all these methods are quick and nearly painless." A podiatrist can remove warts during a regular office visit, and you should be back on your feet the following day.

PART EIGHT
MAKE AN
IMPRESSION

M U S T   R E A D S

Look Your Best in 10 Minutes or Less

Hot date at 8:00—and no time to spare? Here's how to look great without being late

By Brian Boyé

7:50 Splash down lightly. Okay, deep breath. There's no need to rush, especially since you're going to be spending less time in the shower. That's the advice of Manhattan-based skin-care expert Paula Moynahan, M.D. "Keep your showers short and your water tepid," she says. (Remember, short and tepid. Like David Spade.) "Too much hot water depletes the body's moisture balance." The other thing to remember: When washing, avoid common alkaline soaps—they say "soap" right there on the label—which can dry your skin. Instead use nonalcohol shower gels, liquid cleansers, or nonsoap bars, such as Neutrogena, that are gentler on your skin. One product we like: Bulgari's Black shower gel and shampoo ($40). It comes in a tall black tower that looks cool in your shower stall—in case she winds up there next morning.

7:52 Make like *Face/Off*. You may not realize it, but your body is covered with a nasty layer of dead skin. (Your own, we hope.) From the neck up, "use a mild facial scrub to get rid of the dead skin. It will give your face a nice glow," says Fredric Brandt, M.D., a dermatologist practicing in New York City and Miami. Just don't be too aggressive with your scrubbing, he cautions. Too much pressure, and you'll scratch your face and irritate your skin. Tommy Hilfiger's Polished Clean ($14) is a good choice for polishing your mug. Heavier-duty scrubs such as H_2O Plus's Black Ice Invigorating Body Scrub ($14) are available for the neck down. What does all this do? you ask. "When you take dead skin cells off the surface, you stimulate the skin to produce new cells and new collagen," Dr. Brandt says. "That helps give your skin a smooth texture and healthy glow." We're not sure, but we think that's a good thing.

7:53 Cut through the fog. The best time to shave is when the bathroom is still steamed up, which will help soften your beard and make it easier to cut, says Myriam Malka, co-owner of The Art of Shaving, based in New York City. First step: "Before shaving, apply a preshave oil, which protects the skin, softens the beard, and helps the razor glide evenly," Malka says. This is especially important for anyone who tends to look more like Fred than Barney;

dark hair and a heavy beard increase your chances of razor burn and ingrown hairs. Try The Art of Shaving's Pre-Shave Oil ($22). Then lather up with shaving cream. "First shave with the grain, then go against the grain for the closest shave. This helps get rid of ingrown hairs," she explains, "and it will leave your face as smooth as a baby's bottom." And less prone to diaper rash. Malka also suggests using a three-blade razor for a faster shave. Follow it all with an aftershave balm instead of aftershave: Alcohol-free versions like Lab Series for Men Razor Burn Relief Plus ($25) keep your skin moist.

7:54 Spritz into the wind. The key to using cologne is this: Women have a stronger sense of smell than men. What smells good to you smells to her like Joey Buttafuoco—assuming she'd ever let him get within 3 miles of her. To smell just right, spray the fragrance into the air, then walk through the mist. On a first date, try a cologne that's just hit the market—that way, you don't have to worry about reminding her of her ex-boyfriend, the one her cat hated and, oh, if only she had listened. We like Nautica's Latitude Longitude ($45) and Calvin Klein's Contradiction for Men ($45).

7:55 Lock it in. Maybe you think you're too macho to use moisturizer. Perhaps you feel that it's best left to those men who watch *Frasier* and find themselves feeling self-conscious every time someone makes fun of Niles. Well, look: The staff of *Men's Health*, who are very buff men who play sports and land more women than air-traffic controllers land planes, recommend that you use moisturizer. Don't make us come down there, okay? If it's rated at SPF

NEVER A DOH! MOMENT

If you can't sweep her off her feet, you can at least avoid embarrassing yourself. Do this, don't do that.

Check the cash drawer. Call the number on the back of your credit card, and double-check that you're not going to be humiliated in front of her by having the waiter snip the card in half. Also carry at least $80 in cash for tips or cabs, or to impulsively buy her flowers on the street. (You big lug, you!) Pocket a few singles for faster transactions.

Prepare a couple of interesting things to say in case there's an awkward lull in the conversation. Something like "Did you know the word *assassin* stems from the word *hashish,* which Muslim warriors chewed during the Crusades?" This can seamlessly be worked into al-most any conversation, as in "No, I never saw *Erin Brockovich.* But did you know that the word *assassin . . . ?"

Edit your wallet. You lose points for dozens of credit cards, pictures of ex-wives, loose scraps of paper with other women's phone numbers, and that telltale circle shape. This is a date. The less baggage everybody carries, the better.

Inspect your shoes before you leave (because she'll do the same when you arrive). If you don't have time for a full polish, give them a once-over with a shoe-shine brush to remove any dust or grime. If you have I more minute, polish the heels. If you have 2 more, just shine them already.

15 or better, it'll protect you from skin cancer by day, from ugly flakes and wrinkles by night. "Put it on while your face is still wet, and you'll seal in the moisture," Dr. Brandt says. "This draws water from the deeper layers of the skin." Look for moisturizers without oil for a less shiny look; Davidoff Cool Water Function's Cool O_2 Face Shield ($24) fits the description.

7:56 Untangle your tangle. Yo, Elvis, that shiny helmet thing just isn't working. You've got the same problem Scarface had—you're using too much product. "You want to make sure you're using the right amount of hair product—don't overdo it," says Edward Tricomi, co-owner of the Warren-Tricomi Salon in New York City. For fine hair, he suggests a light mist of hair spray on damp hair. "Lightly blow-dry for texture and volume." Next, apply a finishing cream, such as Kiehl's Creme with Silk Groom ($17), to create a natural, thicker appearance. These aren't gels that turn brittle; they're creams that, when dry, still allow her to run her fingers (or toes) through your hair. For curly or frizzy hair, comb in a leave-in conditioner and some of Redken's Rewind Styling Paste ($15). "It smooths the hair and makes it more manageable," Tricomi says. For a bit of extra shine, smooth on a few drops of Aveda's Pure-Fume Brilliant Emollient for Hair ($20). It's a lot better than the Mediocre-Grade-Point-Average Emollient for Hair we used to use.

7:58 Spit and polish (but not necessarily in that order). To ungrit your teeth, take this four-step approach from Ziba Yaghmai, D.D.S., a cosmetic dentist in New York City. First, floss. Second, brush your teeth for longer than 2 minutes. "It's a must," Dr. Yaghmai says, unless you're going for that jack-o'-lantern look later in life. Third, try Colgate's 2-in-1 Toothpaste and Mouthwash gel ($3) for the freshest breath. Finally, attack your tongue, home to all sorts of nasty bacteria that cause bad breath: Do it with a different toothbrush so you don't spread the bacteria around. Your date will thank you for it later. At least that's the plan.

7:59 Hunt for hairs. Okay, guys. It's an ugly fact, but deal with it. The older you are, the more stray hairs you grow. And she'll definitely notice. So before you leave the house, stick your face right up in the mirror and look for them. Then tweeze, cut, or buzz the intruders with a trimmer. Next, move up to the eyebrows. Use a pair of small scissors to trim the flyaways, or risk that Boris Yeltsin look.

8:00 Finger licking, good. They say you can discern a man's wealth by the look of his hands. Particularly if he's giving you the finger when you ask him for a raise. So clean your fingernails. It's even okay to file them so you don't snag your claws on her hose. Buy a simple, functional nail-care kit. Soak your hands in water for a minute, then clean your nails, trim them, and if you're really feeling neat, push your cuticles back with—what else?—a cuticle pusher. Easy does it, though. Too hard, and you'll miss your next start. While you're at it, trim your toenails, too, and you'll never draw blood in a carnal embrace.

Ready? Now get going . . . you're late!

Make Your Wardrobe Measure Up

When it comes to looking great, size matters more than you think.
Here's how to get your clothes and your body to look perfect together

By Amy Donohue

There's no such thing as a small advantage. If a lineman holds his block for an extra 0.2 second, it's the Lombardi trophy, instead of an MRI for the quarterback. Every little edge is a big edge.

The secrets of properly fitting clothes are the ultimate little edge, a set of standards that will help you get more of everything: women, wealth, admiration from strangers. These rules of thumb and waist and foot are solid-gold secrets of style.

OVERCOATS

Most men wear coats that are too big and look sloppy, according to Leon Hall, host of E!'s *Fashion Emergency*.

- Buy a coat that's just one size larger than your suit size. It should follow the contour of your shoulders.
- Avoid padded shoulders.
- The down-to-the-knee fit is a good casual look. For business, go with the traditional midcalf length.

SWEATERS

Different fit rules apply depending on the weight of the sweater.

- Heavy sweaters should be roomy—nice and loose where the arms meet the body, and across the chest.
- Thinner sweaters worn under a jacket should be more form-fitting, and the armholes should be a tad higher.
- Sweaters should fall below your waist to your hipbones. Too short, and you could be mistaken for a figure skater.

EYEGLASSES

Choose frames that de-emphasize the feature an artist would exaggerate to turn you into a caricature.

AVERAGE AGE AT WHICH AMERICANS BELIEVE PHYSICAL ATTRACTIVENESS PEAKS: 38

- Circular Charlie Brown face? Try a horizontal and more rectangular shape.
- Square face, like Bart Simpson's? Ovals will soften your chiseled look.
- An elongated, Jay Leno jaw? Pick wide, angular frames, a squarish pair. They'll add depth to your face.
- Short, wide nose? Look for a bridge that sits high on your schnozz.
- Long, hawklike nose? Try a bridge that sits lower on your blower.
- If you're very fair or blond, the trendy black frames may be too strong for your face. Try a metal frame in gunmetal, silver, or tortoiseshell.

GLOVES

If gloves are tight, they won't keep you warm. They inhibit bloodflow, and the insulation gets the air flattened out of it. Air in the glove is the key to cozy digits.

- One simple fit trick: Put one on and make a fist. There should be no binding or tightness in the fingers. About that fist: Don't punch anybody unless there's no alternative.

SUIT JACKETS AND SPORT COATS

A jacket that fits just so is a great style tool. It covers love handles and abs that are slightly softer than steel.

- The sleeve should come down to that prominent bone at your wrist. Most men wear their jacket sleeves too long, says Alan Flusser, owner of a custom design company in New York City, who knows more about men and style than anybody else in the world. The sleeve should be short enough that $\frac{1}{2}$ inch of your shirt cuff sticks out below it.
- If you have big shoulders or arms, make sure the sleeves fall in straight, smooth lines all the way down. Sometimes big shoulders bulge at the point where the sleeves are sewn to the body of the jacket.
- A jacket should just cover the lower curve of your kiester—with $\frac{1}{2}$ inch to spare. Any more, and you'll look shorter than you are. Any less, and you'll look like you're wearing a busboy's jacket.

PERCENTAGE OF MEN WHO WOULDN'T MIND BEING STUPID, AS LONG AS THEY HAD A PERFECT BODY: **19**

PERCENTAGE OF MEN WHO BELIEVE A PERSON'S PHYSICAL ATTRACTIVENESS IS IMPORTANT FOR HAPPINESS, SOCIAL LIFE, AND ABILITY TO GET AHEAD: **76**

- If you have a big head, choose a jacket cut just a little wider in the shoulders—it'll make your head appear smaller. If you're small-headed, you want the shoulders of your jacket as narrow as they can comfortably be.
- No matter how many buttons your jacket has, one of them is pivotal—the waist button. The waist button should be $\frac{1}{2}$ inch below your natural waist—also known as the smallest part of your torso.
- If you normally carry a billfold or eyeglass case in your inside pocket, put it in there during the test drive.

SHOES AND BOOTS

Shoe sizes vary more from brand to brand than any other clothing item.

- Shop in the afternoon. Your feet swell slightly as the day wears on. Better to have shoes a little big in the morning than a little tight after lunch.
- The ball of your foot should rest easily in the widest part of the shoe, the flex point, so you can bend your foot easily while walking. Make sure there's enough width to move your toes a little.
- No need to "break in" shoes. Leather won't stretch over time; it just expands and contracts with each wearing.
- For dress shoes, be sure you can tie the laces so there's no more than a quarter-inch gap between the sides at the top.
- Buy hiking boots a tad larger than your street shoes. Your feet get a workout climbing all those peaks and may swell a bit.

PANTS

We're convinced that tight pants lead to most of society's problems, including crime. Fight back with the right fit.

- A precise waist fit is tricky, but Flusser suggests sitting down in the pants when you try them on. Since your waist and hips get bigger when you sit, if the pants are too small, you'll be uncomfortable in a sitting position.
- Pants legs should hit the tops of your shoes, with a slight break of material just above the cuffs.
- Pleats should lie flat. If they pull open when you're standing straight, the pants are too tight. Don't ever buy pants and plan to lose the weight to get into them. Studies show that this has never happened.
- Cuffs? Flusser says $1\frac{5}{8}$ inches if you're under 5 feet 10 inches, $1\frac{3}{4}$ inches if you're taller.
- The crease should run straight down over the center of your kneecap and land on the middle of your shoe. If it's outside the middle, it will make you look less sleek than you are.

SHIRTS

The rules are rigid when it comes to dress shirts. Don't just rummage through the stack until you find a 16/34. Buying by the numbers is the reason most men end up wearing dress shirts that are small in the collar and short in the sleeve.

- With the top button closed, you should be able to slide two fingers between your neck and the collar. If this sounds big, it is. But dress shirts almost always shrink in the collar after washing, says Flusser.
- The sleeve has to come to $\frac{1}{2}$ inch below the prominent bone at your wrist—and the sleeve of the jacket you're wearing.
- Beware of tightness in the torso. You should be able to sit down and move your arms freely.
- The cuff has to be tight enough that it doesn't slip down over your hand.

No More Bad-Hair Days

A man's guide to waxing, shaving, plucking, burning, and shocking away unwanted body foliage

By Lou Schuler

I remember my father as one of the great apes. Hair sprouted from the neck of his T-shirts, front and back. With his shirt off, he looked like a snowman standing downwind of a barbershop.

For most of my adult life, I had hairy arms and legs, but my chest hair was minimal. Back hair? None. I congratulated myself on how far I had taken the family gene pool. In just one generation, we'd gone from mountain gorillas to information gatherers.

Then I hit middle age.

Every hair that I'd lost on my head—and we're talking a quorum here—reappeared on my back. On my lats, the stringy bastards. My chest hair turned gray and grew out like a field of birch trees in winter.

PERCENTAGE OF MEN WHO WOULD DESCRIBE THEIR PHYSICAL APPEARANCE AS ABOVE AVERAGE: 43

PERCENTAGE OF MEN WHO ARE SATISFIED WITH HOW ATTRACTIVE THEY ARE: 81

PERCENTAGE OF AMERICANS WHO WOULD CONSIDER ELECTIVE COSMETIC SURGERY TO IMPROVE THEIR APPEARANCE: 19

So I decided to get rid of every single hair on my arms, legs, chest, ears, nose, and back. The question was, how? My experience with body-hair removal consisted of trimming my nose hairs with cuticle scissors.

Which removal methods gave me the best chance of eliminating my hair for good? How much did each one hurt? And how weird was it to walk around with a denuded body?

I sampled every antihair product known to man: razors, tweezers, lasers, chemical depilatories, electrolysis, wax. I even waxed my butt, swear to God. Here's what works, and what I hope you never try.

METHOD: Electrolysis
Where I tried it: Chest

I show up at Andrews Professional Electrolysis in Wescosville, Pennsylvania, hoping owner Dawn Andrews can deforest a significant portion of my chest. This is wishful thinking; electrolysis is a hair-by-hair procedure, way too labor-intensive for large areas.

Still, Andrews gamely offers a demonstration. She works with about a dozen electrically charged needles at a time, which hang over my chest on a small rack as I lie on an exam table. She sticks the needles into individual hair follicles, then goes back and pulls out the executed hairs with a pair of tweezers. There's a little sting as each needle goes in, and a couple of times it feels as if my skin is burning.

Aftermath: Andrews shows me a stack of hairs she has removed in the 45-minute demonstration. It seems like a lot, until I look at my chest. The cleared area doesn't look much different from the uncleared area on my opposite pectoral. I have small red welts across the cleared site, and I later develop a small bruise in one spot.

Assessment: Three weeks later, no hairs seem to have grown back in the tiny area that was electrolyzed. For ears and eyebrows, I'd give it a thumbs-up.

Where to go: To find a licensed electrologist in your area, log on to www.electrology.com.

Cost: $45 per hour, which is long enough to treat several square inches of spare hair growth. You'll probably need two or three sessions to clear an area the size of the chest.

Pain: 😖 😖 😖 (out of 5)

METHOD: Salon Waxing
Where I tried it: Chest (again)

Sherry Povenski, my waxtress at the Jon Thomas Salon and Day Spa in Emmaus, Pennsylvania, starts by rolling hot wax over my chest. The way the

THE MYSTERIES OF MIDDLE-AGE HAIR

I've always assumed there was some evolutionary purpose to this: Clearly, natural selection had determined that I needed hair on my back to protect my lungs and on my butt to protect my colon, but none on top of my head to protect my brain.

But I've been wrong. "I can't think of any evolutionary purpose for hair in those areas," says dermatologist David Vasily, M.D., of the Aesthetica Cosmetic and Laser Center in Bethlehem, Pennsylvania. Dr. Vasily reasons that living to old age is relatively new to the human species, so evolution wouldn't have produced ways to deal with it.

So why all this hair? Because different hair follicles are genetically programmed to activate at specific points in your life. "In some cases, it takes 60 to 70 years for this to happen," says dermatology professor Richard Wagner, M.D., of the University of Texas Medical Branch in Galveston.

The key to the process is the male hormone testosterone, particularly the way in which it converts to another hormone called dihydrotestosterone, the same evil chemical that causes baldness and may be the culprit in prostate cancer, says Dr. Vasily.

Okay, one more question: Why'd the hair on my chin and chest go gray first?

"I don't know, but I believe the same thing happens in silverback gorillas," says Dr. Vasily. "It must have something to do with establishing social status."

Which, if I were a gorilla, would make me feel really good about myself.

—Lou Schuler

---

wax roller tugs on my chest hairs gets the nerve endings good and worked up for the main event: She lays a piece of cloth across the waxed area, and then . . . rrrri-i-i-ippp! She shows me the cloth—dozens of hairs are stuck to it. She starts at about the nipple line and works down, then does the upper chest. I can see why she saved this for last—the closer we get to my throat, the more it hurts.

She wipes off the remaining flecks with GiGi Honnee wax-off, and we're finished; the whole thing takes 20 minutes.

Aftermath: My chest is beet-red immediately after, and that evening it looks like a field of pimples. By the next morning, the irritation is mostly cleared up; and by the end of the following day, my chest is as smooth and clear as my office at 5:00 P.M.

Assessment: About a week later, I can see the first hairs starting to grow back. Three weeks later, about half the hairs are returning, and they seem a little less bristly than before. The other half look like they've learned who's boss. So waxing seems to have one main advantage over shaving: It thins the herd. Plus, the salon experience is nice.

Where to go: Any full-service salon or spa.

Cost: Depends on where you live and the density of the forest you're clearing. A back-and-chest job might be $80.

Pain:

METHOD: Laser

Where I tried it: Back

Too bad I'm not French-Canadian. The combination of very dark hair with very light skin would make me ideal for laser hair removal, says dermatologist David Vasily, M.D., of the Aesthetica Cosmetic and Laser Center in Bethlehem, Pennsylvania. But I'm not a bad candidate. The hair on my back, unlike the stuff that was on my chest before I turned it into a baby's butt, is dark enough for the laser. (People with blond, gray, or red body hair are SOL; the laser needs melanin-rich brown or black hair to do its work.)

Step one is a test run of the laser: First, my skin tones are measured by a handheld device called a spectrophotometer. (Try saying that drunk—or sober.) Then the laser is applied on very small areas of my back to see how my skin reacts.

The next day, before I return to Aesthetica, my wife shaves my back for me—unlike waxing, the laser needs a smooth surface to do its work—rubs it down with alcohol, and then applies an analgesic cream called Emla. But it's not nearly analgesic enough. The technician at Aesthetica fires a laser shot into my back every 10 millimeters, and whenever the laser hits a hair follicle, the sensation is like being stabbed with a hypodermic needle. Around my neckline, where the hairs are thickest, some of the shots are so painful my hips come up off the table I'm lying on. But on the rest of my back, where the hairs are much thinner, it hardly hurts at all.

It takes a little over 2 hours to zap my entire back.

Aftermath: Immediately after, my skin looks and feels as if it's badly sunburned. The technician applies an ice pack along with an anti-inflammatory cream, which I have to reapply three times a day for the next 2 days.

The next day, my back looks as if I lost a dart fight; and 5 days later, I can still see a swath of red dots. Dr. Vasily tells me I'll probably need two more treatments to permanently kill all the follicles back there—a percentage of them would have been dormant at the time I got treated, so they wouldn't have gotten any laser action at all. Plus, others will undoubtedly develop as I get older and hairier.

Assessment: Three weeks later, the scabs are all gone, and my back has absolutely no hair on it—not a single one. If you have the money, this seems like the only way to permanently turn back the clock on large carpets of body hair.

Where to go: A board-certified dermatologist or plastic surgeon.

PERCENTAGE OF MALE PLASTIC-SURGERY PATIENTS WHO HAVE LIPOSUCTION: 28

Cost: Expensive. It's $350 per half-hour session, and you'll need at least three sessions to mow a large patch like your back. The bill can run to $1,200 the first year.

Pain: 🙀 🙀 🙀 🙀 🙀 (in select areas)

METHOD: Tweezers

Where I tried it: Nose and ears

Pluck, pluck, pluck. Two things I learn about myself here: My ears aren't very sensitive (something my wife has been trying to tell me for years, except I don't listen) but my nose is. As soon as I start plucking, it starts running like a mountain creek in spring. My eyes are soon streaming, too. I nearly go through a box of Kleenex and still don't get all of the nose hairs out.

Aftermath: I give up on tweezing the nose hairs and go back to using a pair of cuticle scissors to trim them back.

Assessment: Two weeks later, I need to trim the nose hairs again with the scissors, which takes only a couple of minutes. As for the ear hairs, new ones have popped up, but for some reason, they're never in the same place twice in a row.

Where to go: You can buy tweezers or cuticle scissors at any drugstore.

Cost: $3 for tweezers, $8 for cuticle scissors.

Pain: 🙀 for plucking ears; 🙀 🙀 🙀 🙀 🙀 for plucking nose

METHOD: Depilatory

Where I tried it: Arms

It's fun asking salesclerks where I can find the Nair. It's fun telling my 18-month-old daughter, "Don't touch Daddy's depilatory." It's fun sitting around with the blue goop on my arms for 7 minutes as I watch basketball and get the "I don't know you anymore" look from my wife.

When I wipe it off, I'm pleasantly surprised to see that most of the hair has come off on the towel. The only problem is that the hairs don't come off uniformly—stray tufts remain. I finish these off with a razor.

Aftermath: The day after, I attend a photo shoot with three *Men's Health* workout models. I realize we all have hair-free arms. It occurs to me that we could form a band: Denudo. For this horrible misuse of my God-given language skills, I punish myself by reading *Atlantic Monthly* cover-to-cover.

Assessment: The arm hairs removed with Nair seem to grow back just as fast as the leg hairs I shaved (see the next page). So it's more expensive and messier than shaving, with no advantages I can detect.

Where to go: Any drugstore.

Cost: $4 or so for a bottle of Nair.

Pain: None

METHOD: Shaving

Where I tried it: Legs

You don't realize how much hair you have below the butt until you buzz it all off at once. (I use Wahl clippers.) I could stuff a cat with all that hair on the floor. And I've still missed a bunch of places.

Aftermath: Here's something that bodybuilders, personal trainers, and fitness models figured out a long time ago: If you want to see the muscles you've built, you have to take the hair off the top. You really see the results of all those workouts. Once you get over the weirdness of not having leg hair for the first time since puberty, it's kind of cool.

Assessment: This is as fast, cheap, and easy as hair removal can possibly be.

Where to go: Any drugstore.

Cost: About $5 a month for razors and shaving cream, or $25 for electric clippers. Since I began buzzing my own head hair, I've replaced my clippers every 2 to 3 years.

Pain: None

METHOD: Home Waxing Kit

Where I tried it: Butt

Some reporters make a career out of getting their butts shot off in war zones. I'm effectively ending my career by standing in my bathroom with a small pot of melted wax and a wooden tongue depressor, preparing to pull out my butt hair by the roots.

I use the tongue depressor to slather the wax on my 'tocks, then I pull off the wax. It's not as painful as when I got my chest waxed at the spa, but it's also ridiculously sloppy and inefficient—I have to go back downstairs to reheat the wax several times to get the entire area cleared (the wax solidifies in a couple of minutes), and I never manage to pull off all the wax on the first try.

Aftermath: No residual pain or redness, but 2 days later I still feel completely ridiculous for having waxed my butt. Be a pal and don't tell anybody.

Assessment: The hair grows back about as fast as it did from chest waxing—some pops right back, but other hairs seem to be taking a wait-and-see attitude. Like me, they don't want to go through it a second time.

Where to go: You can get a home waxing kit at any drugstore.

Cost: About $7.

Pain: 😣 😣 😣

PERCENTAGE OF FACELIFTS PERFORMED ON MEN: 7

AVERAGE PRICE OF A FACELIFT: $4,899

The *Men's Health* Guide to Blue Jeans

How to buy the best jeans, look great in them, and make them last

By Kimberly Flynn

Blue jeans are not simply the backbone of your wardrobe but the backbone of your life. They are the uniform for utility: Every useful thing we do has to be done in denim. What's more, the right pair will last longer than many marriages. So pull on something that will suit you. Four men from our office test-drove dozens of pairs of jeans to find the ones that best fit their varied body types, from big and tall to round and small. You've got flaws? Tell us about it. But we're here to say, "Hide 'em, cowboy." Here are the right jeans for every guy.

FOR BIG GUYS

Cuts to look for: Jeans labeled "relaxed" will give you some room in the thighs and legs.

Cuts to avoid: Don't buy baggy jeans—they'll make you look like a rodeo clown.

Favorite pairs: *Guess? UrbanFit ($58).* "The best I tried," says contributing editor Ted Spiker, (6 feet 2 inches, 222 pounds). "Roomy but not baggy. A simple, classic pair that would work with a T-shirt or a sport coat."

DENIM COLOR GUIDE

Stone-Washed

This is the basic blue jean. The denim is washed with pumice stones to soften and fade it. It's a classic and casual look.

Wear with: Anything from a white T-shirt to a cashmere sweater.

Black

Black denim is, uh, black. A computer-help-desk look. Good for guys who wash their clothes semi-annually.

Wear with: X-Files T-shirt. Every day for a year.

Vintage

Vintage jeans are heavily stone-washed, some-times with bleach, to create an old, worn look.

Wear with: An oxford shirt or pullover sweater in a muted color.

Indigo

Indigo jeans haven't been treated. Their dark-blue color makes them suitable for dressier events.

Wear with: Something light for contrast, such as a blue or white shirt.

Antique

Antique jeans are both sanded and washed to make them appear aged.

Wear with: A casual shirt, polo, or pullover. No sport coat, and nothing too dressy.

JEANS DICTIONARY

If the Label Says . . .	It Means . . .
Slim Fit	The jeans are very narrow through the waist, hips, and legs. This cut can be too tight if you're big, and it's best for slender guys with good bodies
Regular Fit	They'll be narrower in the waist and hips but roomier in the seat and thighs, with straight legs. This is the dressiest cut
Relaxed	You'll have extra room in the hips and thighs. These are casual and easy for almost any man to wear
Boot Cut	Flared to ride over high boots or really fat ankles. The jeans also sit low on the waist and are slim through the hips, a tough look for most men to wear well
Carpenter	Inspired by actual work wear, their defining feature is a hammer loop on the leg. They rest at your natural waist and are meant to be fuller than regular fit
Cargo	They come in a variety of cuts, from slim to baggy, but they all have extra pockets on the legs
Baggy	Cut large all over, especially in the seat and hips. Unflattering if you're on the bigger side

Polo Jeans Co. Ralph Lauren Banner ($52). As comfortable as khakis.
Tommy Jeans Freedom ($49). Spiker's wife called the dark blue "slimming."
Nautica Jeans Company Classic ($49). Soft, faded blue. Plenty of butt-and-thigh room.

FOR AVERAGE GUYS

Cuts to look for: Wear almost any style, from slim to baggy, but regular or relaxed cuts are the most flattering and versatile.

Cuts to avoid: You wear a favorite pair of jeans for 10 years, while the average style swing lasts 3. Stick with the classics.

Favorite pairs: *CK Calvin Klein Jeans Original* ($48). "The fit is perfect in the waist and seat," says our production director, Erik Wikane (6 feet, 170 pounds). "They're worth the price."

Levi's Jeans 501 ($50). Plan on a break-in period.

Tommy Jeans Freedom ($49). Rich blue; baggy where you need it.

FOR THIN MEN

Cuts to look for: Regular or slim fit. They'll keep you on your training program.

Cuts to avoid: Anything with tapered legs. They're not flattering to skinny calves and ankles.

Favorite pairs: *AIX Armani Exchange Classic* ($78). "The perfect blend of baggy in the thighs and lower legs and snug in the seat and crotch," says executive editor Peter Moore (5 feet 11 inches, 150 pounds). "These are classic, classy blue jeans."

Diamond Gusset Regular ($40). Comfort jeans.

Gap Vintage ($54). Silky finish.

Edwin American Classic Regular Straight ($78). If you've got bulges, these will show them off.

FOR FIREPLUGS

Cuts to look for: Regular or relaxed fit. Extra room in the thighs and legs.

Cuts to avoid: Big and baggy. They'll draw attention to your lack of a lower half.

Favorite pairs: *Gap Easy Fit* ($36). "Extremely comfortable," says contributing editor Ron Geraci (5 feet 6 inches, 170 pounds), "with the right amount of taper in the legs for a guy my size."

Nautica Jeans Company Easy Fit ($49). Jeans you can dress up.

Diamond Gusset Rugged ($40). Wear 'em cutting wood or to a rock concert.

Rustler Regular ($12). Soft blue, soft fabric.

How to Tip in Every Situation

The smartest ways to show your appreciation

From *The* Men's Health *Real-Life Survival Guide* (Rodale) by Larry Keller, Christian Millman, and the other guys in the trenches at *Men's Health*

Debate his singing or acting all you like, but about this there can be no argument: Frank Sinatra was a tipper extraordinaire. Author Bill Zehme relates the following story in *The Way You Wear Your Hat*, his book about the crooner. A parking lot attendant brings Sinatra's car to him, and Sinatra asks him what his biggest tip ever was. The kid says 100 bucks. Not to be outdone, Sinatra slips him 200, then asks who gave him the C-note. Replies the valet: "You did, sir, last week."

For those of us not blessed with Sinatra's bankroll or his savoir faire, however, who we should tip and how much can be as perplexing as deciphering the tax code.

These days, it seems that everyone who does anything for you has his palm out. "The basic guideline is if the person is a professional, then you do not tip," says *At Ease . . . Professionally* author Hilka Klinkenberg, managing director of Etiquette International, a New York City company that provides advice on international protocol, business etiquette, and entertaining. "Or if the person is a salaried employee, you do not tip." Examples of people who provide services for which you do not tip include airline attendants and personal trainers, though you may want to give the latter something during the holiday season.

Among the people who ought to be tipped—either routinely or during the holidays—are those who provide somewhat invisible services such as vacuuming the halls of your apartment building or delivering the morning newspaper to your door. These people often are overlooked, Klinkenberg explains, as are hotel housekeepers and wine stewards.

Sometimes people feel obligated to leave a gratuity regardless of the service received, but they shouldn't, says *The Art of Tipping* author John Schein, president and founder of Tippers International. "If you don't feel like tipping, you don't have to," he says. It's merely a custom, and a good one, he believes. "We can't get along without service people. How else are you going to let people know the service they provided was satisfactory?"

Tips also make up the bulk of some service-industry-workers' incomes. Still, if you don't think a tip is merited, don't show your displeasure by leaving pennies, advises Klinkenberg. It just makes you look small, she says.

It's not enough to show your displeasure with bad service by stiffing the staff on the tip, Schein says. Your act of protest could be construed as mere forgetfulness or ignorance on your part. For that reason, you should find a person in authority and voice your complaint, he says.

This ought to be done sooner rather than later, Klinkenberg adds. If the service is lousy during a meal, for example, don't wait until you have finished eating to voice your complaint. Act quickly and you can still salvage the evening, she says.

It's important, however, not to use a small tip to punish someone for events beyond his control, Schein says. If your meal was cold or not cooked to your liking, that's the fault of the chef—not the person serving you.

One distinction: Tipping is done after a service is rendered to show your appreciation. Money paid in advance, such as to a maître d' to secure a good table, is not a tip but more akin to a bribe, Schein says.

Klinkenberg is opposed to this practice and says it often doesn't buy the intended result, anyway.

It's not just how much you tip that tells others you're a suave kind of guy. It's how you tip. Here are some pointers.

Be discreet. "It's so tacky when people are flashy and showy about it," Klinkenberg says.

Sinatra was generous but not ostentatious when he tipped. "He never showed off. He would never flash a bill," Zehme quotes one Sinatra pal as saying.

Know when to fold 'em. "Don't hold the bills open," Klinkenberg says. "Fold them in your hand and just say, 'Thank you.'"

Sinatra usually had others in his entourage do the tipping. But if he handed a tip to somebody personally, he folded bills three times, into small squares that could be subtly passed in a handshake, according to Zehme.

Leave the table. If you are entertaining guests at a restaurant, try to pay the bill away from the table, Klinkenberg suggests. "Let the captain or maître d' know beforehand that during coffee and dessert you will be coming to them to pay the bill. Ask if they could please have it ready. Then excuse yourself from the table, pay the bill, relax over dessert and coffee, and leave." This enables you to calculate the tip without fanfare, she says.

YOUR TIP SHEET

Here are guidelines for whom to tip and how much, according to *At Ease . . . Professionally* author Hilka Klinkenberg, managing director of Etiquette International, a New York City company that provides advice on international protocol, business etiquette, and entertaining. Copy it, fold it, and keep it in your wallet at all times.

• Skycap or train porter: $1 per bag; more if your bags are very heavy

• Airport shuttle driver: $1.50 to $2

• Parking valet: $1 to $2

• Taxi driver: 15 to 20 percent, depending on the professionalism of the driver and the cleanliness of the taxi

• Limousine driver: 10 to 20 percent

• Hotel doorman: $1 to $2 for hailing a taxi; $1 for carrying heavy luggage

• Bellman: $1 to $2 per bag; $5 to $10 if your luggage is especially heavy or large; $2 to $5 for special errands

• Room service: 15 percent—$2 minimum—each time (you can give cash or write the amount of the tip on the bill)

• Housekeeper: $1 to $2 per person per night (if you begin your stay late in the week and extend it through the weekend staff changes, leave the tip daily in an envelope marked "Housekeeping"; otherwise, leave one tip at the end of your stay)

• Coat check: $1 per coat

• Bathroom attendant: $1; $2 for special service

• Waiter or waitress: 15 to 20 percent

• Wine steward: $2 to $5 per bottle (if he brings you a special reserved bottle, tip 5 to 10 percent of the cost of the wine, separate from the dinner check)

• Musicians, including strolling players: $1 for a solo artist per request; $2 to $3 for a small group; $5 for larger bands

• Bartender: 15 percent

• Barber or stylist: 15 percent

Parting of the Waves

Is your friendly neighborhood barber really running a chop shop?

By Joe Queenan for *GQ*

I stopped going to barbershops in 1968, the year Richard Nixon was elected president. I'd like to be able to say this action was a protest against the napalming of North Vietnam or the murder of Robert Kennedy, but in fact I stopped going to barbershops for entirely personal reasons. Pointing to the parallel rivulets of flesh gradually asserting themselves on either side of my skull, my barber in Philadelphia told me one morning in November 1968 that I would be bald by the age of 30 and that there was nothing I could do about it. He knew because he was a barber. A rather bald barber.

At the time, it seemed to me that this unpleasant experience was tantamount to visiting a doctor for a routine checkup and being told that I would die of syphilis by age 30, so I jumped out of the chair, tore off the gown, and told the barber to go to hell. I would not set foot in a barbershop for 27 years.

This was not a mature way to handle the situation. Since I did not go bald by age 30 and am not bald now at age 49, there should have come a time in those 27 years when I finally realized I had foolishly allowed a chance remark by an obvious nitwit to cast a gigantic tonsorial shadow over my entire existence. Yet for 27 years, I kept the faith. In my late teens and 20s, I let my hair grow long, occasionally clipping it myself. After I got married, in 1977, my wife cut my hair. Then, once I got my career under way and needed to look presentable, I started getting my hair cut at fashionable unisex hair salons, usually by personable young women.

But for 27 years, I never got my hair cut by a barber, because a barber had once told me I would be bald by the time I was 30, proving that all barbers were dicks. And when I did finally break down and visit a barber, it was as a cheap stunt for a magazine story about getting a deliberately stupid haircut just so I could look like a pathetic slacker. That was in 1995. After the story ran, I started another 27-year exile from the barbershop.

Recently, I had occasion to reassess my position. Although I am quite fond of my hair and like to look my best whenever I appear on shows like *Politically Incorrect*, I am also an unbelievably tight-fisted son of a bitch and hate the thought that I sometimes have to shell out as much as $65 to get a decent haircut. One day I got to discussing this subject with a good friend whose hairdressing bill has risen as high as $90, an outrageous price considering that his hair isn't even in a class with mine. We agreed that the amount of money we were spending on our hair was ridiculous and reflected badly on us as men. We agreed that manly men wouldn't be caught dead shelling out more than $10 for a haircut. We agreed that we had reached a point in our lives where spending a huge amount of money on fancy-schmancy haircuts wasn't going to make much difference one way or the other. In short, we agreed that it was time to reverse course and get back to our roots: the barbershop.

As I made this decision, I could not help feeling a certain bittersweet nostalgia for the many hours I had spent at Eclipse: A Salon for Hair, the Tarrytown, New York, establishment where I had been getting my hair cut once every 2 to 3 months for years. During that period, Heidi, my adroit Norwegian coiffeuse, had done miracles with my graying locks, always cutting them at exactly the length and in exactly the style I requested. At some point, after being shorn by a dowdy male barber, I knew I would have to return to this elegant salon and explain to Heidi that my new policy should not be interpreted as a repudiation of her fine craftsmanship. But with money getting a bit tight and two kids soon heading off to college, I now felt that the $35 to $40 I was regularly forking over for the shampoo, cut, and tip was way out of line.

MY NEW GROOMING PHILOSOPHY

I set out to find the least expensive barber in the tristate area. His name was Gamal, he hailed from Cairo, he was a student at a storefront tonsorial academy on Manhattan's Lower East Side, and he had a mildly receding hairline and a confident demeanor. A haircut would cost me all of $4, and if things worked out I would probably toss in a $1 tip, a generous 25 percent. Did I honestly expect his work to be on a par with Heidi's? I did not. But was Heidi's work likely to be eight times as good as Gamal's? I had my doubts. If Gamal's work was even vaguely professional, I would be more than happy with this new arrangement.

I must confess that as I took my head in my hands, I was consoled by the presence of an ace up my sleeve. I have extremely wavy hair. I have hair that does what it wants when it wants. And I still have a lot of hair. Unlike pathetic men with straight, lifeless hair or men with Rudy Giuliani–type hair (the faux unbald), I do not have to worry that an incompetent barber is going to butcher my hair so completely that I cannot go out in public. Long ago, when clipping my own hair, I learned that a few waves will compensate for a multitude of sins. In other words, if Gamal was even passably competent, I was going to come out of this experience looking pretty damn presentable.

Approximately 90 seconds after Gamal began cutting my hair, it was possible to identify a few serious flaws in my new grooming philosophy. One of the reasons people pay $30 or $40 or even $90 for a haircut is that the person cutting your hair isn't likely to nip the tips of your ears every time he makes what amounts to a matador's pass at the hair on the back of your head. More upscale stylists also tend to sterilize their combs and shears before they start working on your hair and rarely borrow freshly used equipment from a colleague in the next room. And more upscale salons generally do not have a clientele who look as if they are on a work-release program from Alcatraz.

I am not saying that my industrious Egyptian barber actually butchered my hair. True, he did nip my ears a few times with the electric razor. Yes, he nearly garroted me a few times when he whiplashed the clipper cord across the front of my face. Yes, I was terrified he was going to slice off the wart growing on a vein in the back of my head, thus causing me to bleed to death right there in his chair. Yes, he did cut my hair twice as short as I had asked, deliberately clearing out the area surrounding that wart to make it stand out like Mount Rushmore. Yes, he did completely forget that I comb my hair more to the left than to the right. And, yes, he did vainly try to insert a part in a head of hair that had not seen one since Eisenhower was in office. Other than that, Mrs. Lincoln, how did you like the play?

"How long does your course last?" I finally asked him.

"About 4 months," he replied.

"How far along are you?"

"About halfway."

I did not ask whether the teacher had gotten to the part about hair yet.

To be fair, the haircut was not intuitively appalling, at least not on first glance. Split ends? Sure. Slightly uneven sideburns? You betcha. Hair combed in completely the wrong direction? You guessed it. Too much off in the back, too little off in the front? Yes, indeedy. Yet in the end, it was a haircut I could live with, because for 4 bucks, beggars could not be choosers. Especially not manly beggars.

For the next few days, I tried to persuade myself that getting a dirt-cheap spit-and-polish old-fashioned haircut had been a good idea. But eventually the mirror convinced me otherwise. The frivolous pompadour Gamal had erected at the front of my hairline gave me a decidedly retro look, like a flamboyant but untrustworthy character in an unpublished James Ellroy story. And because Gamal had cut my hair as if I were right-faced rather than left-faced, there wasn't an obvious way to brush it anymore.

ACCEPTING DEFEAT

Reluctantly, I admitted to myself that my megatightwad personality had now culminated in a serious tonsorial faux pas. Looking on the bright side, the haircut had cost me only $5, including the tip, so even if I had to go and get another haircut, I would still have shelled out far less than what I usually paid Heidi. So I immediately set out to get my hair surgically repaired.

My next stop was a $7 barbershop on 14th Street in Manhattan. I explained to my barber, whose hair reflected the direct styling influence of the Everly Brothers, that my last haircut had been less than successful, with too much left up front. David was clearly a pro and said he would do what he could. What he did was cut off the pompadour at the front and trim the sides even further, while completely deforesting the back. Meanwhile, he was speaking to his two colleagues in what I took to be Russian. As the haircut proceeded, I realized that every barber, no matter what his training, has a subconscious desire to make his customer look like a member of his own ethnic group. Which meant I was going to end up looking like Vladimir Putin.

The session was thorough, concluding with an eyebrow trim and a razor cut of the neckline. Nevertheless, this compensatory clip job had not been a rip-roaring success. When I got home that night, I realized the haircut needlessly accentuated the fleshy portions of my forehead that had led to my tonsorial hegira of 1968. Worse, I now had those little comb-over-the-forehead bangs that all Russian men seem to resort to in an effort to conceal their receding hairlines.

"You look like George Clooney in his first movie," said a close friend when he saw what David had wrought. "It's the *I, Cloonius* look."

He was right. There was no denying it. Rising the next morning and scrutinizing myself in the mirror, I realized that I now looked like Julius Caesar about 28 dagger punctures into his assassination. This was bad. I tried to live with the haircut for a few days, but it was no use. Belatedly, I admitted to myself that I had betrayed my hair, and so my hair was now exacting its revenge. Human hair comes to expect a certain level of respect, and once it has been mistreated or abused, it can become profoundly disoriented, seditious, and even vindictive. That first haircut had merely confused my hair. The second had utterly traumatized it. My hair no longer knew how to behave. It didn't know whether to curl or bunch or tangle or wave in the breeze or just lie there looking stupid. So it did what double-crossed hair has been doing since the beginning of time: It seceded from my overall appearance. It succumbed to anarchy. It went native.

Shamefacedly, I skulked into a $10-a-head barbershop in the bowels of the New York subway system, slithered into a chair and gave the barber his instructions. In the end, I suspected that when I went back to her, Heidi would be far more receptive to a barely plausible yarn about recreational chemotherapy or imperceptible head trauma than to the admission that I was a grubby skinflint who'd had so little respect for her skills that I'd entrusted my follicular fate to a feckless Egyptian and a barber who looked like an extra from *GoodFellas Go to Moscow*.

"Take it all off," I told the barber, still having trouble believing the scale of cephalic catastrophe I had visited upon myself because of my epic cheapness. "And take your time. I'm not coming back for at least 27 years."

KNOW THIS

You're OK, You're OK

According to a recent study reported in the *American Journal of Psychiatry*, most men think they would get more women if they had 30 pounds more muscle. Not true. When asked to pick the male image they dug most, women didn't choose the big V-shaped hero that men thought they would. They went with a less ripped model. Okay, they didn't choose the guy who looked all soft and cuddly. But there's no need to look like Schwarzenegger. "It's okay to look okay," says the study leader, Harrison G. Pope Jr., M.D., a professor of psychiatry at Harvard Medical School and coauthor of *The Adonis Complex*.

Get Better Interest Rates

High-interest credit cards are for losers. Literally. People who use them lose their money before they even earn it. Are you a loser? No. Scan www.bankrate.com. The site ranks the 25 best credit-card deals daily, based on rates, late fees, and grace periods. Most have interest rates much lower than the national average of 16 percent—including many under 10 percent. Call the bank's toll-free number (listed on the Web site) to see if it will accept a balance transfer from your regular card. Just click on "credit card" and search the links to "best deals." The site also offers advice on such money matters as correcting a false credit report and calculating mortgage payments. Better, it lists nearly 50 banks that offer Internet banking, which will give you one more thing to do when you should be working.

Join the Speeding Club

Tearing up a speeding ticket doesn't make it go away. Turns out the police keep a copy. Who knew? So, assuming you lose in court, let the National Motorists' Association pony up. The group will pay for one ticket a year for members (membership is $29 a year; sign up at www.motorists.org). Smirking at the cop is not covered.

DOES IT WORK?

The Tanita BreathAlert ($30)

This is how it's supposed to work: You blow into a tiny sensor that monitors levels of noxious-smelling sulfur and hydrocarbon gases in your breath. In 3 seconds, the gadget tells you whether you have bad breath.

Great idea, unreliable product. We're unsure whether the machine can detect the difference between good and bad smells. When we tried it, it gave toothpaste breath a strong odor score and garlic breath a neutral score, ruining our date. "The BreathAlert told me some of my patients had horrible breath, even though their breath was fine," says Anthony Dailley, D.D.S., director of the Center for Breath Treatment in San Francisco, who compared the device with his high-tech equipment.

We recommend spending the $30 on something that'll give you more reliable results—like, say, 2,000 Tic-Tacs.

Teflon-Coated Dress Shirt

You'll never forget the time you splashed merlot on your favorite shirt, ruining the punch line of your Dalai Lama joke. You'll never forget because the stain turned it into your favorite painting shirt. The solution? Justwhiteshirts.com sells a Teflon-coated cotton dress shirt that causes spills to bead up and slide right off. It worked when we dumped grape juice on it. But it turns out the coating is good for only 25 washings. So in 15 years or so, you'll need to spend another $55. Go to www.justwhiteshirts.com, or call (800) 221-8595.

Anti-Wrinkle Creams

If you've sneakily been using your partner's anti-wrinkle cream, check the ingredients. An ingredient known as alpha hydroxy acid (AHA) could cause skin aging. Creams containing the acid work by revealing newer layers of skin. But this leaves the fresh flesh unprotected from the damaging effects of ultraviolet rays.

COOL STUFF

Iron Man

Rowenta's Ultra Professional iron ($110)

Say "That thing's all wrinkled!" to a woman, and she'll think you're talking about her face. Say it to a man, and he'll know you're talking about his shirt. After testing a half-dozen topflight irons on an intern's pants (while he was still in them), we picked Rowenta's Ultra Professional (DM-990). It's pricey but much more efficient than less expensive irons. You don't have to press down on it to help it do its job. The jet of steam is strong, and the iron glides smoothly over sleeves and collars. It even turns itself off if you forget.

Steam Heat

Rowenta Steambrush ($20)

Hang your clothes on the hotel shower rod and use this light-enough-to-pack steamer to eliminate wrinkles. Even at home, try steaming. An overly hot iron can damage fabrics.

Bubbly Buddy

Perfect-Pop champagne opener ($50 in silver plate; $40 in chrome)

Opening champagne can be tricky and dangerous, especially by the fourth bottle or so. The foil, the wire thingy, the emergency eye surgery—it all slows down a party. To speed things up, we tried the Perfect-Pop champagne opener at a recent office celebration. We were impressed by both its heft and the speed at which it facilitated our drinking. Pull the wire loop out of the foil,

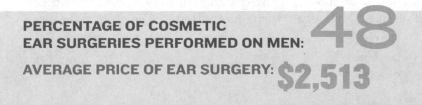

PERCENTAGE OF COSMETIC
EAR SURGERIES PERFORMED ON MEN: 48

AVERAGE PRICE OF EAR SURGERY: $2,513

then fit the Perfect-Pop over the foil, wire cage, and cork. A sharp twist makes the device grip the cork, and a counter-twist loosens the wire cage. Then, point the bottle away from you at a 45-degree angle, and twist clockwise, gently pulling up. Works like a charm. Get it at www.perfectpop.com.

Fuzz Fighter

The Sharper Image Turbo-Groomer 2.0 ($60)

Lots of scientists think they can slow down aging, but we've yet to meet one who's confident he can conquer the nose-hair/ear-hair problem. (Scissors lead to that problem Van Gogh had.) This tool is our best defense so far. Wet the lobe, grab the very bottom with your fingertips, stretch it gently downward, and carefully shave it. The gizmo is available at www.sharperimage.com.

DIY Pearly Whites

Crest Whitestrips ($44 for a box of 56)

White teeth are essential to a fulfilling life—the shiny, happy people inside our television set told us so, and they never lie. The surest way to take the grime off your grin is a bleaching regimen from your dentist. But that costs at least a couple hundred bucks.

For cheaper whiter teeth, stick these disposable adhesive strips to your choppers twice a day for about 30 minutes. Remember that too much bleaching can lead to slightly porous teeth and tooth sensitivity, says dentistry professor Michael Eggert, D.D.S., Ph.D., of the University of Alberta in Edmonton.

Cybereyes

www.eyeglasses.com

There's one downside to looking for a new pair of sunglasses: shopping malls. That's why we like this site. You scan or download an image of your face so you can "try on" more than 9,000 models (priced from $40 to $400) from 74 designers. No digital camera or scanner? Use someone else's head from the site's gallery of pictures. Find a pair, then order it from the site.

WHAT WORKS

It's no accident John Wayne is America's all-time favorite actor. The Duke possessed confidence and charisma matched by few since his days on the silver screen. Follow our simple pointers below and you, too, will turn women's heads, command the respect of your colleagues, and carry yourself with dignity, strength, and confidence. In short, you'll be the man you want to be. Oh, you also want to land a Hollywood role? That part is up to you.

1. Get a really close shave. Unless you're Richard Nixon, you can avoid a 5-o'clock shadow with a little extra vigilance in the morning. After your shower, run a washcloth under warm water and place it over your beard for 30 seconds. Lather with a shaving brush, and scrape in the direction of the grain of your beard. Rinse with warm water, relather, and shave again, this time going against the grain. It's tougher on your skin, though, so moisturize and make sure you haven't used the same blade more than three times.

2. Straighten up. Slouching not only makes you look slow-witted but also can shorten your spine and cause neck pain and breathing difficulty. And if you're hairy, people mysteriously assume you stink.

3. Groom the years away. Short, close-cropped hair makes you look younger, especially if your hair is thinning. Keep your sideburns and the hair on the back of your neck (not to mention your ear hair) meticulously shaved and trimmed.

4. Make an omelette for your skin. Beat two egg whites into a meringue and apply it to your face for 30 minutes. It will tighten your skin and close pores which, we're told, makes you look younger. This temporary face-lift lasts for about 2 hours.

5. Shampoo on the go. The problem with a long-distance relationship is that you look like hell when you get there. Take this with you: a small bottle containing 1 teaspoon of shampoo mixed into 1 cup of water. When you need a shower but don't have the time—or facilities—just pour the mixture in your hair, towel it off, and brush. There's enough shampoo to eliminate that greasy feel but not enough that it'll lather up and need to be rinsed out.

6. Freshen your breath by whetting your whistle. Anchovies and garlic are notorious bad-breath villains, but there's a far more insidious condition responsible for your fetid breath: dry mouth. Saliva normally acts like a cleansing rain, washing away the food particles that bacteria feed upon—the source of much of the smell—while also dissolving odorous sulfur compounds. Snoring all night, talking too much, dehydration, dieting, drinking alcohol, and smoking all conspire to dry out your yap. Solution: Stay hydrated by drinking water. And chew sugarless gum to stimulate your salivary glands.

7. Iron less. Buy some pants hangers and let gravity start working on those creases for you. You'll save time ironing and eliminate all those upper-thigh creases regular hangers can leave.

8. Use a quick wardrobe fix. Are you falling to pieces? We are, all the time. Luckily, you can patch up various clothing disasters in no time.

Stuck zipper. Rub a bar of soap or the lead tip of a pencil along the zipper's teeth. The lubrication will get it moving.

Scuffed shoe. If you're wearing dark-colored pants and shoes, buff away the mark with the inside of your pant leg. Or try coloring in the scuff with a marker. Rub in hand lotion for a quick shine.

Mustard stain. Shout Laundry Wipes ($2 for 12) take out most stains in a couple of seconds. Put a napkin between your shirt and your undershirt so you don't end up with wet spots.

Grease stain. Sprinkle on baking soda to absorb the oil, then brush it off.

Broken glasses. Run a paper clip through the screw hole. Twist the wire around itself a couple of times, then break it off close to the frames to hold your glasses in place.

Torn pants. Put duct or packing tape on the inside of your pants, right against the tear. The tape will hold the material in place until you have time to change. Remember, this is a temporary fix. Duct tape is not a fashion accessory.

9. Treat your pockets well. Shoving a PalmPilot, cell phone, and wad of lottery tickets into your breast pockets will destroy the lay of your suit jacket—permanently, over time. Clear all the crap out of your jacket pockets; they were made to handle the incidental racing form, not travel umbrellas. Get a money clip, too. A fat wallet in your pants pocket will misshape your trousers, and sitting on it can cause back and leg pain.

10. Know the dirt on shirts. Buy fitted dress shirts with high collars; these will frame your tie knot and your face more prominently than lower collars. Then make sure your shirt cuffs peek out below your suit cuffs when your arms hang straight. Finally, go for classic high contrast: dark ties, light shirts.

11. Make your cologne last. If you want it to last past lunch, do more than slap it on your mug. Apply it on your chest, forearms, and neck, too. (You can put it on your slacks and shirt, but test it first on a small patch of material to make sure it doesn't stain.) One other thing: Moisturize. Dry skin does a poor job of retaining fragrances.

12. Preserve your shoes. Before your wing tips were shoes, they were skin, so moisturize them with a water-resistant polish, such as Kiwi's neutral shoe polish. Then clean the leather every few months, using a cleansing cream—Rockport makes a good one—to lift the dirt. And never wear the same pair of shoes 2 days in a row. Leather can become sodden with sweat, so it needs a day to dry out before it goes back on your feet.

13. Sock the holes. Turn your socks inside out before each washing, says Tommye Allred, a product manager for the makers of Gold Toe socks. This will preserve their color and prevent pilling. Also, wear each pair only once between washings. Repeated wearings will mat the fibers and cause them to break down faster.

14. Know what you want to get what you want. Sexless? You're probably indecisive. Women hate indecisiveness because, biologically, it means you'll be the first sheep turned into mutton. To strike the pose of an alpha male, look her in the eye when you're talking to her, always have a plan, and be liberal about saying no—all things wimps don't do.

15. Check up on your IPOs. These days, few initials start the pulse pounding like IPO (except maybe SWBiF). If your broker recommends investing in an initial public offering, do some investigating. In a Cornell University study, IPOs picked by brokers whose companies also underwrote them dropped 15 percent (those picked by brokers whose firms didn't underwrite IPOs rose 42 percent). The bottom line: It's a basic conflict of interest, like asking the Dairy Council what to drink with dinner.

16. Who's the boss? Remember the following rules of power for a smooth ride to the corner office.

Don't trust anyone but yourself. It's not that everyone is out to screw you—although many people probably are—it's that some people are simply incompetent. Always assume they're going to make the kinds of mistakes you would never make.

Seize your opportunities. When you see a genuine opportunity or when you meet someone who can help further your goals, don't be coy. Do everything you can to make the most of the chance. You may get only one or two in your life.

Don't listen to everyone. If you listen to every person who offers advice,

PERCENTAGE OF MALE OFFICE WORKERS WHO NEVER WEAR A SUIT TO WORK: 70

PERCENTAGE OF EXECUTIVES WHO FEEL THAT WORKPLACE ATTIRE HAS BECOME TOO CASUAL: 34.2

NUMBER OF OFFICE WORKERS WHO BELIEVE THAT CASUAL DRESS INCREASES THEIR PRODUCTIVITY: 60

you'll become confused about your own ideas. If you're comfortable with what you're doing, go with it.

Alternate between lion and lamb. Develop a pattern of arbitrarily getting angry. Three out of four times you can be a nice guy, but the fourth time you need to act tough. Otherwise, people will walk all over you.

Be prepared for envy. Envy accompanies success. If a friend is envious, deflect it with humility. If an enemy is jealous, wave your triumph in his face.

17. Make yourself heard. When you ask for a raise or flirt with a waitress, you want to sound as smooth and persuasive as James Earl Jones. But what if your voice squeaks like R2D2's? Then you need to make it more powerful. To do that, try these exercises from Anna Bernstein, owner of Voice Success, a voice-coaching company in New York City.

The Siren: In private, hum back and forth between the bottom and top of your vocal range, like a siren. Repeat the cycle 10 times, once or twice a day. This will help you vary your pitch when speaking, making your voice sound more interesting and emphatic.

The Hum: To keep your voice from cracking unexpectedly during a presentation, warm up by humming a few bars of a song. Make sure you stop before you enter the conference room. Especially if you're humming 'N Sync.

The Tongue Flip: If you mumble or constantly trip up on words, it's usually a sign that your tongue is getting jumbled up with your lips and teeth when you talk. Improve your enunciation with this exercise: Place the tip of your tongue in front of your upper lip. Flick your tongue to the inside of your top teeth and back. Do this as fast as you can for a few minutes each day. (Your girlfriend will also thank you.)

18. Make a big deal over dinner. Hosting a successful business dinner takes more than springing for the large shake. You have to do all you can to make sure the contract ends up in your hand and not in the soup.

Make him drool. Negotiating is about making impressions. Before you pick a place, call your client's secretary to find out his favorite food. Choose a restaurant that serves it (find good restaurants at www.zagats.com).

Make your server happy. A week before the meeting, make two reservations—one for that night and one for the big dinner. At your first dinner, tip more than 30 percent; then tell the server how important the next dinner is.

Mingle at the bar. Order a drink that shows you're confident and knowledgeable, like Maker's Mark bourbon on the rocks, says Raymond Foley, publisher of *Bartender* magazine. Stick to one.

Position yourself. Sit directly across from the decision maker, and keep your shoulders up. Leaning back or slumping shows disinterest—or superiority. He won't take kindly to either.

Order meat. Filet mignon is a power dinner, says *Power Etiquette* author Dana May Casperson. It's also a tender cut—meaning you won't splash him with bloody juice by sawing at it.

Come in under budget. You have a spending limit; he wants to blow it. To keep your job without looking cheap, have the place design a special wine list within your price range. He'll never know.

Make the deal over dessert. Arrange a "stay away" code with the server— such as tugging on your ear. That'll give you 15 uninterrupted minutes to close the deal. Offer your client chocolate; it'll improve his mood.

Negotiate smart. When the client makes a good offer, don't give in. Grunt an inquisitive "Hmm?" This negotiation tactic subconsciously makes people sweeten the deal.

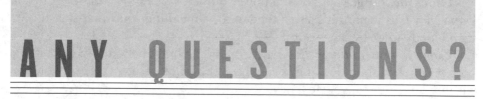

ANY QUESTIONS?

Face Time

Women always seem to wash their faces at night. Should I?

—J. M., Liguori, Mo.

If your skin is oily or acne-prone, wash your face before you go to bed, says dermatologist D'Anne Kleinsmith, M.D., of West Bloomfield, Michigan. That will remove the oils that penetrate your skin when you lie with your face pressed into a pillow for 8 hours. But the most important time to wash your face isn't before you go to bed or first thing in the morning—it's after you exercise. Perspiration is man's biggest acne aggravator (besides prom night). If your skin is dry and can handle only one washing a day, wash your face with soap after you work out, and just rinse it with water before bed.

A Soapy Shave

I ran out of shaving cream, so I had to use soap to shave. I actually got a better shave. Is it okay to shave with soap every day?

—R. D., Montreal

Absolutely. Shaving cream is just soap that's processed into a foamier form, so one really works as well as the other, says *Your Skin: An Owner's Guide* author Joseph Bark, M.D. You'll produce the best results with one of the rich, creamy brands your wife uses, such as Aveeno or Dove. They have moisturizers, so they won't dry your skin. Leave the deodorant soaps for other body parts. Zest may make your armpits tingle, but it's much too harsh for your face.

AVERAGE NUMBER OF HAIRS LOST BY A BALDING MAN DAILY: 200

NUMBER OF VISIBLE HAIRS ON AN AVERAGE GUY'S HEAD: 100,000

PERCENTAGE OF BALDING THAT CAN BE CHALKED UP TO HEREDITY: 95

Footwear Formality

What kind of shoes can I wear with a tuxedo? I don't want to look too casual, but do I have to wear those goofy "evening shoes"?

—M. A., Olympia, Wash.

You may already have something in your closet that you can wear with a tuxedo, says Dan McCampbell, men's fashion director at Saks Fifth Avenue in New York City. "With a tuxedo, it's important to keep your shoes simple and elegant," he says. Traditional choices are velvet slip-ons or patent leather lace-ups, but for men who hate wearing such dressy shoes, there are less fussy options. Plain black leather slip-ons (make sure they're well-shined) or your simplest, most classic black dress shoes will look fine with a tuxedo. What doesn't work: wing tips. "Anything with detailing or perforated leather isn't appropriate for formal wear," says McCampbell. "And shoes with thick soles or square toes look wrong with a classic tuxedo."

Stain Solutions

One of my light-brown nubuck shoes has a grease stain on it. I've tried detergent and scrubbing with a suede eraser and brush to get it out, but neither worked. Any other suggestions?

—E. R., Durham, N.C.

Grease on a shoe is like grease on a politician's hand: You can't get rid of it completely, but you can try to cover it up. Here are tips from Henry Goldsmith, associate professor at the Fashion Institute of Technology in New York City.

Iron it out. Put tissue paper, dull side down, over the stain. Set the iron for cotton, no steam, and run it over the damaged area. "The paper will help absorb the grease. Keep changing the position of the paper so you always get a fresh spot," says Goldsmith.

Steam it out. Turn on the shower and then run the shoe, stain side down, through the steam until the suede gets damp. The moisture loosens debris on the stain's surface. Then use a suede brush to buff the area.

Paint over it. If all else fails, the only way to salvage it is to spray paint the shoe to match the color of the stain. Goldsmith recommends Nu-Life Color Spray, sold at shoemaker's shops. Before spraying, cover the heel with masking tape.

Browbeating

I have bushy eyebrows. How can I keep them neat and thin?

—P. D., Dade City, Fla.

Brow trimming should be part of a man's haircut," says Carmine Minardi, owner of Minardi Salon in New York City. "The stylist should also trim your sideburns and use a clipper on those fine hairs on your earlobes." If brow trimming isn't included in the cost of the cut, do it yourself.

1. Comb your brows straight up with a fine comb.
2. Use a small pair of scissors—Minardi likes $4\frac{1}{2}$-inch haircutting scissors—to trim hairs that extend above the brow line.
3. Thin the brows by laying the comb flat against your skin so that the brow hairs stick up through the teeth of the comb. Cut the hairs right down to the comb. "The comb is about $\frac{1}{4}$-inch thick," says Minardi, "so it's impossible to cut the hair too short." Or to accidentally give yourself an eyebrow Mohawk.

Tie Tips

Why do some ties cost $20 and others $100? How do I know if a tie is a good one?

—M. M., Brooklyn, N.Y.

You pay more for more durable construction of both the lining and the outer material, according to Gerald Andersen, executive director of the Neckwear Association of America. You should use the following checkpoints to find a quality noose.

The pattern. Make sure patterns and colors are evenly printed. You can spot a cheap tie if the colors run together or overlap like the ink on a misprinted comic page.

The fabric. Do more than just feel it to make sure the material isn't rough or stiff. Check the label. The nicest and most durable silks come from Italy, Korea, and China.

The length. Manufacturers who make the best ties don't skimp on material. Quality ties are at least 55 inches long (about Gary Coleman's height), so there's plenty of fabric for any size man and any style knot.

The lining. Good ties are fully lined from the bottom of the tie to where the knot would be. If the lining extends only 6 to 8 inches from the bottom, the tie might lose its shape quickly.

Credits

The glycemic-index values for 14 of the foods listed on pages 59 and 60 are from the book *The Glucose Revolution* by Jennie Brand Miller, Ph.D.; Thomas M. S. Wolever, M.D., Ph.D.; Stephen Colagiuri, M.D.; Anthony Leeds, M.D.; and Kaye Foster-Powell. © 1996, 1998, 1999 by Jennie Brand Miller, Ph.D.; Thomas M. S. Wolever, M.D., Ph.D.; Stephen Colagiuri, M.D.; Anthony Leeds, M.D.; and Kaye Foster-Powell. Appears by permission of the publisher, Marlowe & Company, a Division of the Avalon Publishing Group, Inc.

The questions in "How Are You Doing" on page 90 were adapted from *Fighting for Your Marriage: Positive Steps for Preventing Divorce and Preserving a Lasting Love* by Howard Markman, Scott Stanley, and Susan L. Blumberg, quiz on pages 5 and 6. © 1994 by Jossey-Bass, Inc. This material is used by permission of Jossey-Bass, Inc., a subsidiary of John Wiley & Sons, Inc.

Commit to Yourself on page 169 was excerpted from *Leading with the Heart* by Mike Kryzewski and Donald T. Phillips. © 2000 by Mike Kryzewski. Reprinted by permission of Warner Books, Inc.

Interpreting DocSpeak (Hint: "Good" Means "Bad") on page 238 was reprinted, with the permission of Simon & Schuster, from *The Hypochondriacs Guide to Life. And Death* by Gene Weingarten. Illustrations by Bob Staake. © 1998 by Gene Weingarten.

Fire in the Hole on page 242 was excerpted from *Staying at the Top of Your Game: A Man's Guide to Peak Performance* by Timothy Gower. © 1999 by Hearst Communications, Inc. Reprinted with permission.

Statistics in the sidebars on pages 271, 273, and 285 are courtesy of the American Society of Plastic Surgeons.

Parting of the Waves on page 279 was reprinted with the permission of Joe Queenan. This article originally appeared in GQ in December 2000.

Index

Underscored page references indicate boxed text. **Boldface** references indicate photographs.